国际经典内科学教科书

第 10 版
Cecil Essentials of Medicine
希氏内科学精要
中英双语版

原　著　**Edward J. Wing, MD, FACP, FIDSA**
Former Dean of Medicine and Biological Sciences
Professor of Medicine
Warren Alpert Medical School of Brown University, Providence, Rhode Island

Fred J. Schiffman, MD, MACP
Sigal Family Professor of Humanistic Medicine
Vice Chair, Department of Medicine
Warren Alpert Medical School of Brown University, Providence, Rhode Island

中英双语版　编辑委员会　主任委员　王　辰

—— 第 8 分册 ——

肌肉骨骼与结缔组织疾病

主　译　栗占国　李梦涛

北京大学医学出版社

XISHI NEIKEXUE JINGYAO (DI 10 BAN) DI 8 FENCE JIROU GUGE YU JIEDI ZUZHI JIBING (ZHONGYING SHUANGYU BAN)

图书在版编目（CIP）数据

希氏内科学精要：第10版.第8分册，肌肉骨骼与结缔组织疾病：汉、英／（美）爱德华·温（Edward J. Wing），（美）弗雷德·谢夫曼（Fred J. Schiffman）原著；栗占国，李梦涛主译．－－北京：北京大学医学出版社，2024.11.－－ISBN 978-7-5659-3258-8

Ⅰ.R5

中国国家版本馆CIP数据核字第2024S7U167号

北京市版权局著作权合同登记号：图字：01-2024-4518

Elsevier (Singapore) Pte Ltd.
3 Killiney Road, #08-01 Winsland House I, Singapore 239519
Tel: (65) 6349-0200; Fax: (65) 6733-1817

Cecil Essentials of Medicine, Tenth Edition
Copyright © 2022 by Elsevier, Inc. All rights are reserved, including those for text and data mining, AI training, and similar technologies.
Publisher's note: Elsevier takes a neutral position with respect to territorial disputes or jurisdictional claims in its published content, including in maps and institutional affiliations.
Previous editions copyrighted 2016, 2010, 2007, 2004, 2001, 1997, 1993, 1990, and 1986.
ISBN-13: 978-0-323-72271-1

This translation of Cecil Essentials of Medicine, Tenth Edition by Edward J. Wing and Fred J. Schiffman was undertaken by Peking University Medical Press and is published by arrangement with Elsevier (Singapore) Pte Ltd.

Cecil Essentials of Medicine, Tenth Edition by Edward J. Wing and Fred J. Schiffman 由北京大学医学出版社进行翻译，并根据北京大学医学出版社与爱思唯尔（新加坡）私人有限公司的协议约定出版。

《希氏内科学精要（第10版）第8分册 肌肉骨骼与结缔组织疾病（中英双语版）》（栗占国 李梦涛 主译）
ISBN: 978-7-5659-3258-8
Copyright © 2024 by Elsevier (Singapore) Pte Ltd. and Peking University Medical Press.
All rights reserved. No part of this publication may be reproduced or transmitted in any form or by any means, electronic or mechanical, including photocopying, recording, or any information storage and retrieval system, without permission in writing from Elsevier (Singapore) Pte Ltd. and Peking University Medical Press.

注　意

本译本由北京大学医学出版社独立完成。相关从业及研究人员必须凭借其自身经验和知识对文中描述的信息数据、方法策略、搭配组合、实验操作进行评估和使用。由于医学科学发展迅速，临床诊断和给药剂量尤其需要经过独立验证。在法律允许的最大范围内，爱思唯尔、译文的原文作者、原文编辑及原文内容提供者均不对译文或因产品责任、疏忽或其他操作造成的人身及（或）财产伤害及（或）损失承担责任，亦不对由于使用文中提到的方法、产品、说明或思想而导致的人身及（或）财产伤害及（或）损失承担责任。

Published in China by Peking University Medical Press under special arrangement with Elsevier (Singapore) Pte Ltd. This edition is authorized for sale in the People's Republic of China only, excluding Hong Kong SAR, Macau SAR and Taiwan. Unauthorized export of this edition is a violation of the contract.

希氏内科学精要（第10版）第8分册　肌肉骨骼与结缔组织疾病（中英双语版）

主　　译：栗占国　李梦涛
出版发行：北京大学医学出版社
地　　址：（100191）北京市海淀区学院路38号　北京大学医学部院内
电　　话：发行部 010-82802230；图书邮购 010-82802495
网　　址：http://www.pumpress.com.cn
E-mail：booksale@bjmu.edu.cn
印　　刷：北京信彩瑞禾印刷厂
经　　销：新华书店
策划编辑：高　瑾
责任编辑：高　瑾　　责任校对：靳新强　　责任印制：李　啸
开　　本：889 mm×1194 mm　1/16　印张：10.25　字数：376千字
版　　次：2024年11月第1版　2024年11月第1次印刷
书　　号：ISBN 978-7-5659-3258-8
定　　价：80.00元

版权所有，违者必究

（凡属质量问题请与本社发行部联系退换）

中英双语版 编辑委员会

主任委员

王　辰

委　　员（按姓氏笔画排序）

王　洁	王伊龙	王建祥	巴　一	代华平	宁　光	宁晓红	朱　兰
任景怡	刘海鹰	李小鹰	李梦涛	李雪梅	杨爱明	张福杰	郑金刚
房静远	赵　晶	赵明辉	郝　伟	姜　辉	栗占国	贾继东	夏维波
黄　慧	黄晓军	曹　彬	彭　斌	潘　慧

第 1 分册　内科学概论·呼吸与危重症医学·术前和术后照护

　　　　　　主译　王　辰　代华平　赵　晶　黄　慧

第 2 分册　心血管疾病

　　　　　　主译　郑金刚　任景怡

第 3 分册　肾脏疾病

　　　　　　主译　李雪梅　赵明辉

第 4 分册　胃肠疾病·肝脏与胆道系统疾病

　　　　　　主译　房静远　杨爱明　贾继东

第 5 分册　血液疾病

　　　　　　主译　黄晓军　王建祥

第 6 分册　肿瘤疾病

　　　　　　主译　王　洁　巴　一

第 7 分册　内分泌疾病与代谢疾病·女性健康·男性健康·骨与骨矿物质代谢疾病

　　　　　　主译　宁　光　朱　兰　姜　辉　夏维波　潘　慧

第 8 分册　肌肉骨骼与结缔组织疾病

　　　　　　主译　栗占国　李梦涛

第 9 分册　感染性疾病

　　　　　　主译　刘海鹰　张福杰　曹　彬

第 10 分册　神经疾病·老年医学·缓和医疗·酒精和物质使用

　　　　　　主译　彭　斌　王伊龙　李小鹰　宁晓红　郝　伟

医学名词审定指导

任慧玲　李晓瑛　冀玉静　张燕舞　李军莲

中英双语版 序言

让我国医学生与国际医学生站在同一起跑线上的首要之事，是为其提供具有世界先进水平的标准教材。我们应争取使每一位医学生都能接触到内容经典、充分代表现代医学水平的国际权威原文教材并力求准确翻译，提供原文与中文双语对照版本，使医学生和医生在学习中形成双语医学词语、概念、概念间逻辑及由此构成的医学知识体系。在这样的思想驱动下，国际经典内科学教科书《希氏内科学精要（第10版）》中英双语版应运而生。

《希氏内科学》原著以其论述严谨准确、系统全面，被誉为"标准的内科学参考书"。自1927年首次出版以来，在内科学领域渐享世界级声誉，成为全球众多优秀医学院校，包括哈佛医学院、斯坦福大学医学院、约翰斯·霍普金斯大学医学院、牛津大学医学部、剑桥大学医学院、墨尔本大学医学院、新加坡国立大学医学院及多伦多大学医学院等普遍采用的内科学参考书。首版《希氏内科学精要》则诞生于1986年，旨在凝炼其全本的精华和要点，以最为简洁明确的方式向以医学生为主体的医学界精辟传达《希氏内科学》的核心信息，包括书中所体现出的人文精神。此后，每版精要本都力求凝炼地反映当时最新医学成果和医疗实践指南，愈来愈成为各国医学生、住院医师、专培医师及教师学习和传授内科学的主要教本，在世界医学教材体系中居引领地位。《希氏内科学》和《希氏内科学精要》两个版本不仅在英语国家被广泛使用，更被翻译为葡萄牙语、西班牙语、希腊语、意大利语、日语、简体中文版，为全球医学界广泛采用。

中国的医学生、住院医师、专培医师需要培养国际专业信息获取能力。将精要本原文引进并准确翻译，以中英文对照的形式呈现，便于读者进行双语对照阅读和学习，使之在学习理解国际标准医学内容的同时，学习好中英文医学词语，为国际医学交流打好基础。相信此举对于提高我国的医学教育水平，培养国际型医学人才至为有益。

《希氏内科学精要》精练地涵盖了内科学的所有主要领域，包括心血管疾病、呼吸疾病与危重症、消化疾病、肾脏疾病、内分泌和代谢疾病、风湿疾病、血液疾病、肿瘤、感染性疾病、神经与老年疾病等，构建了较为系统的知识体系。在翻译引进过程中，我们遵循将相关内容集中的原则，将原书按系统器官拆分为十个分册，使其更具有专科阅读的对应性，以更加灵活轻便的形式为读者提供多样化的阅读选择。

为确保译文质量，我们在译者遴选上采取了严谨的标准。从《希氏内科学（第26版）》翻译团队中择优选取责任心强、译文优质的译者，同时吸纳了临床医学专业"101"计划核心教材的编者团队。每个分册均由主译专家带领各自译者团队完成翻译、审校、交叉互审、通审四级审校工作。这些译者具备扎实的英语与专业能力，他们在翻译过程中，深入理解原文，准确阐述作者思想，并多角度审视译文的准确性、流畅性与风格一致性，确保译文的忠实性、规范性与可读性，在不同的语言和文化间架起坚实的桥梁。尤其值得称赞的是，对原著中疏漏或不够完善之处，译文中以"译者注"的形式加以适当解释和说明，使译文内容在忠实于原著的基础上更为准确。

本书读者定位于具有一定学习能力和基础的高等医学院校医学专业8年制、5年制学生以及相关医学专业人员，可作为医务人员的内科学参考书、住院医师规范化培训和专科医师规范化培训辅导教材、研究生入学考试辅导教材、内科学教师参考书、内科学各专科医师复习回顾其他专科知识的重要读本。

呼吸与危重症医学教授
中国医学科学院院长
北京协和医学院校长
2024年11月

对学习者教科书重要。
对学医者内科学重要。
世界上的内科学教科书，
首推《希氏内科学精要》。

中文是中国医生主要执业用语。
英文是国际医学交流的主要文字。
学习医学，当以双语对应阅读为好。
如此，可获纵横国际之效。

本书力求有助于此。

In Memoriam

Thomas E. Andreoli, MD

Dr. Thomas Andreoli, along with Drs. Lloyd Hollingsworth (Holly) Smith, Jr., Fred Plum, and Charles C.J. Carpenter, was one of the four founding editors of *Cecil Essentials of Medicine*. He served as editor for editions one through eight before he passed away on April 14, 2009. Dr. Andreoli was born in the Bronx, New York, in 1935, attended Catholic primary and high schools, and graduated from St. Vincent College and the Georgetown School of Medicine. He trained as a resident at Duke University under legendary Chair of Medicine Dr. Eugene Stead, who recognized him as a brilliant physician and scientist and encouraged his research career. Dr. Andreoli received his research training at the NIH and then in the laboratory of Dr. Tosteson at Duke. His research focused on the biochemical and biophysical properties of renal tubular cell membranes and their role in water and electrolyte transport. He made fundamental discoveries on the normal renal physiology, illuminating the way to subsequent work by many others on renal health and disease. His research was recognized with numerous awards and election to honorific societies both in the United States and in Europe. Dr. Andreoli also served as editor of *The American Journal of Physiology: Renal Physiology* and Editor in Chief of *Kidney International*.

Tom's national prominence and leadership qualities were recognized early in his career when he became head of Nephrology at the University of Alabama in Birmingham. There he helped faculty and trainees develop outstanding research, organized clinical services, and created a hemodialysis program to build one of the outstanding Divisions of Nephrology in the country. In 1979, Dr. Andreoli was appointed Chair of the Department of Internal Medicine at the University of Texas, Houston, where he assembled an outstanding faculty focused on research, clinical care, and teaching. In 1988, he accepted the position as Chairman of Internal Medicine at the University of Arkansas School of Medicine, a position he held until his death. There he again assembled a distinguished faculty who were outstanding researchers but also dedicated to outstanding clinical care and teaching. Morning report and clinical rounds with Dr. Andreoli were rigorous and riveting, focusing on the individual patient, not only their diagnoses and treatment but also on each patient's personal concerns and well-being. Dr. Andreoli was revered by medical students, his house staff, faculty, and colleagues, and I (EJW) personally can attest to what he regarded as his most cherished role—the mentorship and education of the next generation of physicians.

One of Dr. Andreoli's great interests was *Cecil Essentials of Medicine*, for which he was the editor/chief editor for eight of its ten editions, an interest that reflected his commitment to the education of students, house staff, and other physicians in the "essentials" of Internal Medicine.

Dr. Andreoli was devoted to his family. He was married to Elizabeth Berglund Andreoli from 1987 until his death. He was previously married to Dr. Kathleen Gainor Andreoli, mother of his three children and their ten grandchildren. Being of Italian ancestry and from Bronx, New York, it is not surprising that Dr. Andreoli was a passionate fan of the New York Yankees, Italian opera, which he could sing in Italian, and Frank Sinatra.

Dr. Andreoli's legacy lives on in his numerous previous students, house staff, colleagues, and in this book.

缅 怀

托马斯·安德里奥利博士

托马斯·安德里奥利（Thomas E. Andreoli）博士携手李奥德·霍灵斯沃斯·史密斯［Lloyd Hollingsworth（Holly）Smith］博士、弗雷德·普拉姆（Fred Plum）博士和查尔斯·卡彭特（Charles C.J. Carpenter）博士同为《希氏内科学精要》的创始编者。他在2009年4月14日去世前，曾担任该书第1至第8版的编者。安德里奥利博士于1935年出生于美国纽约布朗克斯区，就读于天主教小学和中学，后毕业于圣文森特学院和乔治城大学医学院。他在杜克大学医学院接受住院医师培训期间师从著名内科主任尤金·斯特德（Eugene Stead）博士，后者将其视为杰出的医生和科学家，并鼓励他投身科研事业。安德里奥利博士在美国国立卫生研究院接受科研训练后，前往杜克大学托斯特森（Tosteson）博士的实验室继续深造。他重点研究肾小管细胞膜的生化和生物物理特性及其在水和电解质转运中所发挥的作用。他在正常肾脏生理学方面的重要发现为后续关于肾脏健康和疾病的研究铺平了道路。安德里奥利博士的研究工作荣获多个学术奖项，并入选美国和欧洲的多个荣誉学会。他还担任《美国生理学杂志：肾脏生理学篇》（The American Journal of Physiology: Renal Physiology）的编辑以及《国际肾脏杂志》（Kidney International）的主编。

安德里奥利博士担任阿拉巴马大学伯明翰分校肾脏病学系主任后不久，即因其杰出领导力而赢得全美业内声誉。他帮助本校师生们取得科研突破，负责临床业务的组织实施，并因开创血液透析业务而使该科跻身全美顶级肾脏内科之列。1979年，安德里奥利博士被任命为得克萨斯大学休斯敦分校内科学系主任，他在该系组建了一支科研、临床诊疗和教学并重的优秀教职团队。自1988年起，他担任阿肯色大学医学院内科学系主任，直至辞世。在这里他再次组建了一支卓越的教职团队，他们不仅科研工作出色，临床诊疗和教学工作也出类拔萃。安德里奥利博士带领的晨会报告和查房非常严谨而引人入胜，不仅尽心竭力于每位患者的诊断和治疗，还关注到他们每个人的个体情况和福祉。安德里奥利博士深受医学生、住院医师、教职人员和同事的崇敬，我（EJW）可以证明，他最珍视的角色当属培养和教育下一代医生。

安德里奥利博士对《希氏内科学精要》倾注了满腔热忱，先后担任了该书10版中8版的编者/主编，践行他为医学生、住院医师和其他各科医生们传授内科学"精要"的承诺。

安德里奥利博士高度重视家庭。他与第二任妻子伊丽莎白·伯格兰德·安德里奥利（Elizabeth Berglund Andreoli）的婚姻从1987年延续到辞世。他与第一任妻子凯瑟琳·盖娜·安德里奥利（Kathleen Gainor Andreoli）博士育有三个子女和十个孙辈。作为意大利裔和纽约布朗克斯人，安德里奥利博士是纽约洋基队、意大利歌剧（他能用意大利语演唱）和美国著名歌手、演员、主持人弗兰克·辛纳屈（Frank Sinatra）的忠实拥趸。安德里奥利博士将永远被他的众多学生、住院医师和同事怀念，并因本书而流芳百世。

In Memoriam

Charles C.J. Carpenter, MD

Dr. Charles C.J. Carpenter joined Drs. Thomas Andreoli, Lloyd Hollingsworth Smith, Jr., and Fred Plum as a founder of *Cecil Essentials of Medicine*. He served as editor for seven editions and was followed in that role by Dr. Ivor Benjamin and then Dr. Edward Wing. Sadly, Chuck passed away on March 19, 2020, surrounded by his wife and children. He was Professor Emeritus of Medicine at The Warren Alpert Medical School of Brown University and Physician-in-Chief Emeritus at The Miriam Hospital.

Chuck was born in Savannah, Georgia, on January 5, 1931. He attended college at Princeton and medical school at Johns Hopkins where he also did his house staff training, including chief residency, and then joined the Johns Hopkins faculty. With his young family, he travelled to Calcutta, India, where he carried out landmark studies for the treatment of cholera.

Before coming to Brown in 1986, he was Chair of Medicine at Baltimore City Hospital and Case Western Reserve University.

His contributions to medical science and clinical care were many. While in Calcutta, using basic scientific evidence coupled with practical approaches, Dr. Carpenter developed "oral rehydration therapy" to address the cholera epidemic there. This treatment has saved millions of lives. While at Case, one of his innovations was to develop the nation's first Division of Geographic Medicine because of his strong belief that all physicians should be medical citizens of the world. In 1987, as he became deeply involved in the clinical management of persons living with HIV, he initiated a unique program in which Brown University faculty and trainees assumed responsibility for all HIV care in the Rhode Island State prison system.

Dr. Carpenter served as Chairman of the American Board of Internal Medicine and President of the Association of American Physicians. He has been a member of the NIH AIDS Executive Committee, the National Advisory Allergy and Infectious Diseases Council, and the USPHS AIDS Task Force. He was Chair of the Antiretroviral Treatment Panel of the International AIDS Society-USA and authored their recommendations on antiretroviral treatment. He also served as Chair of the Treatment Committee to evaluate the President's Emergency Plan for HIV/AIDS Relief. He became the director of the Brown University International Health Institute and the director of the Lifespan/Brown Center for AIDS Research with several Boston hospitals.

Throughout his career, Dr. Carpenter was the recipient of many international, national, and regional awards, accepting each with characteristic humility. With both small and large groups of learners, Chuck made certain that every member of his team was well educated, and each felt that they contributed to the well-being of their patients. His ability to sit calmly at the bedside, hold the patient's hand, comfort them, and listen in a genuinely focused way, influenced so many physicians. He was truly grateful for the opportunity to care for those less fortunate than he, and the feeling of being privileged to do so was clearly transmitted to all. Dr. Carpenter was a wonderful blend of profound compassion combined with the adherence to scholarship and teaching. Sir William Osler wrote that physicians should "Do the kind thing and do it first." Chuck lived by this precept. Vigor and insight characterized his approach to clinical and ethical challenges, always with younger colleagues at his side. In a recent tribute to him, many emphasized that Dr. Carpenter dedicated his life to his patients, many of whom were the most vulnerable members of society. We hope that we will have some of his strength and use his example as our compass as we are challenged to reduce suffering and improve the health of all for whom we are responsible.

He is survived by his wife of 61 years, Sally; three sons, Charles, Murray, and Andrew; and seven grandchildren.

缅 怀

查尔斯·卡彭特博士

查尔斯·卡彭特（Charles C.J. Carpenter）博士与托马斯·安德里奥利（Thomas E. Andreoli）博士、李奥德·霍灵斯沃斯·史密斯（Lloyd Hollingsworth Smith）博士和弗雷德·普拉姆（Fred Plum）博士共同开创了《希氏内科学精要》。他共担任了7版的编者，嗣后由艾弗·本杰明（Ivor Benjamin）博士和爱德华·温（Edward Wing）博士接任。查尔斯·卡彭特博士于2020年3月19日在妻子和子女们的陪伴下辞世。他曾担任布朗大学沃伦·阿尔珀特医学院的内科学系名誉教授和米里亚姆医院的名誉主任医师。

查尔斯·卡彭特博士于1931年1月5日出生于美国佐治亚州萨凡纳市。他在普林斯顿大学获得学士学位后进入约翰斯·霍普金斯大学医学院，并完成了包括住院总医师在内的住院医师培训，随后加入了约翰斯·霍普金斯大学的教职团队。他曾携妻子和年幼的孩子前往印度加尔各答，在当地对霍乱的治疗进行了具有里程碑意义的研究工作。

在1986年入职布朗大学之前，他曾担任巴尔的摩市医院和凯斯西储大学医学院的内科学主任。

他在医学科学研究和临床诊疗领域建树颇多。在加尔各答期间，基于基础科学证据及临床实践，查尔斯·卡彭特博士开创了"口服补液疗法"以遏制当地的霍乱疫情。这一疗法拯救了数百万人的生命。秉承医生无国界的世界公民理念，他在凯斯西储大学做了一项开创性工作，建立了美国首个地缘医学部（研究地理环境因素对人体健康和疾病影响的学科）。1987年，他深度参与人类免疫缺陷病毒（HIV）携带者的临床管理，并发起了一个独特的项目——由布朗大学教职团队和医学生们承担罗德岛州监狱系统内所有艾滋病相关诊疗工作。

查尔斯·卡彭特博士曾担任美国内科医师委员会主席和美国医师协会主席。他曾是美国国立卫生研究院艾滋病行政委员会、美国国家过敏与传染病咨询委员会以及公共卫生服务部艾滋病工作组的成员。他还曾担任国际艾滋病学会-美国分会抗逆转录病毒治疗组主席，并撰写了抗逆转录病毒治疗建议。他还担任过艾滋病治疗委员会主席，该委员会负责评估美国总统防治艾滋病紧急救援计划；曾担任布朗大学国际健康研究所所长，以及大学与多家波士顿当地医院合办的生命周期/布朗大学艾滋病研究中心主任。

查尔斯·卡彭特博士在职业生涯中获得过诸多国际性、全美和地区性奖项，同时展现其谦逊品格。无论学员人数多寡，查尔斯·卡彭特博士都会确保人人都能受到良好教育，并让他们感到自己也对患者的健康做出了贡献。他能够安静地坐在病床边，握住患者的手，安慰他们，并全神贯注地听取患者倾诉，这一举动深深地感染了许多医生。他十分珍视诊治不幸染病者的机会，并且能够将这种殊荣感传递给所有人。查尔斯·卡彭特博士完美地融汇了对患者的宅心仁厚与对学术和教学的坚守。威廉·奥斯勒（William Osler）爵士曾写道，医生应该"行善事，为人先"，而这正是查尔斯·卡彭特博士一生奉行的信条。他在面对临床和伦理挑战时充满活力和洞察力，始终重视提携年轻同事。许多人的悼词中都重点指出，查尔斯·卡彭特博士将毕生致力于患者福祉，其中许多人属于社会上最弱势群体。我们希望，在我们面临减少患者痛苦及改善其健康状况的挑战时，能够拥有他的力量，并以他为榜样获得指引。

查尔斯·卡彭特博士与妻子萨丽（Sally）共度了61年的婚姻时光，育有查尔斯（Charles）、穆雷（Murray）和安德鲁（Andrew）三子以及七个孙辈。

ABOUT THE EDITORS

Dr. Edward J. Wing was an editor of *Cecil Essentials of Medicine*, editions 8 and 9, and is the lead editor of edition 10. He graduated from Williams College in 1967 and from the Harvard Medical School in 1971. He was a resident in Internal Medicine at the Peter Bent Brigham and completed an Infectious Diseases Fellowship at Stanford University. Joining the faculty at the University of Pittsburgh in 1975, he focused his NIH-funded research on mechanisms of cell-mediated immunity as well as various clinical aspects of Infectious Diseases. From 1990 to 1998, the University and UPMC appointed him as Physician-in-Chief at Montefiore Hospital, then Chief of Infectious Diseases, and finally Interim Chair of Medicine.

In 1998, Dr. Wing became Chair of Medicine at Brown University (1998–2008) where he consolidated the department across hospitals, practice plans, and training programs. As Dean of Medicine and Biological Sciences at Brown University (2008–2013) he strengthened ties with affiliated hospitals (Lifespan and Care New England), increased research, and oversaw the construction of a new medical school building. International exchange programs with medical schools in Kenya, the Dominican Republic, and Haiti were established during his years as chairman and dean. Dr. Wing has cared for patients with HIV since the beginning of the epidemic in outpatient clinics. He continues to be active in research, clinical care, and teaching.

Dr. Fred J. Schiffman, who along with Dr. Edward Wing is editor of *Cecil Essentials of Medicine,* 10th edition, attended Wagner College and then the New York University School of Medicine, from which he graduated in 1973. He performed his early house staff training at Yale-New Haven Hospital and then spent two years at the National Cancer Institute. He returned to Yale as Chief Medical Resident followed by a hematology fellowship. He became Medical Director of Yale's Primary Care Center before coming to Brown University in 1983, where he has been a leader in the medical residency program as well as Associate Physician-in-Chief at The Miriam Hospital.

Dr. Schiffman holds The Sigal Family Professorship in Humanistic Medicine at The Warren Alpert Medical School of Brown University. His scholarly interests include the structure and function of the human spleen and the intersection of the arts and medical care. He has directed or championed many projects and programs, including those that encourage and reinforce wellness and resilience in patients, families, and caregivers. He began a novel program that places medical students and physicians with other nonmedical professionals as they share in the viewing of works of art in the Museum of the Rhode Island School of Design. Dr. Schiffman recently led a Brown University edX course entitled, "Artful Medicine: Art's Power to Enrich Patient Care," with worldwide participation. Dr. Schiffman has also edited texts on hematologic pathophysiology, consultative hematology, and the anemias.

原著主编

爱德华·温（Edward J. Wing）博士是《希氏内科学精要》第 8 版和第 9 版的编者，以及第 10 版的主编。他先后于 1967 年和 1971 年毕业于威廉姆斯学院和哈佛医学院。他曾在彼得·本特·布里格姆医院任内科住院医师，后在斯坦福大学完成了传染病学的专科医师（Fellowship）课程。自 1975 年加入匹兹堡大学医学院以来，他通过美国国立卫生研究院资助的研究项目，探索细胞介导免疫的机制以及传染病学各领域的临床诊疗工作。1990—1998 年期间，他先后被匹兹堡大学及其医学中心任命为蒙特菲奥里医院的主任医师、传染病科主任，后担任内科临聘主任。

1998 年起，温博士担任布朗大学医学院的内科主任（1998—2008 年）。在此期间，他在不同医院、实践计划和培训项目间对内科进行整合。在担任布朗大学医学与生物科学院院长（2008—2013 年）期间，他加强了与各附属医院（Lifespan 医院和 Care New England 医院）间的联系，提升了科研工作的水准，并为医学院建成了一座新楼。在担任主任和院长期间，他还建立了与肯尼亚、多米尼加共和国和海地的医学院的国际交流项目。温博士自艾滋病流行初期便在门诊诊治艾滋病患者，并始终工作在科研、临床和教学一线。

弗雷德·谢夫曼（Fred J. Schiffman）博士与爱德华·温（Edward Wing）博士共同担任《希氏内科学精要》第 10 版的主编。他就读于瓦格纳学院，随后进入纽约大学医学院，并于 1973 年毕业。他在耶鲁大学附属纽黑文医院接受早期住院医师培训，随后在美国国家癌症研究所工作了两年。回到耶鲁大学后，他担任住院总医师，然后完成了血液学专科医师课程，随后成为耶鲁初级保健中心医学主任。他于 1983 年入职布朗大学，领导医学住院医师项目并担任米里亚姆医院的副主任医师。

谢夫曼博士担任布朗大学沃伦·阿尔珀特医学院人文医学系的西格尔家庭医学教授。他的学术兴趣涵盖人体脾脏的结构和功能，以及艺术与医疗的交叉融合。他主持或参与了许多项目和计划，其中包括许多旨在鼓励和加强患者、家人和医护人员的福祉与康复能力的项目。他所创办的一个新项目可以让医学生和医生与其他非医学专业人士一起，共同欣赏罗德岛设计学院博物馆的艺术作品。谢夫曼博士近期还主持了布朗大学名为"艺术与医学：艺术赋能患者照护"的 edX 课程，此课程的参与者来自全球多个国家。谢夫曼博士还出版了有关血液病理生理学、血液科会诊和贫血的著作。

原著者名单

Jinnette Dawn Abbott, MD
Rajiv Agarwal, MD
Marwa Al-Badri, MD
Hyeon-Ju Ryoo Ali, MD
Jason M. Aliotta, MD
Khaldoun Almhanna, MD, MPH
Mohanad T. Al-Qaisi, MD
Zuhal Arzomand, MD
Akwi W. Asombang, MD, MPH
Su N. Aung, MD, MPH
Christopher G. Azzoli, MD
Christina Bandera, MD
Debasree Banerjee, MD
Mashal Batheja, MD
Jeffrey J. Bazarian, MD, MPH
Selim R. Benbadis, MD
Ivor J. Benjamin, MD, FAHA, FACC
Eric Benoit, MD
Marcie G. Berger, MD
Clemens Bergwitz, MD
Nancy Berliner, MD
Jeffrey S. Berns, MD
Pooja Bhadbhade, DO
Ratna Bhavaraju-Sanka, MD
Tanmayee Bichile, MD
Ariel E. Birnbaum, MD
Charles M. Bliss, Jr., MD
Andrew S. Blum, MD, PhD
Bryan J. Bonder, MD
Russell Bratman, MD
Glenn D. Braunstein, MD
Alma M. Guerrero Bready, MD
Richard Bungiro, PhD
Anna Marie Burgner, MD, MEHP
Jonathan Cahill, MD
Andrew Canakis, DO
Benedito A. Carneiro, MD, MS
Brian Casserly, MD
Abdullah Chahin, MD, MA, MSc
Philip A. Chan, MD
Kimberle Chapin, MD
William P. Cheshire, Jr., MD
Waihong Chung, MD, PhD
Emma Ciafaloni, MD

Joaquin E. Cigarroa, MD
Michael P. Cinquegrani, MD
Andreea Coca, MD, MPH
Harvey Jay Cohen, MD
Scott Cohen, MD, MPH
Beatrice P. Concepcion, MD, MS
Nathan T. Connell, MD, MPH
Maria Constantinou, MD
Roberto Cortez, MD
Timothy J. Counihan, MD, FRCPI
Anne Haney Cross, MD
Cheston B. Cunha, MD, FACP
Joanne S. Cunha, MD
Susan Cu-Uvin, MD
Noura M. Dabbouseh, MD
Kwame Dapaah-Afriyie, MD, MBA
Erin M. Denney-Koelsch, MD
Andre De Souza, MD
An S. De Vriese, MD, PhD
Neal D. Dharmadhikari, MD
Leah Dickstein, MD
Don Dizon, MD, FACP, FASCO
Robyn T. Domsic, MD, MPH
Kim A. Eagle, MD
Michael G. Earing, MD
Pamela Egan, MD
Wafik S. El-Deiry, MD, PhD, FACP
Mitchell S. V. Elkind, MD, MS
Tarra B. Evans, MD
Michael B. Fallon, MD
Dimitrios Farmakiotis, MD
Francis A. Farraye, MD
Ronan Farrell, MD
Panayotis Fasseas, MD, FACC
Mary Anne Fenton, MD
Fernando C. Fervenza, MD, PhD
Sean Fine, MD
Arkadiy Finn, MD
Timothy Flanigan, MD
Brisas M. Flores, MD
Andrew E. Foderaro, MD
Theodore C. Friedman, MD, PhD
Joseph Metmowlee Garland, MD, AAHIVM

Eric J. Gartman, MD
Abdallah Geara, MD
Raul Macias Gil, MD
Timothy Gilligan, MD, FASCO
Michael Raymond Goggins, MB BCh BAO, MRCPI
Geetha Gopalakrishnan, MD
Vidya Gopinath, MD
Susan L. Greenspan, MD, FACP
Osama Hamdy, MD, PhD
Johanna Hamel, MD
Sajeev Handa, MD, SFHM
Mitchell T. Heflin, MD, MHS
Robert G. Holloway, MD, MPH
Christopher S. Huang, MD
Zilla Hussain, MD
T. Alp Ikizler, MD
Iris Isufi, MD
Carlayne E. Jackson, MD
Paul G. Jacob, MD, MPH
Matthew D. Jankowich, MD
Niels V. Johnsen, MD, MPH
Jessica E. Johnson, MD
Rayford R. June, MD
Tareq Kheirbek, MD, ScM, FACS
Alok A. Khorana, MD, FACP, FASCO
Sena Kilic, MD
David Kim, MD
James Kleczka, MD
James R. Klinger, MD
Patrick Koo, MD, ScM
Pooja Koolwal, MD
Mary P. Kotlarczyk, PhD
Nicole M. Kuderer, MD
Awewura Kwara, MD
Jennifer M. Kwon, MD, MPH
Richard A. Lange, MD, MBA
Jerome Larkin, MD
Alfred I. Lee, MD, PhD
Daniel J. Levine, MD
David E. Lewandowski, MD
Kelly V. Liang, MD, MS
Kimberly P. Liang, MD, MS
David R. Lichtenstein, MD

扫描二维码了解更多信息

Douglas W. Lienesch, MD
Geoffrey S.F. Ling, MD, PhD
Ester Little, MD, FACP
Yi Liu, MD
Nicole L. Lohr, MD, PhD
John R. Lonks, MD, FACP, FIDSA, FSHEA
Gary H. Lyman, MD, MPH
Jeffrey M. Lyness, MD
Shane Lyons, MD, MRCPI, MRCP(UK)
Diana Maas, MD
Talha A. Malik, MD, MSPH
Sonia Manocha, MD
Susan Manzi, MD, MPH
Frederick J. Marshall, MD
F. Dennis McCool, MD
Russell J. McCulloh, MD
Kelly McGarry, MD, FACP
Eavan Mc Govern, MD, PhD
Robin L. McKinney, MD
Anthony Mega, MD
Shivang Mehta, MD
Douglas F. Milam, MD
Maria D. Mileno, MD
Abhinav Kumar Misra, MBBS, MD
Orson W. Moe, MD
Niveditha Mohan, MBBS
Larry W. Moreland, MD
Alan R. Morrison, MD, PhD
Steven F. Moss, MD
Christopher J. Mullin, MD, MHS
Sinéad M. Murphy, MB, BCh, MD, FRCPI
Sagarika Nallu, MD, FAAP, FAAN, FAASM
Javier A. Neyra, MD, MSCS
Ghaith Noaiseh, MD

Thomas A. Ollila, MD
Steven M. Opal, MD
Biff F. Palmer, MD
Jen Jung Pan, MD, PhD
Anna Papazoglou, MD
Aric Parnes, MD
Nayan M. Patel, DO, MPH
Ari Pelcovits, MD
Mark A. Perazella, MD
Michael F. Picco, MD, PhD
Kate E. Powers, DO
Laura A. Previll, MD, MPH
Nilum Rajora, MD
Adolfo Ramirez-Zamora, MD
John Reagan, MD
Rebecca Reece, MD
Harlan Rich, MD, AGAF, FACP
Jennifer H. Richman, MD
Lisa R. Rogers, DO
Ralph Rogers, MD
Michal G. Rose, MD
James A. Roth, MD
Sharon Rounds, MD
Jason C. Rubenstein, MD
Abbas Rupawala, MD
Jenna Sarvaideo, DO
Ramesh Saxena, MD, PhD
Fred J. Schiffman, MD, MACP
Ruth B. Schneider, MD
Kristin A. Seaborg, MD
Anil Seetharam, MD
Stuart Seropian, MD
Jigme Michael Sethi, MD
Sanjeev Sethi, MD, PhD
Elizabeth Shane, MD
Esseim Sharma, MD

Shani Shastri, MD, MPH
Barry S. Shea, MD
Lauren Shevell, MD, MPH
Joseph A. Smith, Jr., MD
Robert J. Smith, MD
Davendra P.S. Sohal, MD, MPH
Christopher Song, MD, FACC
Thomas Sperry, MD
Jeffrey M. Statland, MD
Emily M. Stein, MD
Jennifer L. Strande, MD, PhD
Rochelle Strenger, MD
Thomas R. Talbot, MD, MPH
Christopher G. Tarolli, MD, MSEd
Yael Tarshish, MD
Pushpak Taunk, MD
Philip Tsoukas, MD
Allan R. Tunkel, MD, PhD
Jeffrey M. Turner, MD
Zoe G.S. Vazquez, MD
Stacie A. F. Vela, MD
Paul M. Vespa, MD, FCCM, FAAN, FANA, FNCS
Wanpen Vongpatanasin, MD
Marcella D. Walker, MD
Eunice S. Wang, MD
Sharmeel K. Wasan, MD
Thomas J. Weber, MD
Brandon J. Wilcoxson, MD
Edward J. Wing, MD, FACP, FIDSA
Ellice Wong, MD
John J. Wysolmerski, MD
Rayan Yousefzai, MD
Thomas R. Ziegler, MD
Rebecca Zon, MD

ACKNOWLEDGMENTS

Dr. Schiffman and I wish to thank first of all, the authors of the 128 chapters that make up the tenth edition of *Cecil Essentials of Medicine*. They have worked diligently to compose the material for each chapter and apply their mastery as they added the newest information, in clear language, to the text. Their efforts are apparent in the excellence of the book, and we are immensely grateful for their work. We wish to also thank Marybeth Thiel, Jennifer Ehlers, and Dan Fitzgerald from Elsevier who guided and supported our work as editors and whose expertise has made this volume possible. Finally, we are always thankful to our wives, Dr. Rena Wing and Ms. Gerri Schiffman, without whose love, support, and especially humor, this book would not have happened.

致 谢

谢夫曼博士和我首先要致谢《希氏内科学精要》第 10 版全书 128 章的各位作者。感谢他们精益求精地撰写每一章节，并运用其专业知识，以简明的语言将前沿资讯呈现在书中。正是他们的辛勤努力确保了本书的卓越地位，对他们唯有由衷的感激。我们还要感谢爱思唯尔出版集团的玛丽贝丝·蒂尔（Marybeth Thiel）、詹妮弗·埃勒斯（Jennifer Ehlers）和丹·菲茨杰拉德（Dan Fitzgerald），他们对本书的编辑工作给予了指导和支持，其专业水准保障了本书的完稿。最后，要特别感谢我们的妻子——蕾娜·温（Rena Wing）博士和盖瑞·谢夫曼（Gerri Schiffman）女士，对她们的爱和支持，特别是积极乐观的心态始终心存感激，她们为本书的圆满完成发挥了不可或缺的作用。

总目录

第 1 分册

第 1 篇　内科学概论　Introduction to Medicine
第 2 篇　呼吸与危重症医学　Pulmonary and Critical Care Medicine
第 3 篇　术前和术后照护　Preoperative and Postoperative Care

第 2 分册

心血管疾病　Cardiovascular Disease

第 3 分册

肾脏疾病　Renal Disease

第 4 分册

第 1 篇　胃肠疾病　Gastrointestinal Disease
第 2 篇　肝脏与胆道系统疾病　Diseases of the Liver and Biliary System

第 5 分册

血液疾病　Hematologic Disease

第 6 分册

肿瘤疾病　Oncologic Disease

第 7 分册

第 1 篇　内分泌疾病与代谢疾病　Endocrine Disease and Metabolic Disease
第 2 篇　女性健康　Women's Health
第 3 篇　男性健康　Men's Health
第 4 篇　骨与骨矿物质代谢疾病　Diseases of Bone and Bone Mineral Metabolism

第 8 分册

肌肉骨骼与结缔组织疾病　Musculoskeletal and Connective Tissue Disease

第 9 分册

感染性疾病　Infectious Disease

第 10 分册

第 1 篇　神经疾病　Neurologic Disease
第 2 篇　老年医学　Geriatrics
第 3 篇　缓和医疗　Palliative Care
第 4 篇　酒精和物质使用　Alcohol and Substance Use

第 8 分册
肌肉骨骼与结缔组织疾病

第8分册译者名单

主　译

栗占国　李梦涛

译　者（按姓氏笔画排序）

王　俐	中国科学技术大学附属第一医院	金月波	北京大学人民医院
厉小梅	中国科学技术大学附属第一医院	周佳鑫	中国医学科学院北京协和医院
田新平	中国医学科学院北京协和医院	赵　征	中国人民解放军总医院第一医学中心
朱华群	北京大学人民医院	赵久良	中国医学科学院北京协和医院
孙　兴	北京大学人民医院	赵萌萌	中国医科大学附属第一医院
李　茹	北京大学人民医院	栗占国	北京大学人民医院
李梦涛	中国医学科学院北京协和医院	贾　园	北京大学人民医院
李谦华	中山大学孙逸仙纪念医院	徐　东	中国医学科学院北京协和医院
杨娉婷	中国医科大学附属第一医院	黄　璨	中国医学科学院北京协和医院
何　菁	北京大学人民医院	靳尚宜	中国医学科学院北京协和医院
张　婷	浙江大学医学院附属第二医院	薛　静	浙江大学医学院附属第二医院
罗　贵	中国人民解放军总医院第一医学中心	戴　冽	中山大学孙逸仙纪念医院

第 8 分册目录

肌肉骨骼与结缔组织疾病　Musculoskeletal and Connective Tissue Disease

1. Approach to the Patient With Rheumatic Disease, 4
   风湿性疾病患者的接诊，5

2. Rheumatoid Arthritis, 12
   类风湿关节炎，13

3. Spondyloarthritis, 26
   脊柱关节炎，27

4. Systemic Lupus Erythematosus, 36
   系统性红斑狼疮，37

5. Systemic Sclerosis, 58
   系统性硬化症，59

6. Systemic Vasculitis, 72
   系统性血管炎，73

7. Crystal Arthropathies, 84
   晶体性关节病，85

8. Osteoarthritis, 96
   骨关节炎，97

9. Nonarticular Soft Tissue Disorders, 106
   非关节软组织疾病，107

10. Rheumatic Manifestations of Systemic Disorders and Sjögren's Syndrome, 114
    系统性疾病的风湿性表现和干燥综合征，115

索引 Index，128

CECIL ESSENTIALS OF MEDICINE

Musculoskeletal and Connective Tissue Disease

Musculoskeletal and Connective Tissue Disease

1. **Approach to the Patient With Rheumatic Disease, 4**
2. **Rheumatoid Arthritis, 12**
3. **Spondyloarthritis, 26**
4. **Systemic Lupus Erythematosus, 36**
5. **Systemic Sclerosis, 58**
6. **Systemic Vasculitis, 72**
7. **Crystal Arthropathies, 84**
8. **Osteoarthritis, 96**
9. **Nonarticular Soft Tissue Disorders, 106**
10. **Rheumatic Manifestations of Systemic Disorders and Sjögren's Syndrome, 114**

肌肉骨骼与结缔组织疾病

1　风湿性疾病患者的接诊，5

2　类风湿关节炎，13

3　脊柱关节炎，27

4　系统性红斑狼疮，37

5　系统性硬化症，59

6　系统性血管炎，73

7　晶体性关节病，85

8　骨关节炎，97

9　非关节软组织疾病，107

10　系统性疾病的风湿性表现和干燥综合征，115

1

Approach to the Patient With Rheumatic Disease

Niveditha Mohan

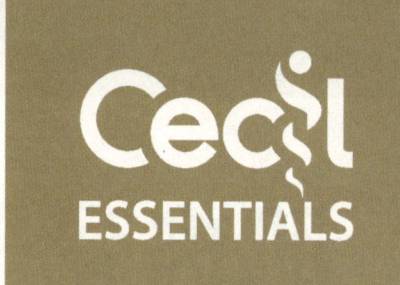

INTRODUCTION

Rheumatic diseases encompass a range of musculoskeletal and systemic disorders that involve the joints and periarticular tissues in addition to other organ systems in the body. Differentiating localized from systemic processes, executing logical diagnostic procedures, and embarking on appropriate therapeutic courses demand careful clinical evaluation. The medical history and physical examination are paramount in this process. Laboratory tests are more confirmatory than diagnostic. Confirmation or exclusion of systemic connective tissue disease on the basis of laboratory results is unreliable and therefore unwise.

MUSCULOSKELETAL HISTORY

A logical approach to musculoskeletal complaints is indispensable to arriving at the correct diagnosis. Features in the medical history that are useful for distinguishing different types of arthritis are listed in Tables 1.1 and 1.2. The first step is to confirm that the complaint originates from the musculoskeletal system and is not referred pain caused by other organ system pathology (e.g., left shoulder pain due to cardiac disease). The next step is to define whether the problem is articular or extra-articular based on the history and clinical presentation.

Demographic data provide useful information. The age of the patient can point to a specific rheumatic disorder. The spondyloarthropathies are more commonly diagnosed in young men, systemic lupus erythematosus (SLE) in young women, gout in middle-aged men and postmenopausal women, and osteoarthritis in the older population. Asymmetrical pain and swelling in the knees have different connotations in a 70-year-old patient than in a 20-year-old patient.

Immune status may affect the diagnosis of rheumatic disease. Immunocompromised patients should be evaluated for infectious arthritis. Patients with human immunodeficiency virus (HIV) infection may have a severe form of Reiter syndrome or a sudden flare of psoriasis or psoriatic arthritis.

The patient's history provides the basis for differentiating inflammatory from noninflammatory arthropathies. Inflammatory arthritis is characterized by pain at rest, morning stiffness (typically greater than 60 minutes), gelling phenomenon (i.e., stiffening of joints after inactivity), and joint tenderness associated with other signs of inflammation such as swelling, erythema, and warmth. In osteoarthritis and nonarthritic musculoskeletal problems, pain usually does not occur at rest and is precipitated or worsened by activity. Some osteoarthritic joints are stiff initially but are improved with activity. The onset of disease is abrupt in crystal-induced arthritis, less so in septic arthritis, and slow and insidious in most other disorders.

Patterns of joint involvement are typical of certain disorders: monoarthritis (one joint), as in septic or crystal-induced arthritis; pauciarthritis or oligoarthritis (two to four joints), as in Reiter syndrome or psoriatic arthritis; and polyarthritis (five or more joints), as in rheumatoid arthritis or SLE. Symmetry, migratory features, large versus small joint involvement, and axial versus appendicular locations are characteristic features of specific diseases and should be sought in the patient's history. Enthesopathy (i.e., disease at the attachment of tendons or ligaments to bone) can indicate a spondyloarthropathy.

Constitutional features such as fatigue, weight loss, and fever are seen in systemic autoimmune disease and infection but not in localized conditions. A thorough review of systems can provide clues to the primary diagnosis by defining associated systemic syndromes. Although there are many exceptions to these demographic and clinical generalizations, they provide helpful starting points when a patient is being evaluated for the first time.

PHYSICAL EXAMINATION

On physical examination, active and passive range of motion in all joints should be carefully assessed, and tenderness, swelling, warmth, erythema, deformity, and joint effusions should be evaluated (Fig. 1.1). Patients are frequently unaware of detectable joint abnormalities, including deformity and effusion, which are signs of joint disease. Reported pain may be referred from another site, which can be determined by examination. Pain in the knee is often a sign of hip disease and may be reproduced on examination of the hip. Palpable synovitis (i.e., thickening of the synovial membrane) is helpful in diagnosing inflammatory arthritides such as rheumatoid arthritis.

Different diseases have distinctive patterns of joint involvement, which provide critical diagnostic information. For example, prominent disease of distal interphalangeal joints is seen in psoriasis and inflammatory osteoarthritis. Wrist and metacarpophalangeal involvement are almost universal in rheumatoid arthritis but rare in osteoarthritis. Examination of the axial skeleton may reveal diminished lumbar flexion, decreased rotational motion of the spine, and decreased chest expansion, features of ankylosing spondylitis and other spondyloarthropathies. Patients may report symptoms in only a single joint, but finding additional affected joints on physical examination can change the entire evaluation.

Because rheumatic diseases may involve any organ system, a complete physical examination should be performed for all patients.

风湿性疾病患者的接诊

张婷 译　薛静 赵征 审校　李梦涛 通审

引言

风湿性疾病包括一系列肌肉骨骼和系统性疾病，累及关节和关节周围组织以及其他器官系统。鉴别局部或系统性病变、展开合理的诊断流程、给予恰当的治疗需要细致的临床评估。在这一过程中，病史和体格检查至关重要。实验室检查更多是有助于确认而非直接诊断。仅仅基于实验室检查的结果确认或排除系统性结缔组织病是不可靠且不明智的。

肌肉骨骼病史

针对肌肉骨骼主诉展开合理的评估是获得正确诊断必不可少的。表1.1和表1.2列出了病史中有助于区分不同类型关节炎的特征。首先确认症状源自肌肉骨骼系统，而非其他器官系统病变引起的牵涉痛（如心脏疾病引起的左肩痛）。其次根据病史和临床表现确定是关节病变还是关节外病变。

人口学数据可提供有用的信息。患者的年龄可以指向特定的风湿性疾病。脊柱关节病常见于年轻男性，系统性红斑狼疮（SLE）常见于年轻女性，痛风多见于中年男性和绝经后女性，骨关节炎则多见于老年人。膝关节不对称的疼痛和肿胀在70岁患者和20岁患者具有不同的提示意义。

免疫状态可能影响风湿性疾病的诊断。免疫功能低下的患者应评估感染性关节炎的可能。感染了人类免疫缺陷病毒（HIV）的患者可能出现严重的赖特综合征，或者出现银屑病或银屑病关节炎的突然发作。

患者的病史是区分炎症性和非炎症性关节病的基础。炎症性关节炎的特征是休息时疼痛、晨僵（通常大于60 min）、胶着现象（即静息后关节僵硬）、关节压痛伴有其他炎症表现如肿胀、发红和皮温升高。在骨关节炎和非关节炎性肌肉骨骼病变中，疼痛通常不会在休息时出现，而是在活动时加剧或恶化。但有些骨关节炎患者的关节起初很僵硬，而活动后会有所改善。晶体诱发的关节炎急性起病，化脓性关节炎起病急性程度较之略缓，而其他大多数关节炎起病缓慢而隐匿。

关节受累的模式是某些疾病的典型特征：单关节炎（1个关节）见于化脓性关节炎或晶体诱发的关节炎；少关节炎或寡关节炎（2～4个关节）见于赖特综合征或银屑病关节炎；多关节炎（大于等于5个关节）见于类风湿关节炎或SLE。对称性、游走性、大关节或小关节受累、中轴或外周关节受累是特定疾病的典型特征，应在病史中寻找。附着点病（即肌腱或韧带在骨骼附着部位的疾病）可提示脊柱关节病。

全身性症状如疲劳、体重减轻和发热可见于系统性自身免疫性疾病和感染，但不会在局部病变时出现。通过全面的系统回顾发现相关系统性症状时，可以为主要诊断提供线索。尽管这些人口统计学特征和临床表现结论存在诸多例外，但它们为首次评估患者时提供了有益的切入点。

体格检查

在体格检查中，应细致评估所有关节的主动和被动活动范围，并评估是否存在压痛、肿胀、皮温升高、发红、关节畸形和关节积液（图1.1）。患者通常不会意识到关节的异常征象如关节畸形和关节积液，而这些都是关节疾病的表现。患者主诉的疼痛可能来自其他部位，这可以通过查体明确。膝关节的疼痛常常在检查髋关节时也会出现，因此也可能是髋关节疾病的表现。可触及的滑膜炎（即滑膜增厚）有助于诊断炎症性关节炎如类风湿关节炎。

不同的疾病有不同的关节受累模式，可提供关键的诊断信息。例如，远端指间关节显著受累可见于银屑病和炎症性骨关节炎。腕和掌指关节受累在类风湿关节炎中普遍存在，但在骨关节炎中罕见。中轴骨骼查体发现腰椎屈曲受限、脊柱旋转运动减少、胸廓扩张度下降，这些是强直性脊柱炎和其他脊柱关节病的特征。患者可能仅报告单个关节的症状，但在体格检查时发现还存在其他关节受累就会改变整个疾病的评估。

由于风湿性疾病可能累及任何器官系统，应对所

Alopecia and funduscopic changes (in SLE), uveitis (in spondyloarthropathy and juvenile arthritis), conjunctivitis (in reactive arthritis), sicca symptoms (in Sjögren's syndrome), oral and other mucous membrane ulcers (in reactive arthritis, SLE, and Behçet syndrome), lymphadenopathy (in SLE and Sjögren's syndrome), and cutaneous lesions (in psoriasis, dermatomyositis, scleroderma, SLE, and vasculitides) should be considered. Recurrent otorhinolaryngologic complaints, such as sinusitis, should raise suspicion for granulomatosis with polyangiitis (i.e., Wegener's granulomatosis). Lesions of psoriasis in the scalp, umbilicus, and anal crease, thickening of the skin on the fingers in scleroderma, and mucous membrane ulcers are often overlooked.

The lung examination may find evidence of interstitial fibrosis (in scleroderma, SLE, rheumatoid arthritis, and myositis), and a cardiac evaluation may reveal aortic insufficiency (in SLE and spondyloarthropathy), pulmonary hypertension (in systemic sclerosis), or evidence of cardiomyopathy (in systemic sclerosis, myositis, and amyloidosis). Pleural and pericardial rubs may be detected in SLE. Hepatosplenomegaly (in SLE and rheumatoid arthritis) and abdominal distention (in scleroderma) are also valuable clinical clues.

Muscle examination may reveal weakness from myositis, neuropathy (in vasculitis and SLE) or myopathy (in steroid myopathy). A complete neurologic examination may reveal carpal tunnel syndrome, peripheral neuropathy such as mononeuritis multiplex (i.e., asymmetrical sensory or motor neuropathy seen in many vasculitides), and central nervous system disease (in SLE and vasculitis). Recurrent miscarriages, livedo reticularis, Raynaud's phenomenon, and recurrent thrombotic events indicate antiphospholipid antibody syndrome.

The onset of systemic rheumatic diseases is usually insidious, and the clinical course is prolonged. However, presentation sometimes can be acute depending on the organ system involved. The initial evaluation must determine whether diagnosis and treatment of the patient's problem requires urgent attention. Infectious processes need immediate treatment. Acute joint inflammation, fever, and systemic signs such as chills, night sweats, and leukocytosis provide supporting evidence for infection. Gouty arthritis may share some or all of these clinical features, but its onset tends to be more abrupt. Inflammation extending beyond the margins of the joint is characteristic of septic arthritis and is otherwise seen only in crystal disease. Nonarticular processes such as cellulitis, septic bursitis, tenosynovitis, and phlebitis may mimic infectious arthritis. Analysis of synovial fluid is the key to diagnosis.

Acute nerve entrapment or spinal cord compression, tendon rupture, and fractures may occur in the absence of obvious trauma. Spinal cord compression may be the result of a herniated disk or vertebral subluxation. Tendon rupture may occur in inflammatory arthritides, particularly in the wrist of patients with rheumatoid arthritis. Pelvic and other insufficiency fractures may be seen in patients with osteoporosis or osteomalacia.

Patients with SLE or systemic vasculitis may have central or peripheral nervous system disease, including brain and peripheral nerve infarcts, glomerulonephritis, inflammatory or hemorrhagic lung disease, coronary artery involvement, intestinal infarcts, and digital infarcts. Threatened digit loss may also be seen in cases of scleroderma due to severe Raynaud's and vasculitis. Renal crisis may occur in scleroderma, with vasculopathy leading to renal infarcts, azotemia, microangiopathy, and severe hypertension. Acute blindness is a potential complication of giant cell arteritis, and the diagnosis requires urgent therapy even before confirmatory biopsy.

Acute inflammatory myositis should be promptly treated because it may progress rapidly and involve the respiratory musculature. In some cases, major organ involvement may be occult. When systemic disease is suggested, the patient's lungs and kidneys should be carefully evaluated.

TABLE 1.1 Clinical Features That Are Helpful in the Evaluation of Arthritis

- Age, sex, ethnicity, family history
- Pattern of joint involvement
- Monoarticular, oligoarticular, polyarticular
- Large versus small joints
- Symmetry
- Insidious versus rapid onset
- Inflammatory versus noninflammatory pain (e.g., morning stiffness, gelling, night pain)
- Constitutional symptoms and signs (e.g., fever, fatigue, weight loss)
- Synovitis, bursitis, tendinitis
- Involvement of other organ systems (e.g., rash, mucous membrane lesions, nail lesions)
- Arthritis-associated diseases (e.g., psoriasis, inflammatory bowel disease)
- Anemia, proteinuria, azotemia
- Erosive joint disease

TABLE 1.2 Differentiating Features of Common Arthritides

Disease	Demographics	Joints Involved	Special Features	Laboratory Findings
Gout	Men, postmenopausal women	Monoarticular or oligoarticular	Podagra, rapid onset of attack, polyarticular gout, tophi	SF: Crystals, high WBC count, >80% PMNs
Septic arthritis	Any age	Usually large joints	Fever, chills	SF: High WBC count, >90% PMNs, culture
Osteoarthritis	Increases with age	Weight-bearing, hands		Noninflammatory SF
Rheumatoid arthritis	Any age, predominantly women ages 20–50 yr	Symmetrical, small joints disease	Rheumatoid nodules, extra-articular	SF: High WBC count, >70% PMNs
Reactive arthritis (Reiter syndrome)	Young males	Oligoarticular, asymmetrical	Urethritis, conjunctivitis, skin and mucous membranes	SF: Moderate WBC count, >50% PMNs
Spondyloarthropathy	Young to middle-aged men	Axial skeleton, pelvis (sacroiliac joints)	Uveitis, aortic insufficiency, enthesopathy	
Systemic lupus erythematosus	Women in childbearing years	Hands, knees	Nonerosive joint disease, autoantibodies, mostly mononuclear; multiorgan disease	SF: Low to moderate WBC count, almost 100% have antinuclear antibodies

PMNs, Neutrophils; *SF*, synovial fluid; *WBC*, white blood cell.

有患者进行全面的体格检查。应关注脱发和眼底改变（SLE）、葡萄膜炎（脊柱关节病和幼年型关节炎）、结膜炎（反应性关节炎）、干燥症状（干燥综合征）、口腔和其他黏膜溃疡（反应性关节炎、SLE和白塞综合征）、淋巴结肿大（SLE和干燥综合征）和皮肤病变（银屑病、皮肌炎、硬皮病、SLE和血管炎）。反复出现耳鼻咽喉症状如鼻窦炎，应怀疑肉芽肿性多血管炎（即韦格纳肉芽肿病）。头皮、脐和肛周皱褶处的银屑病皮损，硬皮病患者手指皮肤增厚和黏膜溃疡常被忽视。

肺部检查可能发现间质纤维化的证据（硬皮病、SLE、类风湿关节炎和肌炎），心脏评估可能提示主动脉瓣功能不全（SLE和脊柱关节病）、肺动脉高压（系统性硬化症）或心肌病（系统性硬化症、肌炎和淀粉样变性）证据。SLE中可能检测到胸膜和心包摩擦音。肝脾肿大（SLE和类风湿关节炎）和腹胀（硬皮病）也是有价值的临床线索。

肌肉检查可发现肌炎、神经病变（血管炎和SLE）或肌病（类固醇性肌病）引起的肌无力。全面的神经系统检查可能会发现腕管综合征、周围神经病变如多发性单神经炎（即多种血管炎中出现的不对称感觉或运动神经病变）和中枢神经系统疾病（SLE和血管炎）。复发性流产、网状青斑、雷诺现象和反复血栓事件提示抗磷脂综合征。

系统性风湿性疾病的起病通常是隐匿的，临床病程迁延。但是，临床表现有时可能是急性的，这取决于受累的器官系统。初始评估必须明确患者的问题是否需要紧急诊断和治疗。感染需要立即治疗。急性关节炎症、发热和全身性表现如寒战、盗汗和白细胞增多为感染提供了支持证据。痛风性关节炎可能具有部分或所有上述临床表现，但其发作往往更突然。炎症范围超出关节边界是化脓性关节炎的典型表现，除此之外这种情况仅见于晶体诱发的关节炎。非关节病变如蜂窝织炎、化脓性滑囊炎、腱鞘炎和静脉炎等可能表现出感染性关节炎的症状。滑液分析是诊断的关键。

急性神经卡压或脊髓压迫、肌腱断裂和骨折可能在没有明显创伤的情况下发生。脊髓压迫可能由椎间盘突出或椎体脱位造成。肌腱断裂可能发生于炎症性关节炎，特别是类风湿关节炎患者的腕关节。骨盆和其他不全骨折可见于骨质疏松症或骨软化症患者。

SLE或系统性血管炎患者可能出现中枢或周围神经系统病变（包括脑和周围神经梗死）、肾小球肾炎、炎症性或出血性肺病、冠状动脉受累、肠梗死和指趾梗死。在硬皮病患者中，严重的雷诺现象和血管炎可能导致指趾坏死。硬皮病可能出现肾危象，血管病变可导致肾脏梗死、氮质血症、微血管病变和严重高血压。急性失明是巨细胞动脉炎的潜在并发症，甚至在活检确诊前就需要紧急治疗。

急性炎症性肌炎应及时治疗，因其可能快速进展并累及呼吸肌。在某些情况下，主要器官受累可能较为隐匿。当考虑系统性疾病时，应仔细评估患者的肺和肾脏。

表1.1 有助于评估关节炎的临床特征

年龄、性别、种族、家族史
关节受累模式
　单关节、寡关节、多关节
　大关节 vs. 小关节
　对称性
　隐匿起病 vs. 急性起病
　炎症性疼痛 vs. 非炎症性疼痛（如晨僵、胶着、夜间疼痛）
全身症状和体征（如发热、疲乏、体重减轻）
滑膜炎、滑囊炎、肌腱炎
其他器官系统受累（如皮疹、黏膜病变、指甲病变）
关节炎相关疾病（如银屑病、炎症性肠病）
贫血、蛋白尿、氮质血症
侵蚀性关节疾病

表1.2 常见关节炎鉴别特征

疾病	人口统计学特征	受累关节	特殊表现	实验室检查
痛风	男性，绝经后女性	单关节或寡关节	累及第一跖趾关节的足痛风，急性起病，多关节痛风，痛风石	SF：晶体，WBC计数高，>80% PMN
化脓性关节炎	任何年龄	通常大关节	发热、寒战	SF：WBC计数高，>90% PMN，培养
骨关节炎	随年龄增加	承重关节，手		非炎症性SF
类风湿关节炎	任何年龄，20～50岁女性多见	对称性、小关节受累	类风湿结节，关节外表现	SF：WBC计数高，>70% PMN
反应性关节炎（赖特综合征）	年轻男性	寡关节，非对称性	尿道炎、结膜炎、皮肤和黏膜受累	SF：WBC计数中等量，>50% PMN
脊柱关节病	青中年男性	中轴骨，骨盆（骶髂关节）	葡萄膜炎，主动脉瓣关闭不全，附着点病	
系统性红斑狼疮	育龄期女性	手，膝	非侵蚀性关节炎，自身抗体，几乎100%抗核抗体阳性；多脏器受累（译者注：原文"几乎100%抗核抗体阳性"和"多数为单个核细胞"排位有误）	SF：WBC计数低-中等量，多数为单个核细胞

PMN，中性粒细胞；SF，滑液；WBC，白细胞。

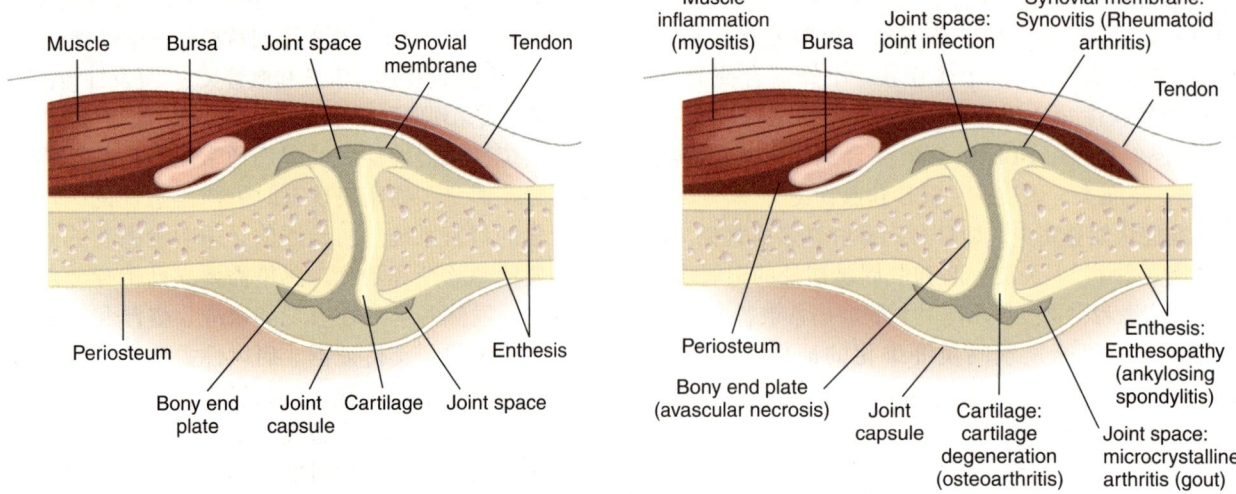

Fig. 1.1 Anatomic structures of the musculoskeletal system *(left)*. Locations of musculoskeletal disease processes *(right)*. (From Gordon DA: Approach to the patient with musculoskeletal disease. In Bennett JC, Plum F, editors: Cecil textbook of medicine, ed 20, Philadelphia, 1996, WB Saunders, p 1440.)

TABLE 1.3	Classification of Synovial Effusions by Synovial White Blood Cell Count			
Group	Sample Diagnoses	Appearance	Synovial Fluid WBC Count (MM³)[a]	PMN Cells (%)
Normal		Clear, pale yellow	0–200	<10
I. Noninflammatory	Osteoarthritis; trauma	Clear to slightly turbid	50–2000 (600)	<30
II. Mildly inflammatory	Systemic lupus erythematosus	Clear to slightly turbid	100–9000 (3000)	<20
III. Severely inflammatory (noninfectious)	Gout	Turbid	2000–160,000 (21,000)	≈70
	Pseudogout	Turbid	500–75,000 (14,000)	≈70
	Rheumatoid arthritis	Turbid	2000–80,000 (19,000)	≈70
IV. Severely inflammatory (infectious)	Bacterial infections	Very turbid	5000–250,000 (80,000)	≈90
	Tuberculosis	Turbid	2500–100,000 (20,000)	≈60

PMNs, Neutrophils; *WBC*, white blood cell.
[a]Range, with mean values in parentheses.

LABORATORY TESTING

Synovial fluid analysis is an important part of the evaluation of arthritis (Table 1.3). It helps to distinguish between inflammatory and noninflammatory arthritis, and results can be diagnostic of infectious arthritis or crystal disease.

Synovial fluid consists of an ultrafiltrate of plasma plus hyaluronic acid that is secreted by synovial lining cells. Evaluation of synovial fluid should include a cell count and differential, examination for sodium urate and calcium phosphate dehydrate crystals, Gram stain, and culture. Synovial fluid glucose and protein levels are not useful tests. Synovial fluid examination should be performed for all acute arthritides and all situations in which joint infection is likely. It should be performed at least once to evaluate chronic inflammatory arthritis. Aspiration and analysis of fluid before therapy are essential for appropriate decision making.

Although autoantibodies are often considered the hallmark of rheumatic diseases, their utility in diagnosing individual patients is much less than commonly assumed. Although almost 95% of patients with SLE have antinuclear antibodies (ANAs), as do most patients with scleroderma and autoimmune myositis, the proportion of patients with other rheumatic diseases who have positive test results is much lower. Conversely, 15% to 25% of healthy persons have ANAs, sometimes in high titers, when commercial test kits are used. Older persons and patients with nonrheumatic systemic diseases such as malignancies and nonrheumatic autoimmune diseases such as thyroiditis or hypothyroidism have even higher frequencies of ANAs.

The very low specificity of a positive ANA result in the absence of clinical findings for an autoimmune disorder precludes its use as a screening test for disease in the general population. Other autoantibodies may be more useful and are discussed in subsequent chapters.

Rheumatoid factor is found in approximately 80% of patients with rheumatoid arthritis but also found in other rheumatic diseases, chronic infection, neoplasia, and almost any disease state that can cause chronic hyperglobulinemia. Neither positive nor negative test results are diagnostic, and the results should be interpreted only in the clinical context. Although the specificity of the rheumatoid factor is low, it does predict more aggressive joint disease and extra-articular joint manifestations.

Antibodies to cyclic citrullinated peptides are helpful in diagnosing rheumatoid arthritis because they have a high specificity (>90%). Their sensitivity varies from about 50% to 75%. Antibody tests should be ordered and repeated only if they can help in making the diagnosis, assessing the prognosis, or altering the treatment plan.

Tests for acute phase proteins, C-reactive protein, and the erythrocyte sedimentation rate are nonspecific, but positive results suggest an inflammatory disease. In some cases, such as in patients with giant cell

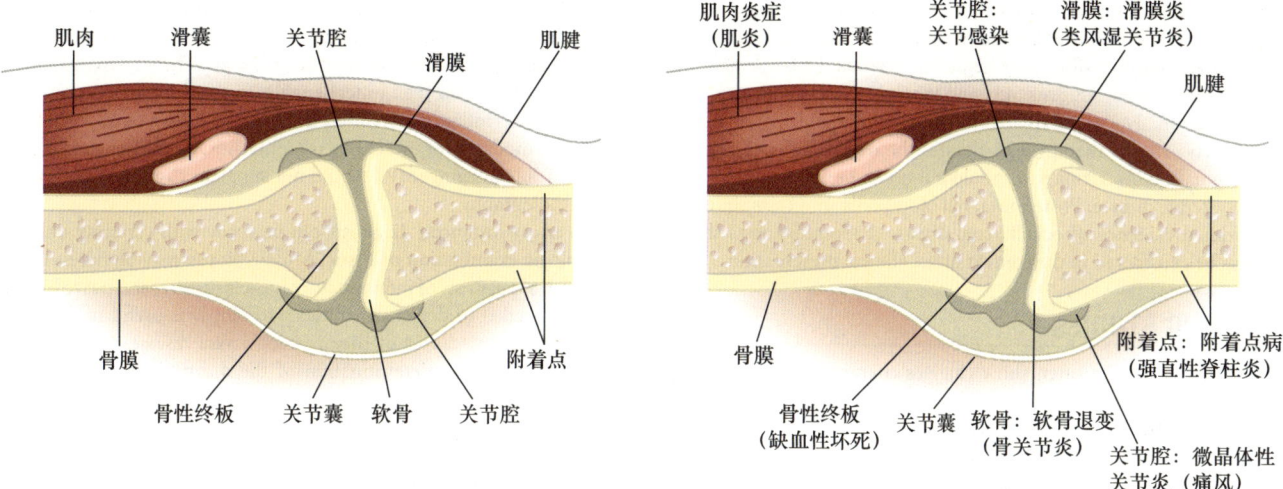

图1.1 肌肉骨骼系统解剖结构（左）和肌肉骨骼疾病累及部位（右）（引自 Gordon DA：Approach to the patient with musculoskeletal disease. In Bennett JC, Plum F, editors: Cecil textbook of medicine, ed 20, Philadelphia, 1996, WB Saunders, p 1440.）（译者注：原文右图骨膜箭头标注位置有误）

表1.3 根据滑液白细胞计数的滑液分类				
类型	标本诊断	外观	滑液 WBC 计数（/mm³）ª	PMN（%）
正常		清，淡黄	0～200	<10
Ⅰ.非炎症性	骨关节炎；外伤	清至微混	50～2000（600）	<30
Ⅱ.轻度炎症	SLE	清至微混	100～9000（3000）	<20
Ⅲ.重度炎症（非感染）	痛风	混浊	2000～160 000（21 000）	≈70
	假性痛风	混浊	500～75 000（14 000）	≈70
	类风湿关节炎	混浊	2000～80 000（19 000）	≈70
Ⅳ.重度炎症（感染）	细菌感染	非常混浊	5000～250 000（80 000）	≈90
	结核	混浊	2500～100 000（20 000）	≈60

PMN，中性粒细胞；WBC，白细胞。
ª 范围，括号内为均值

实验室检查

滑液分析是关节炎评估的重要组成部分（表1.3）。它有助于区分炎症性关节炎和非炎症性关节炎，其结果可以诊断感染性关节炎或晶体性关节炎。

滑液由血浆超滤液和滑膜衬里细胞分泌的透明质酸组成。滑液评估应包括细胞计数和分类、尿酸钠和脱水磷酸钙晶体的检查、革兰氏染色和培养。滑液葡萄糖和蛋白质水平改变临床意义不大。对于所有急性关节炎和可能发生关节感染的情况都应进行滑液检查。对于慢性炎症性关节炎应至少进行一次关节滑液的评估。治疗前对滑液进行抽吸和分析是做出适当决策的关键。

尽管自身抗体通常被认为是风湿性疾病的标志，但它们在风湿病个体患者临床诊断时的作用要远低于预期。几乎95%的SLE患者抗核抗体（ANA）阳性，大多数硬皮病和自身免疫性肌炎患者也是如此，而其他风湿性疾病患者检测结果呈阳性的比例要低得多。相反，当使用商业检测试剂盒时，15%～25%的健康人也会出现ANA阳性，甚至有时呈高滴度阳性。老年人、非风湿性系统性疾病如恶性肿瘤、非风湿性自身免疫性疾病如甲状腺炎或甲状腺功能减退症患者，ANA阳性比例更高。

在没有自身免疫性疾病临床表现的情况下，ANA阳性的特异性非常低，因此不能用作一般人群的疾病筛查试验。其他自身抗体可能更有意义，将在后续章节中讨论。

类风湿因子见于大约80%的类风湿关节炎患者，但也见于其他风湿性疾病、慢性感染、肿瘤以及几乎任何可引起慢性高球蛋白血症的疾病状态。阳性或阴性检测结果均不具有诊断意义，结果应结合具体临床情况进行解读。虽然类风湿因子的特异性较低，但它可以预测更具侵袭性的关节疾病和关节外表现。

抗环瓜氨酸肽抗体有助于诊断类风湿关节炎，具有高特异性（>90%）。其敏感性约为50%～75%。只有当抗体检测有助于诊断、评估预后或调整治疗方案时，才应安排测定和复查。

急性期蛋白、C反应蛋白和红细胞沉降率并不特异，但阳性结果提示炎症性疾病。在某些情况下，例如巨细胞动脉炎和风湿性多肌痛患者，这些检查可能

arteritis and polymyalgia rheumatica, these tests may be useful for the diagnosis and monitoring the course of disease and therapy. Anemia may suggest chronic disease or hemolytic anemia. Leukopenia, especially lymphopenia, suggests SLE, and thrombocytosis indicates active inflammation. Leukocytosis may reflect inflammation or infection, and glucocorticoid therapy also elevates the neutrophil cell count by demargination. Urinalysis should always be performed in patients with systemic disease. Proteinuria, red blood cells, and casts should be considered evidence of occult renal disease. Laboratory tests should always be considered in the context of the clinical presentation.

IMAGING STUDIES

Radiographic studies often show changes characteristic of particular diseases. In patients with established rheumatoid arthritis, radiographs may demonstrate classically erosive disease of the small joints of the wrists, the ulnar styloid, the metacarpophalangeal and proximal interphalangeal joints, and the small joints in the foot. The erosions are bland and nonreactive. In contrast, erosive psoriatic arthritis causes a sclerotic reaction, and the patient may have characteristic telescoping of joints, also called *pencil-in-cup lesions.* Large erosions with overhanging sclerotic margins and even juxta-articular tophi may be seen in gout.

In ankylosing spondylitis, sacroiliitis is observed on pelvic radiograph films and has high diagnostic specificity. Syndesmophytes (i.e., calcification of the outer rim of the annulus fibrosis), bridging osteophytes, calcification of spinal ligaments, and a typical bamboo spine in the late stages are seen on lumbar and chest radiographs. Joint space narrowing, bony spurs, and sclerosis are seen in osteoarthritis. Chondrocalcinosis is a common finding. It may be asymptomatic or may lead to crystal arthritis (i.e., pseudogout). In acute arthritis, radiographs are much less helpful because bony changes take time to develop; only in septic joint disease is destruction observed in the early stages.

Imaging modalities such as magnetic resonance imaging (MRI), radionuclide scans, ultrasound, and computed tomography are often useful in assessing diseases of bones, joints, muscle, and soft tissues. Ultrasound may be used to detect synovial cysts, especially Baker cysts of the knee, and it is being used more frequently in the outpatient setting to guide procedures.

MRI is the procedure of choice for evaluating early avascular necrosis of bone, especially the hips, and for meniscal or rotator cuff disease. MRI is preferred for evaluating intervertebral disk disease with radiculopathy and spinal stenosis, and it is useful for assessing solid lesions of bone and joints, including neoplastic lesions. The sensitivity of MRI for detecting edema (i.e., water) enables evaluation of infectious and noninfectious inflammatory muscle diseases. MRI is a sensitive but not a specific modality for evaluating osteomyelitis, properties shared with radionuclide imaging. MRI should not supplant clinical evaluation or plain radiography.

In many instances, diagnosis can be made with certainty only by pathologic examination of tissue. Muscle biopsy may be necessary to establish a diagnosis of inflammatory muscle disease, and nerve biopsy may be needed to detect vasculitis. Skin biopsy is useful in differentiating the many causes of rheumatologic skin disease. Renal biopsy is often needed for determination of the diagnosis, treatment, and prognosis.

SUMMARY

The evaluation of arthritis begins with a detailed history consisting of the location and pattern of joint involvement, differentiation of inflammatory from mechanical and other causes, and a thorough review of systems to determine the nonarticular systemic features. The patient's age and sex, family history, medication history, and coexisting medical conditions have a bearing on the diagnosis and treatment plan. Radiographic and laboratory studies, particularly synovial fluid analysis, provide confirmatory and sometimes diagnostic information.

For a deeper discussion of these topics, please see Chapter 241, "Approach to the Patient with Rheumatic Disease," in *Goldman-Cecil Medicine*, 26th Edition.

SUGGESTED READINGS

Felson DT: Epidemiology of the rheumatic diseases. In Koopman WJ, editor: Arthritis and allied conditions, ed 13, Baltimore, 1997, Williams & Wilkins, p 3.

Gordon DA: Approach to the patient with musculoskeletal disease. In Goldman L, Bennett JC, editors: Cecil textbook of medicine, ed 21, Philadelphia, 2000, WB Saunders, pp 1472–1475.

Sergent JS: Approach to the patient with pain in more than one joint. In Kelley WN, Harris Jr ED, Ruddy S, et al, editors: Textbook of rheumatology, ed 5, Philadelphia, 1997, WB Saunders, p 381.

有助于诊断以及监测疾病和治疗过程。贫血可能提示慢性疾病或溶血性贫血。白细胞减少，尤其是淋巴细胞减少提示 SLE；血小板增多提示活动性炎症。白细胞增多可能反映炎症或感染，糖皮质激素治疗通过动员边缘池内白细胞进入循环池，导致中性粒细胞计数升高。系统性疾病患者应进行尿液分析。蛋白尿、红细胞尿和管型尿应视为隐匿性肾病的证据。应始终结合临床表现解读实验室检查。

影像学检查

放射学检查通常可显示特定疾病的特征性改变。在确诊的类风湿关节炎患者中，放射平片可显示腕部小关节、尺骨茎突、掌指关节和近端指间关节以及足部小关节的典型侵蚀性改变。这种侵蚀不伴有反应性增生。相反，侵蚀性银屑病关节炎会引起硬化增生反应，患者可能出现特征性的关节套叠，也称为"笔套征"。痛风患者可见大面积糜烂伴边缘悬空硬化，甚至出现关节旁痛风石。

在强直性脊柱炎患者中，骨盆平片可显示骶髂关节炎，诊断特异性高。腰椎平片和胸片可见韧带骨赘（即纤维环外缘钙化）、桥接骨赘、脊柱韧带钙化以及晚期典型的脊柱竹节样改变。关节间隙狭窄、骨刺和硬化可见于骨关节炎。软骨钙质沉着是常见表现。它可能无症状，也可能导致晶体性关节炎（即假性痛风）。在急性关节炎中，平片的用处不大，因为骨骼变化需要时间才能显现；只有化脓性关节病在早期阶段即可观察到骨破坏。

磁共振成像（MRI）、放射性核素扫描、超声和计算机断层成像等成像方式通常有助于评估骨骼、关节、肌肉和软组织疾病。超声可用于检测滑膜囊肿，尤其是膝关节腘窝（贝克）囊肿，并且在门诊中被越来越多地用于指导操作。

MRI 是评估早期骨缺血性坏死，特别是髋关节缺血性坏死、半月板或肩袖疾病的首选检查，也是评估椎间盘疾病伴神经根病和椎管狭窄的首选检查，亦可用于评估骨和关节的实质病变，包括肿瘤性病变。MRI 检测水肿（即水分）的敏感性使其可用于评估感染性和非感染性的炎症性肌肉疾病。MRI 评估骨髓炎时敏感但不特异，其性质与放射性核素成像相同。MRI 不应取代临床评估或放射平片。

在很多情况下，只有通过组织病理检查才能确定诊断。肌肉活检是诊断炎症性肌病的必要手段，神经活检可能是检测血管炎的必要手段。皮肤活检有助于鉴别多种风湿性皮肤病变。肾活检通常有助于确定诊断、治疗和预后。

总结

关节炎评估应从详细的病史开始，包括关节受累位置和模式、炎症与机械性和其他原因的鉴别、全面系统回顾以明确关节外全身性表现。患者年龄和性别、家族史、用药史和共患病可影响诊断和治疗方案。影像学和实验室检查，特别是滑液分析，可提供确认信息，有时还直接具有诊断价值。

有关此专题的深入讨论，请参阅 Goldman-Cecil Medicine 第 26 版第 241 章"风湿性疾病患者接诊"。

推荐阅读

Felson DT: Epidemiology of the rheumatic diseases. In Koopman WJ, editor: Arthritis and allied conditions, ed 13, Baltimore, 1997, Williams & Wilkins, p 3.

Gordon DA: Approach to the patient with musculoskeletal disease. In Goldman L, Bennett JC, editors: Cecil textbook of medicine, ed 21, Philadelphia, 2000, WB Saunders, pp 1472–1475.

Sergent JS: Approach to the patient with pain in more than one joint. In Kelley WN, Harris Jr ED, Ruddy S, et al, editors: Textbook of rheumatology, ed 5, Philadelphia, 1997, WB Saunders, p 381.

Rheumatoid Arthritis

Larry W. Moreland, Rayford R. June

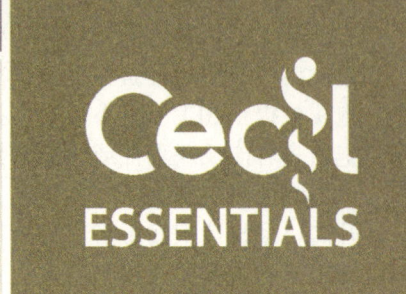

DEFINITION

Rheumatoid arthritis (RA) is a chronic, systemic, inflammatory disorder that is characterized by symmetrical joint pain and swelling, morning stiffness, and fatigue. RA has a variable disease course, often with periods of exacerbations and, less frequently, disease quiescence. Outcomes range from rarely seen remitting disease to severe disease that produces disability and, for some patients, premature death.

Without treatment, most patients have progressive joint damage and significant disability within a few years. Since the introduction of methotrexate in 1985 and tumor necrosis factor-α (TNF-α) inhibitors in the 1990s, there has been a change in the treatment paradigm; many conventional and biologic therapies are now available to effectively treat this previously debilitating chronic disease.

EPIDEMIOLOGY

RA is a worldwide problem with a prevalence in Europe and North America of 0.5% to 1% of the adult population and an annual incidence of 25 to 50/100,000. RA is at least twice as common in women as in men and has a higher prevalence in specific patient populations such as the Pima and Chippewa Native Americans, with a respective prevalence of 5.3% and 6.8%. The disease affects individuals at any age, but most common age of onset is between 50 and 60 years. RA is uncommon among men younger than 45 years of age, but the incidence rises steeply with increasing age. Poor prognostic factors include high disease activity with many joints involved, increased inflammatory markers, high titers of rheumatoid factor (RF) and/or cyclic citrullinated peptides (CCP) antibodies, tobacco use, and erosions on radiographs. With the advent of new therapies, disease severity has decreased over time with less marked radiographic damage and fewer major orthopedic surgeries including joint replacements. However, despite these advances, work-related disability rates remain high for patients with RA. Numerous studies have demonstrated increased mortality rates for patients with RA compared with the general population, with a relative risk of 1.3. The increased mortality rate is more pronounced in males than in females with RA and is attributed to infectious complications and cardiovascular disease.

ETIOLOGY AND GENETICS

The specific underlying cause of RA (i.e., triggers in the susceptible host) is unknown. As for most autoimmune diseases, RA is thought to result from a complex interaction of genetic and environmental factors. RA may consist of multiple environmental stimuli leading to a common clinical presentation. There is not a known single mechanism of initiation or perpetuation. Various environmental triggers such as smoking, obesity, silica exposure, mineral oil, and organic solvents have been associated with the development of RA. Smoking has the most impact, particularly on CCP antibody–positive disease; CCP-positive disease has a more distinct presentation and epidemiology than CCP-negative disease.

An individual's genetic profile also plays a critical role in the susceptibility to and severity of RA. Supporting a genetic component, studies have revealed a 9% to 15% concordance in monozygotic twins that is approximately four times greater than the rate in dizygotic twins. RA is a polygenetic disease with over 100 susceptibility loci reported. The genes with the greatest impact lie in the class II major histocompatibility (MHC) locus, accounting for approximately 60% of the genetic risk for RA. A specific sequence on the HLA-DR haplotype involved in antigen recognition is called the *shared epitope*, which is strongly associated with severe RA and extra-articular manifestations. Multiple mutations in various alleles can then cause changes in the peptide binding grove leading to decreased self-tolerance. Although important, the shared epitope does not fully explain RA because it also occurs in only 25% to 35% of the white population whereas the chance of developing RA in shared-epitope carriers is only 1 in 25 (4%). Non-MHC and HLA genetic associations primarily involve pathways within $CD4^+$ T cells and pathways affecting T- and B-cell interactions, cellular proliferation, and cytokine signaling pathways.

The interplay between environmental and genetic factors is most clearly seen with the increased risk of RA associated with smoking and the MHC class II loci. The exact association between the two is unclear, but research has shown that the bacteria in periodontal and mucosal lung disease, which are increased with smoking, can promote citrullination of bacteria leading to antibodies against multiple different citrullinated peptides. Anti-CCP antibodies are associated with aggressive disease.

For a deeper discussion of these topics, please see Chapter 248, "Rheumatoid Arthritis," in *Goldman-Cecil Medicine*, 26th Edition.

PATHOLOGY AND PATHOGENESIS

RA is a heterogeneous disease with a complex pathogenesis. RA is a clinical diagnosis presenting as a single clinical phenotype, but the underlying pathogenic immunologic genotype is more often than not unique. Instead, several signaling pathways often lead to the same clinical presentation.

Synovial membrane inflammation characterizes RA. Specific processes that lead to this inflammation and cellular proliferation are loss of tolerance, cytokine production, and autoantibody production. Several cytokine signaling pathways are involved with the predominant cytokines interleukin-1 (IL-1), IL-6, TNF-α, and granulocyte-macrophage colony-stimulating factor (GM-CSF)

类风湿关节炎

朱华群 译 李茹 戴冽 审校 栗占国 通审

定义

类风湿关节炎（RA）是一种以对称性关节肿痛、晨僵及疲劳为主要特征的慢性、系统性炎症性疾病。RA 患者的疾病过程表现不一，常伴疾病活动，完全缓解者较少。预后也存在差异，从少见的疾病缓解到严重致残，甚至早亡。

未经治疗的 RA 患者，多数在数年内即可出现进行性关节损伤和功能障碍。然而，自 1985 年甲氨蝶呤以及 20 世纪 90 年代肿瘤坏死因子-α（TNF-α）拮抗剂问世以来，RA 的治疗模式发生了变革。许多传统和生物治疗方法已用于这一慢性致残性疾病。

流行病学

RA 是一种全球性疾病，在欧洲和北美的成人患病率为 0.5%～1%，年发病率为（25～50）/10 万。女性的 RA 患病率至少为男性的 2 倍。在特定的人群中，如 Pima 和 Chippewa 印第安人，RA 患病率分别高达 5.3% 和 6.8%。该病可在任何年龄发病，但最常见的发病年龄在 50～60 岁之间。45 岁以下男性罹患 RA 并不常见，但随着年龄增长，RA 发病率明显上升。预后不良因素包括高疾病活动度伴多关节受累、炎症标志物升高、高滴度类风湿因子（RF）和（或）抗环瓜氨酸肽（CCP）抗体阳性、吸烟以及出现放射学上的骨侵蚀。随着新型治疗方法的出现，该病的严重程度逐渐降低，放射学损伤逐渐减少，包括关节置换术等主要骨科手术数量也越来越少。然而，尽管取得了这些进展，RA 仍存在较高的工作相关致残率。大量调查显示，与一般人群相比，RA 患者死亡率增加，相对危险度为 1.3。男性 RA 患者死亡率增加比女性更为显著，原因在于感染并发症和心血管疾病。

病因和遗传学

RA 具体的潜在病因（即易感宿主的触发因素）尚不清楚。与大多数自身免疫性疾病一样，RA 被认为是遗传和环境因素复杂相互作用的结果。RA 可能是由多种环境刺激而致。目前尚无单一的机制解释 RA 的发生和发展。各种环境诱因，如吸烟、肥胖、二氧化硅暴露、矿物油和有机溶剂等，均与 RA 的发展有关。其中，吸烟对于抗 CCP 抗体阳性患者影响最大；相比于抗 CCP 抗体阴性患者，抗 CCP 抗体阳性患者的临床表现和流行病学特征更为鲜明。

个体的遗传特征在 RA 的易感性和严重程度中起着关键作用。遗传研究表明，同卵双胞胎的共同患病率为 9%～15%，大约是异卵双胞胎的 4 倍。RA 是一种多基因遗传疾病，据报道存在 100 多个易感位点。其中，影响最大的基因是 II 类主要组织相容性（MHC）基因座，约占 RA 遗传风险的 60%。HLA-DR 单体型上参与抗原识别的特定序列被称为共享表位，它与 RA 严重程度和关节外表现密切相关。各种等位基因的多重突变可引起肽结合区发生变化，导致自身耐受性降低。尽管共享表位很重要，但其无法完全解释 RA 的发病机制。原因在于共享表位只出现在 25%～35% 的白种人群中，而携带共享表位者发生 RA 的概率仅为 1/25（4%）。非 MHC 和 HLA 遗传关联主要涉及 $CD4^+$ T 细胞内通路、影响 T 和 B 细胞相互作用及细胞增殖的通路、细胞因子信号通路等。

环境和遗传因素间相互作用最明显的体现，是 RA 发病风险增加与吸烟和 MHC II 类位点的相关性。两者之间的确切联系尚不清楚，但研究表明，牙周和黏膜性肺病中的细菌随着吸烟而增加；吸烟可促进细菌的瓜氨酸化，从而产生针对多种不同瓜氨酸肽的抗体。抗 CCP 抗体与 RA 侵袭性病变有关。

有关此专题的深入讨论，请参阅 *Goldman-Cecil Medicine* 第 26 版第 248 章"类风湿关节炎"。

病理学及发病机制

RA 是一种发病机制复杂的异质性疾病。尽管 RA 在临床上表现为单一的临床表型，但潜在的致病免疫基因型往往不是单一的。反之，多种信号通路常导致相同的临床表现。

滑膜炎是 RA 的特征性表现。导致这种炎症和细胞增殖的具体过程包括耐受性丧失、细胞因子产生以及自身抗体生成。多种细胞因子信号通路参与 RA 疾病进展，主要包括外周血和滑膜中的细胞因子白介素-1（IL-1）、IL-6、TNF-α 和粒细胞-巨噬细胞集落刺激

detected within the synovium and peripheral blood. As mentioned, in anti-CCP–positive disease, the initial site of inflammation may be in the periodontal mucosa and lung. Many advances have been made in understanding the cell-cell interactions and cytokine signaling, but little is known about the loss of tolerance and role of regulatory T cells in disease onset and propagation. Many insights into the pathogenesis of RA have resulted from analyzing the responses to cytokine inhibition (i.e., IL-1, TNF-α, and IL-6) and to specific T- and B-cell–directed therapies. For instance, TNF-α blockade therapies were initially developed for other diseases but then found to be very effective for RA.

The process of synovial inflammation and proliferation is initiated by an interaction between antigen-presenting cells (APCs) and $CD4^+$ T cells. APCs display complexes of class II MHC molecules and peptide antigens that bind to specific receptors on the T cells. Clonal expansion of T-cell subsets occurs with an appropriate second signal, or co-stimulation, delivered by the APC to the T cell. Activated T_H1 and T_H17 T-cell subsets predominate in synovial tissues. These cell types stimulate synovial macrophages to secrete proinflammatory cytokines such as IL-1, TNF-α, GM-CSF, and IL-6 to activate inflammatory pathways.

In addition to cellular and cytokine processes, the humoral immune system is also involved in the pathogenesis of RA. The autoantibodies found most frequently in patients with RA are immunoglobulin M (IgM), RF, and anti-CCP. Positive RF and anti-CCP testing is associated with aggressive, erosive RA, and these autoantibodies are found in serum sometimes years before patients develop signs of RA. Although a causal link has not been confirmed, CCP antibodies, combined with genetic and environmental factors (e.g., smoking, periodontal disease), are involved in the development of RA. It is not known yet how to prevent RA in people with high risk for developing it.

RA pathogenesis occurs in stages. In the induction phase, the anatomy of the synovial lining within the articular joint enables recruitment of inflammatory cells. Cigarette smoke, bacterial products, viral components, and other environmental stimuli may amplify this process and promote a dysregulated immune system. A genetic propensity for autoreactivity may initiate a then irreversible pathway to RA.

The destructive phase, which can be antigen dependent or independent, involves mesenchymal elements such as fibroblasts and synoviocytes. Bone erosions result from local differentiation and activation of osteoclasts, whereas cartilage damage appears to be caused by proteolytic enzymes produced by synoviocytes, macrophages, and synovial fluid neutrophils. Counter-regulatory mechanisms (e.g., soluble TNF-α receptors, suppressive cytokines through regulatory T cells, protease inhibitors, natural cytokine antagonists) are not produced in high enough levels, leading to a loss of tolerance.

Cytokines, which are hormone-like proteins that regulate many immune cell functions, have been implicated in synovial inflammation. The inflammatory milieu of the joint is dominated by proinflammatory factors produced by macrophages and fibroblasts, especially in the synovial intimal lining. In addition to the four cytokines mentioned previously (IL-1, IL-6, GM-CSF and TNF-alpha), many other cytokines and chemokines have been identified at the protein and mRNA level within the synovium.

Joint damage in RA results from proliferation of the synovial intimal layer forming a pannus that overgrows, invades, and destroys adjacent cartilage and bone (Fig. 2.1). Fibroblast-like synoviocytes

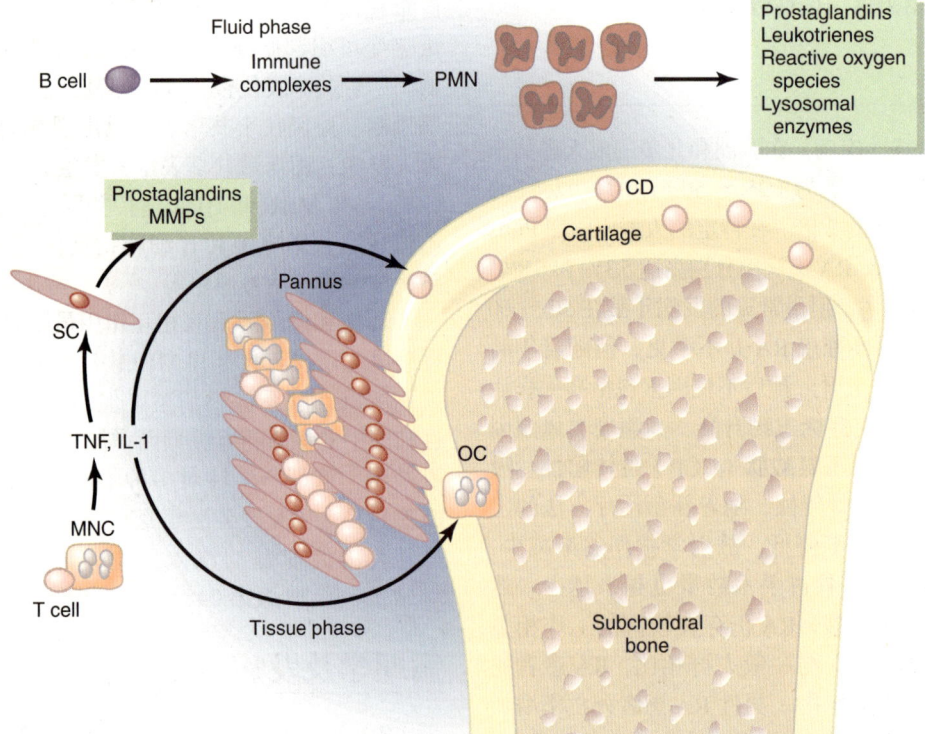

Fig. 2.1 Pathogenetic events in rheumatoid arthritis. The proliferative synovial pannus invades at the bone-cartilage interface. Interleukin-1 (IL-1) and tumor necrosis factor-α (TNF-α) activate synovial cells (SC) to produce prostaglandins and matrix metalloproteinases (MMPs). In the synovial fluid, polymorphonuclear leukocytes (PMN), activated by immune complexes and complement, produce mediators of inflammation and destruction. *CD,* Chondrocytes; *MNC,* mononuclear cell; *OC,* osteoclast.

因子（GM-CSF）。如前所述，在抗 CCP 抗体阳性患者中，炎症的初始部位可能在牙周黏膜和肺部。在 RA 中，尽管细胞间相互作用和细胞因子信号传导方面的研究取得了许多进展，但关于免疫耐受失调和调节性 T 细胞在疾病发生和发展中的作用仍知之甚少。通过分析细胞因子（即 IL-1、TNF-α 和 IL-6）抑制剂和靶向特异性 T 细胞和 B 细胞的治疗反应，促进了对 RA 发病机制的深入认识。例如，TNF-α 抑制剂最初是为其他疾病研发的，但后来发现对 RA 患者非常有效。

滑膜炎症和增殖的过程是由抗原提呈细胞（APC）和 CD4⁺ T 细胞之间的相互作用启动的。APC 表达 MHC Ⅱ类分子，与抗原肽形成复合物，并与 T 细胞上的特定受体结合。T 细胞亚群的克隆性扩增需要适当的第二信号传导，即由 APC 传递给 T 细胞的共刺激信号。活化的 Th1 和 Th17 T 细胞亚群在滑膜组织中占主导地位。这些细胞刺激滑膜巨噬细胞分泌促炎细胞因子，如 IL-1、TNF-α、GM-CSF 和 IL-6，以活化炎症通路。

除了细胞和细胞因子通路外，体液免疫系统也参与了 RA 的发病机制。RA 患者中最常见的自身抗体是免疫球蛋白 M（IgM）、RF 和抗 CCP 抗体。RF 和抗 CCP 抗体阳性与进展性、侵蚀性 RA 相关，这些自身抗体有时在患者出现 RA 症状前数年就存在于血清中了。虽然因果关系尚未得到证实，但抗 CCP 抗体与遗传和环境因素（如吸烟、牙周病）共同参与了 RA 的发展。关于如何在高风险人群中预防 RA 的发生，目前尚未可知。

RA 的发病是分阶段的。在疾病诱导阶段，关节内滑膜衬里层能招募炎症细胞。吸烟、细菌产物、病毒片段和其他环境刺激可能会放大这一过程，促进免疫系统的失调。自身免疫反应的遗传易感性可能启动这一不可逆的 RA 进程。

在抗原依赖性或非依赖性的疾病破坏阶段，成纤维细胞和滑膜细胞等间充质细胞参与其中发挥作用。骨侵蚀由破骨细胞的局部分化和激活引起，而软骨损伤由滑膜细胞、巨噬细胞和滑液中性粒细胞产生的蛋白溶解酶所致。负反馈调节机制（如可溶性 TNF-α 受体、调节性 T 细胞产生的抑制性细胞因子、蛋白酶抑制剂、天然细胞因子拮抗剂）的产生水平不足，最终导致免疫耐受丧失。

细胞因子是类激素蛋白，可以调节多种免疫细胞功能，参与滑膜炎症反应。巨噬细胞和成纤维细胞产生的促炎因子，尤其在滑膜内层产生的炎症因子，形成了关节的炎症微环境。除了前述提到的 4 种细胞因子（IL-1、IL-6、GM-CSF 和 TNF-α）外，还有许多其他的细胞因子和趋化因子已在滑膜蛋白水平和 mRNA 水平上被鉴定出来。

RA 的关节损伤是由滑膜内层增生形成血管翳过度生长、侵入和破坏相邻软骨和骨造成的（图 2.1）。成

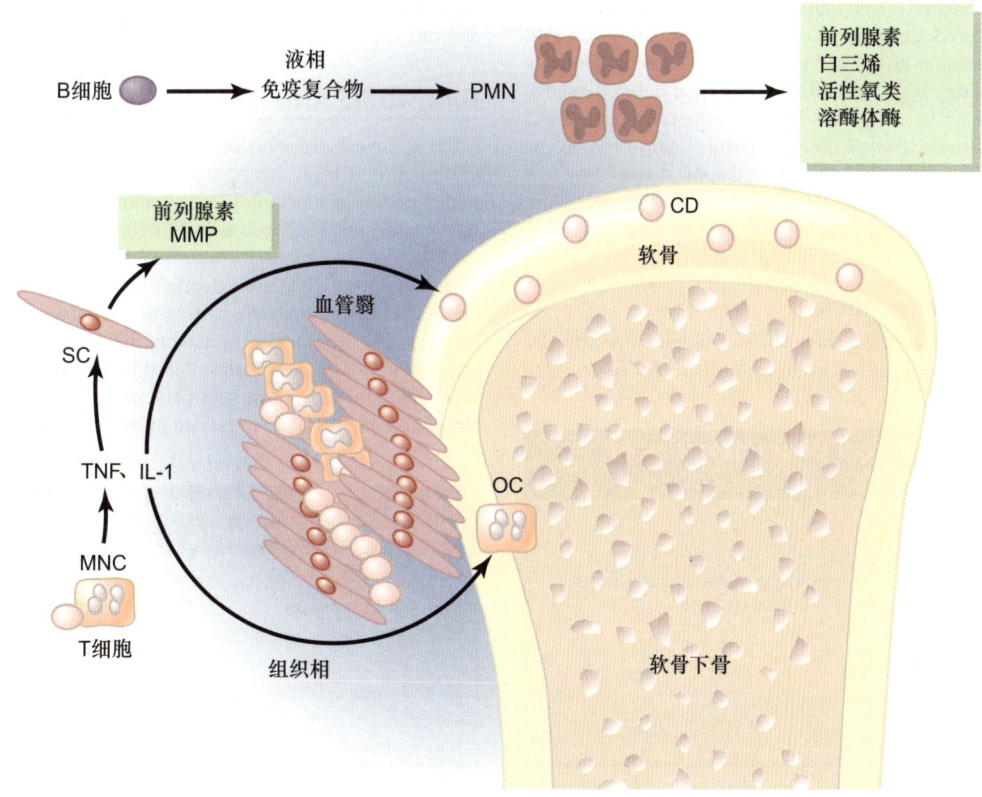

图 2.1　类风湿关节炎的发病机制。增生的滑膜血管翳在骨-软骨界面处侵入。白细胞介素 -1（IL-1）和肿瘤坏死因子 -α（TNF-α）激活滑膜细胞（SC）产生前列腺素和基质金属蛋白酶（MMP）。在滑液中，免疫复合物和补体激活多形核白细胞（PMN）产生炎症和骨破坏介质。CD：软骨细胞；MNC：单核细胞；OC：破骨细胞

and macrophages are the predominant cellular components of the invading pannus of the synovium. Extracellular matrix damage resulting from synovial expansion is caused by several families of enzymes, including serine proteases, cathepsins, and matrix metalloproteinases.

❖ For a deeper discussion of these topics, please see Chapter 248, "Rheumatoid Arthritis," in *Goldman-Cecil Medicine*, 26th Edition.

CLINICAL PRESENTATION

Articular Manifestations

RA manifests with a symmetrical polyarthritis that typically starts with the small joints of the hands and feet and can progress to the synovium of the wrists, elbows, shoulders, knees, and ankles. Patients have an insidious onset of inflammatory symptoms, which are fatigue, pain, and stiffness that is worse with inactivity and is improved with movement. Prolonged morning stiffness, usually lasting more than 1 hour, is a classic feature of RA (Table 2.1). Often, warm water and heat will also relieve this stiffness. Any diarthrodial (synovial) joint may be involved, including the apophyseal (spinal), temporomandibular, and cricoarytenoid joints. Involved joints are swollen, warm, and tender, and they may have effusions. The synovium, which is normally a few cell layers thick, becomes palpable on examination (i.e., synovitis).

Without treatment, RA progresses in some patients to joint destruction and deformity. Erosive lesions of bone and cartilage often are visible radiographically at the margins of bone and cartilage, the sites of synovial attachment. Not all patients with RA have erosive disease, with only 40% of patients in many present-day studies having radiographic erosions. Tenosynovitis (i.e., inflammation of tendon sheaths) leads to tendon malalignment, stretching or shortening and exacerbates joint subluxation.

Joint deformities leading to functional disability occur in RA after long-standing joint disease. Common deformities are ulnar deviation at the metacarpophalangeal joints and volar subluxation at those joints and at the wrists. Flexion and extension contractures in the proximal and distal interphalangeal (PIP and DIP) joints of the fingers lead to the characteristic swan-neck deformity (i.e., flexion contracture at the DIP joint and hyperextension at the PIP joint) or boutonnière deformity (i.e., flexion contracture at the PIP and hyperextension at the DIP joint).

Synovitis at the wrists can lead to median nerve compression and carpal tunnel syndrome. Carpal tunnel syndrome can often be the first sign of RA. Rarely, long-standing cervical spine disease may lead to C1-C2 subluxation and life-threatening spinal cord compression. Rupture of synovial fluid from the knee into the calf (i.e., Baker cyst) may mimic deep vein thrombosis or imitate cellulitis.

Extra-articular Manifestations

RA is a systemic disease in which there can be multiple extra-articular manifestations, particularly in severe uncontrolled RA (Table 2.2).

Constitutional symptoms are common with disease onset and flares; these symptoms include fatigue, low-grade fever, weight loss, and myalgia. Extra-articular manifestations are more common in RF-positive patients and some epidemiologic studies have shown a decrease in extra-articular manifestations associated with newer treatments and improved disease control.

The most common extra-articular manifestation of RA is rheumatoid nodules, which can occur in 30% to 40% of patients. These are grossly palpable nodules on the skin at pressure points along extensor surfaces, especially at the elbows. Rheumatoid nodules are associated with RF positivity and tobacco use and can also occur in the lungs, pleura, pericardium, sclerae, and other sites, including the heart in rare cases. In the eyes, RA commonly is associated with keratoconjunctivitis sicca with coexistent Sjögren's syndrome and less often with scleritis and episcleritis.

Lung involvement in RA can present as interstitial lung disease and may include pleuropericarditis, producing inflammatory exudative pleural and pericardial effusions. The cardiovascular effects of RA can range from long-term inflammation leading to accelerated coronary artery disease to pericarditis to small and medium-sized vasculitis. The vasculitis of RA can produce cutaneous lesions (e.g., ulcers, skin necrosis) and mononeuritis multiplex.

RA patients often have common hematologic manifestations such as anemia of chronic disease and thrombocytosis with uncontrolled disease and early presentation. Patients with RA also have an increased incidence of lymphoma. Larger granular lymphocyte (LGL) leukemia is a specific form of chronic leukemia associated with RA. Often LGL can present as Felty syndrome (i.e., rheumatoid arthritis, splenomegaly, and neutropenia). This rare complication can be accompanied by leg ulcers and vasculitis.

Medication side effects should also be considered as extra-articular manifestations of RA. Rheumatoid nodules can be precipitated by methotrexate with a syndrome called methotrexate nodulosis and must be differentiated from uncontrolled RA. TNF-α inhibitors, the most common biologic agent for RA, are associated with skin psoriasis and can also cause drug induced lupus.

DIAGNOSIS AND DIFFERENTIAL DIAGNOSIS

RA is a clinical diagnosis based on a thorough history and physical examination. Classic symptoms include morning stiffness associated with synovitis of small joints in a symmetrical fashion. No single diagnostic test enables a diagnosis of RA to be made with certainty. Instead, the diagnosis depends on the accumulation of characteristic symptoms, signs, laboratory data, and radiologic findings. There are no diagnostic criteria for RA but rather a pattern of clinical features and laboratory tests that aid the clinician in making the diagnosis. Classification criteria are useful in guiding the clinical diagnosis of RA and also create clear guidelines for classifying patients in research studies. The RA classification criteria were updated in 2010 to include anti-CCP testing

TABLE 2.1 Clinical Characteristics of Rheumatoid Arthritis
Morning stiffness or gelling
Symmetrical joint swelling
Predilection for wrists and proximal interphalangeal, metacarpophalangeal, and metatarsophalangeal joints
Erosions of bone and cartilage
Joint subluxation and ulnar deviation
Inflammatory joint fluid
Carpal tunnel syndrome
Baker cyst

TABLE 2.2 Extra-articular Features of Rheumatoid Arthritis
Rheumatoid nodules: subcutaneous, pulmonary, sclera
Interstitial lung disease
Vasculitis, especially skin and peripheral nerves
Pleuropericarditis
Scleritis and episcleritis
Leg ulcers
Felty syndrome

纤维样滑膜细胞和巨噬细胞是侵袭性滑膜血管翳的主要细胞成分。滑膜增生导致的细胞外基质损伤是由多个酶家族成员引起的，包括丝氨酸蛋白酶、组织蛋白酶和基质金属蛋白酶。

❖ 有关此专题的深入讨论，请参阅 Goldman-Cecil Medicine 第26版第248章"类风湿关节炎"。

临床表现

关节表现

RA 表现为对称性多关节炎，通常始于手和足的小关节，可进展至腕、肘、肩、膝和踝关节。患者炎症症状呈隐匿发作，表现为疲劳、疼痛和僵硬，静息时加重，活动后改善。长时间的晨僵（通常持续超过 1 h），是 RA 的典型表现（表 2.1）。温水和热敷常可以减轻晨僵。任何运动（滑膜）关节均可受累，包括棘突关节（脊柱）、颞颌关节和环杓关节。受累关节表现为肿胀、皮温升高、压痛，并可能有积液。正常情况下只有数层细胞厚度的滑膜，变得于查体时可被触及（即滑膜炎）。

一些未经治疗的 RA 患者可能出现关节破坏和畸形。放射学上常可见骨和软骨的侵蚀性病变发生在骨和软骨的边缘，即滑膜附着部位。并非所有 RA 患者都有侵蚀性病变，目前的研究中，只有 40% 的患者出现放射学上的骨侵蚀。腱鞘滑膜炎（即腱鞘炎）可导致肌腱排列紊乱、过伸或缩短，并加剧关节半脱位。

长期关节病变导致 RA 患者出现关节畸形，最终引起功能障碍。常见的畸形包括掌指关节的尺侧偏斜、掌指关节和腕关节半脱位。手指近端和远端指间（PIP 和 DIP）关节的屈曲和伸直挛缩导致特征性的天鹅颈畸形（即 DIP 关节的屈曲挛缩和 PIP 关节的过伸），或纽扣花畸形（即 PIP 关节的屈曲挛缩和 DIP 关节的过伸）。

腕关节滑膜炎可导致正中神经卡压和腕管综合征。腕管综合征常可作为 RA 的首发表现。长期颈椎病变可能导致 C1～C2 半脱位及危及生命的脊髓压迫，但这种情况罕见。膝关节滑液经破裂进入腓肠肌形成的腘窝囊肿（即贝克囊肿），类似深静脉血栓形成或蜂窝织炎的表现。

关节外表现

RA 是一种系统性疾病，尤其是在严重的未控制的 RA 患者中，可能出现多种关节外表现（表 2.2）。全身症状常见于疾病的起病初期和复发时，包括疲劳、低热、体重减轻和肌痛。RF 阳性的患者关节外表现更为常见。一些流行病学研究表明，随着新型治疗方法的问世及疾病的改善，关节外表现的发生率在逐渐下降。

类风湿结节是 RA 最常见的关节外表现，可发生在 30%～40% 的患者中，为关节伸面受压部位（尤其是肘部）可触及的皮下结节。类风湿结节与 RF 阳性和吸烟有关，也可发生在肺部、胸膜、心包、巩膜，罕见情况下还可出现在心脏等其他部位。在眼部，RA 常因伴有干燥综合征而出现干燥性角结膜炎，巩膜炎和巩膜外层炎少见。

RA 的肺部受累可表现为间质性肺病，也可出现胸膜心包炎，进而导致炎性渗出性胸腔和心包积液。其心血管受累可表现为长期炎症加速冠状动脉性心脏病发生，导致心包炎及中小血管炎。RA 血管炎可引起皮肤病变（如溃疡、皮肤坏死）和多发性单神经炎。

RA 患者经常会出现一些常见血液系统表现，如慢性病贫血和血小板增多症。这些症状在疾病未控制的情况下以及疾病早期更明显。RA 患者淋巴瘤的发生率也较高。大颗粒淋巴细胞（LGL）白血病是与 RA 相关的一种特殊类型的慢性白血病。通常 LGL 可以表现为 Felty 综合征（即类风湿关节炎、脾大和粒细胞减少症）。这种罕见的并发症可能伴有腿部溃疡和血管炎。

药物副作用也应被视为 RA 的关节外表现。甲氨蝶呤可能会引发类风湿结节，称为甲氨蝶呤结节（作者观点），须与未控制的 RA 相鉴别。TNF-α 抑制剂是 RA 治疗最常用的生物制剂，与皮肤银屑病相关，还可能诱发药物性狼疮。

诊断和鉴别诊断

RA 是在详细病史采集和体格检查基础上做出的临床诊断。其典型症状包括晨僵伴对称性小关节滑膜炎。尚无单一的诊断方法能明确 RA 的诊断。相反，RA 诊断取决于典型症状、体征、实验室和放射学指标的综合评判。RA 没有统一的诊断标准，而临床特征和实验室检查有助于临床医生做出诊断。分类标准有助于指导 RA 的临床诊断，也为研究中患者的分类提供了明确的指南。RA 的分类标准于 2010 年进行了更新，纳入了抗环瓜氨酸肽抗体（anti-CCP）检测，旨在识别早期

表 2.1　RA 的临床表现
晨僵或胶着感
对称性关节肿胀
好发于腕、掌指关节、近端指间关节和跖趾关节
骨和软骨侵蚀
关节半脱位和尺侧偏斜
炎性关节积液
腕管综合征
贝克囊肿

表 2.2　RA 的关节外表现
类风湿结节：皮下、肺、巩膜
间质性肺病
血管炎，尤其是皮肤、外周神经
胸膜心包炎
巩膜炎和巩膜外层炎
腿部溃疡
Felty 综合征

TABLE 2.3 2010 ACR/EULAR Classification Criteria for Rheumatoid Arthritis

For patients who have at least 1 joint with definite synovitis and for whom the synovitis is not better explained by another disease.

A. Joint involvement (0–5 points)
  1 large joint (0)
  2–10 large joints (1)
  1–3 small joints (with or without involvement of large joints) (2)
  4–10 small joints (or without involvement of large joints) (3)
  >10 joints (with involvement of at least 1 small joint) (5)
B. Serology (0–3 points)
  Negative RF and negative anti-CCP (0)
  Low-positive RF or low-positive anti-CCP (2)
  High positive RF or high positive anti-CCP (3)
C. Acute phase reactants (0–1 points)
  Normal CRP and normal ESR (0)
  Abnormal CRP or abnormal ESR (1)
D. Duration of symptoms (0–1 points)
  <6 weeks (0)
  ≥6 weeks (1)

A score of at least 6 of 10 points is needed for the classification of definite rheumatoid arthritis.

ACR, American College of Rheumatology; *CCP*, cyclic citrullinated peptide; *CRP*, C-reactive protein; *ESR*, erythrocyte sedimentation rate; *EULAR*, European League Against Rheumatism; *RF*, rheumatoid factor.
Aletaha D, Neogi T, Silman AJ, et al: 2010 Rheumatoid arthritis classification criteria: an American College of Rheumatology/European League Against Rheumatism collaborative initiative, *Arthritis Rheum* 62:2569-2581, 2010.

and were designed to capture early RA (Table 2.3). Multiple studies have shown that prompt diagnosis and treatment are important to prevent disease progression, joint deformities, and disability. With the advent of specific diagnostic testing such as CCP testing and incorporation into the new classification criteria for early RA, both clinical practice and research settings have seen significant advancements with earlier treatment for patients with subsequently improved outcomes.

The differential diagnosis for RA is broad and includes viral arthritis (e.g., parvovirus, rubella, hepatitis B and C), thyroid disorders, sarcoidosis, reactive arthritis, psoriatic arthritis, Sjögren's syndrome, systemic lupus erythematosus (SLE), bacterial endocarditis, rheumatic fever, calcium pyrophosphate disease (CPPD), chronic tophaceous gout, polymyalgia rheumatica, erosive osteoarthritis, and fibromyalgia syndrome. A history and physical examination, including a thorough review of systems, persistence over time (with 6 weeks being on the most recent classification criteria; see Table 2.3), and available diagnostic testing guide the clinician in making the diagnosis. Initial laboratory tests in the evaluation should include a complete blood count, comprehensive metabolic panel, erythrocyte sedimentation rate, C-reactive protein, uric acid, RF, anti-CCP, ANA by indirect immunofluorescence, and hepatitis B and C testing. Additional tests such as viral serologies and autoantibody testing should be guided by the clinical presentation.

RF is an antibody (typically IgM but also IgG or others) that binds to the Fc fragment of IgG. RF and IgG join to form immune complexes that are detectable in the serum of 70% to 80% of patients with RA over the course of the disease. However, RF is not specific for RA and frequently occurs in patients with SLE, Sjögren's syndrome, infective endocarditis, sarcoidosis, lung and liver diseases (including infections such as hepatitis B and C), and also in healthy individuals. In an individual patient, the RF titer does not correlate with disease activity, but high titers are associated with severe erosive arthritis and extra-articular disease. The finding of RF in serum alone does not establish a diagnosis of RA, but it can help to confirm the clinical impression. RF does not need to be repeatedly tested once the diagnosis is made.

Anti-CCP antibodies are a more specific marker for RA than RF. Anti-CCP antibodies are antibodies directed at citrullinated peptides and can be tested with one diagnostic test. Anti-CCP antibodies in the presence of at least one swollen joint have a high specificity (>95%) for RA. Compared to RF, CCP antibodies have improved specificity (96% vs. 86%), with similar sensitivity (67% vs. 70%) for RA. These antibodies can be detected several years before the development of clinical RA, and they are associated with severe RA outcomes, including radiographic joint damage and a poor prognosis. Because of their specificity for RA, anti-CCP antibodies are useful in differentiating RA from other conditions positive for RF, including Sjögren's syndrome, infection, and hepatitis.

Acute phase reactants, such as the erythrocyte sedimentation rate and C-reactive protein, are usually elevated in active inflammation but are not sensitive or specific for the diagnosis of RA. These tests are useful for differentiating RA from noninflammatory conditions such as osteoarthritis or fibromyalgia. However, even when there is clear clinical evidence of joint inflammation, the values for acute phase reactants may be normal. Inflammation in RA often leads to anemia of chronic disease and thrombocytosis.

Synovial fluid analysis is usually not necessary when there is a clear chronic inflammatory polyarthritis. Arthrocentesis should be performed to rule out infection or crystalline arthropathy in monoarthritis if only a single joint is involved. Synovial fluid analysis is nonspecific but can support the diagnosis by showing inflammatory joint fluid with cell counts between 2000 and 100,000. Radiographs, although not part of the 2010 RA classification criteria, may show characteristic periarticular osteopenia, marginal joint bone erosions, and uniform joint space narrowing in a symmetrical distribution. Often radiographs will be normal in early RA but can serve as a baseline to assess disease progression over time.

For a deeper discussion of these topics, please see Chapter 242, "Laboratory Testing in the Rheumatic Diseases," Chapter 243, "Imaging Studies in the Rheumatic Diseases," Chapter 247, "Bursitis, Tendinitis, and Other Periarticular Disorders and Sports Medicine," and Chapter 248, "Rheumatoid Arthritis," in *Goldman-Cecil Medicine*, 26th Edition.

TREATMENT

The ultimate goals for managing RA are to reduce pain and discomfort, prevent joint deformities, and maintain normal physical and social function. Although there is no cure for RA, remission can be maintained in a subset of patients. Treatment begins with effective communication between the physician and patient regarding the nature of the disease and the goals of treatment.

Nonpharmacologic therapeutic options include reduction of joint stress, often through physical and occupational therapy. Local rest of an inflamed joint can reduce joint stress, as can weight reduction, splinting, and the use of walking aids. Vigorous activity should be avoided during disease flares. Full range of motion of joints, however, should be maintained by a graded exercise program to prevent contractures and muscle atrophy. Physical therapy improves muscle strength, decreases joint stress, and maintains joint mobility. Occupational therapy can provide various appliances to protect joints and make daily activities easier.

表 2.3　2010 ACR/EULAR RA 分类标准
对于至少有 1 个关节存在明确滑膜炎且滑膜炎不能用其他疾病解释。 A. 关节受累情况（0～5 分） 　　1 个大关节（0） 　　2～10 个大关节（1） 　　1～3 个小关节（有或无大关节受累）（2） 　　4～10 个小关节（或无大关节受累）（3） 　　＞10 个关节（至少有 1 个小关节受累）（5） B. 血清学（0～3 分） 　　RF 阴性和抗 CCP 抗体阴性（0） 　　RF 低滴度阳性或抗 CCP 抗体低滴度阳性（2） 　　RF 高滴度阳性或抗 CCP 抗体高滴度阳性（3） C. 急性期反应物（0～1 分） 　　CRP 和 ESR 正常（0） 　　CRP 或 ESR 异常（1） D. 症状持续时间（0～1 分） 　　＜6 周（0） 　　≥6 周（1） 总分≥6 分（满分 10 分）可分类诊断为 RA

ACR：美国风湿病学会；CCP：环瓜氨酸肽；CRP：C 反应蛋白；ESR：红细胞沉降率；EULAR：欧洲抗风湿病联盟；RF：类风湿因子。
Aletaha D，Neogi T，Silman AJ，et al: 2010 Rheumatoid arthritis classification criteria: an American College of Rheumatology/European League Against Rheumatism collaborative initiative，Arthritis Rheum 62: 2569-2581，2010.

RA 患者（表 2.3）。多项研究表明，及时诊断和治疗对预防疾病进展、关节畸形和残疾至关重要。随着诸如抗 CCP 抗体等特异性诊断方法的出现及将其纳入新的早期 RA 分类标准，临床实践和研究都取得了重大进展，患者能更早接受治疗，预后也得以改善。

RA 的鉴别诊断范围广泛，包括病毒性关节炎（如细小病毒、风疹病毒、乙型和丙型肝炎病毒感染）、甲状腺疾病、结节病、反应性关节炎、银屑病关节炎、干燥综合征、系统性红斑狼疮（SLE）、细菌性心内膜炎、风湿热、焦磷酸钙沉积病（CPPD）、慢性痛风石性痛风、风湿性多肌痛、侵蚀性骨关节炎和纤维肌痛综合征等。通过对患者的详细病史采集和全面体格检查，包括全面的系统回顾，了解症状持续时间（现行分类标准为 6 周以上；见表 2.3）以及进行必要的诊断性检查，可帮助临床医生进行诊断。初次实验室评估应包括全血细胞计数、生化、红细胞沉降率、C 反应蛋白、尿酸、RF、抗 CCP 抗体、ANA（间接免疫荧光法检测）以及乙型和丙型肝炎的检测。其他病毒血清学和自身抗体检测等辅助检查根据临床表现酌情考虑。

类风湿因子（RF）是一种可与 IgG 的 Fc 片段结合的抗体（通常为 IgM 型，但也可为 IgG 型或其他类型）。RF 和 IgG 结合形成免疫复合物，在 70%～80% 的 RA 患者血清中可检测到。然而，RF 并非 RA 的特异性指标，在 SLE、干燥综合征、感染性心内膜炎、结节病、肺和肝脏疾病（包括如乙型和丙型肝炎等感染）患者中经常出现，在健康个体中也可存在。在 RA 患者中，RF 滴度与疾病活动度无关，但高滴度 RF 与严重的侵蚀性关节炎和关节外病变相关。仅通过血清中发现 RF 不能确诊 RA，但有助于确定临床诊断的方向。一旦确诊为 RA，无需反复检测 RF。

抗 CCP 抗体是比 RF 更特异的 RA 标志物。抗 CCP 抗体是针对瓜氨酸肽的抗体，可通过诊断性试验进行检测。在至少有一个关节肿胀的患者中，抗 CCP 抗体具有很高的 RA 特异性（＞95%）。与 RF 相比，抗 CCP 抗体在 RA 中的特异性更高（96% vs. 86%），而敏感性相近（67% vs. 70%）。这些抗体在临床 RA 发病前数年即可被检测到，且与重症 RA 相关，包括放射学关节破坏和不良预后。由于抗 CCP 抗体的 RA 特异性，其有助于 RA 与 RF 阳性的其他疾病相鉴别，包括干燥综合征、感染和肝炎。

急性期反应物，如红细胞沉降率和 C 反应蛋白，在活动性炎症中通常会升高，但它们对 RA 的诊断既不敏感也不特异。这些检查有助于将 RA 与骨关节炎或纤维肌痛等非炎症性疾病区分开来。然而，即便有明显的临床关节炎症证据，急性期反应物也可能正常。RA 中的炎症常可导致慢性病贫血和血小板增多症。

当存在明确的慢性炎症性多关节炎时，通常不需要进行滑液分析。若仅有单关节受累，应进行关节穿刺以排除单关节炎中的感染或晶体性关节病。滑液分析并无特异性，但如果表现为细胞计数为 2000～100 000 的炎性关节液，可支持 RA 的诊断。虽然 X 线检查不在 2010 年 RA 分类标准内，但其特征性的关节周围骨质疏松、边缘性关节骨侵蚀和非对称分布的均匀性关节间隙狭窄有助于 RA 诊断。通常，早期 RA 患者的 X 线检查结果正常，但可作为基线数据，用以评估疾病随时间的进展。

有关此专题的深入讨论，请参阅 *Goldman-Cecil Medicine* 第 26 版第 242 章 "风湿性疾病的实验室检测"、第 243 章 "风湿性疾病的影像学研究"、第 247 章 "滑囊炎、腱鞘炎和其他关节周围疾病及运动医学" 以及第 248 章 "类风湿关节炎"。

治疗

RA 治疗的最终目标是减轻疼痛和不适、预防关节畸形，并保持正常的机体和社会功能。尽管 RA 无法治愈，但相当一部分患者的病情可以得到缓解。治疗始于医生和患者就疾病的性质和治疗目标的共同决策。

非药物治疗包括减轻关节压力，常通过物理疗法和作业治疗来实现。炎性关节的局部制动可减轻关节压力，减重、夹板固定和助行器的使用也可达到此效果。在疾病发作期应避免关节剧烈活动。然而，应通过分级锻炼计划保持关节的全范围活动，以预防挛缩和肌肉萎缩。物理疗法可提高肌肉力量、降低关节压力并维持关节活动度。作业疗法可提供各种器具以保护关节，并使关节日常活动更为轻便。

TABLE 2.4 Conventional Disease-Modifying Antirheumatic Drugs

Conventional Agents	Toxicities
Azathioprine	Infection, nausea, bone marrow suppression, fever, pancreatitis
Baricitinib, tofacitinib (targeted synthetic oral DMARD)	Infection rate similar to biologic DMARDs; bone marrow and hepatic toxicity, hyperlipidemia, contraindicated with biologics
Hydroxychloroquine	Retinal toxicity, requires ophthalmologic monitoring
Leflunomide	Bone marrow and hepatic toxicity; cholestyramine washout if toxic; contraindicated in pregnancy
Methotrexate[a]	Oral ulcers, nausea, bone marrow suppression, pneumonitis; contraindicated in pregnancy and severe coexistent lung disease; hepatotoxicity
Sulfasalazine	Nausea, bone marrow suppression

DMARDs, Disease-modifying antirheumatic drugs.
[a]Initial recommended DMARD in moderate to severe RA.

TABLE 2.5 Biologic Disease-Modifying Antirheumatic Drugs

Biologic Agent	Targeted Mechanism
Adalimumab, certolizumab, etanercept, golimumab, infliximab	Cytokine directed, anti-TNF-α
Anakinra	Cytokine directed, anti-IL-1
Sarilumab, tocilizumab	Cytokine directed, anti-IL-6
Abatacept	T-cell directed, inhibits co-stimulation
Rituximab	B-cell directed, anti-CD20

IL, interleukin; *TNF*, tumor necrosis factor.

Pharmacologic Approach

Studies have revealed that disease-modifying antirheumatic drug (DMARD) therapy early in the course of RA slows disease progression more effectively than delayed therapy. Early RA is currently defined as within 6 months of diagnosis and established RA as greater than 6 months. A targeted approach at the extent of disease activity should be used to minimize joint inflammation. Effective treatment with DMARDs can improve signs, symptoms, and radiographic progression, even in long-standing disease. The inflammation of RA should be controlled as completely as possible, as soon as possible, and for as long as possible. Conventional DMARDs and biologic DMARDs prevent disease progression and disability.

Disease Activity

Establishing a diagnosis of RA enables the clinician to determine treatment and also counsel the patient regarding future disease course, need for treatment, and prognosis. Intensity of treatment is guided by the extent of disease activity. As mentioned, RA involves the diarthrodial joints but the exact pattern of joint involvement is patient specific. More joints involved means worse disease and is associated with worse outcomes of disease. Disease activity can be defined by multiple different disease activity tools that combine input from physical exam with counting the number of swollen and tender joints, patient input on their global assessment of RA disease activity, not just pain, and laboratory tests showing evidence of inflammation, most commonly by ESR and CRP. The goal of treatment should be absence of joint inflammation. When the diagnosis is made, the patient should be treated in consultation with a rheumatologist, if available, to use specialized disease activity measurements with a goal to minimize joint inflammation towards remission or low disease activity. These disease activity measures include the DAS28 (disease activity measuring involvement of 28 joints), ESR/CRP, CDAI (Clinical Disease Activity Index), SDAI (Simple Disease Activity Score), RAPID3 (Disease Activity Score developed from short and simple questionnaire), and PASDAS (PAS Disease Activity Score based on a weighted index that includes 7 components).

Conventional Disease-Modifying Antirheumatic Drugs

Many DMARDs are available for treating RA. All conventional DMARDs have a slow onset, taking 1 to 6 months to become fully effective, and they need close monitoring for toxicity (Table 2.4). Once the diagnosis of RA is made, a DMARD should be initiated.

Methotrexate is universally used as the initial DMARD in patients with early RA because of its established efficacy and known toxicity profile (evidence from multiple randomized controlled trials). It can be administered once weekly by the oral or parenteral route. Known side effects to monitor for include oral ulcers, nausea, hepatotoxicity, cytopenias, and pneumonitis. If contraindications to methotrexate exist such as chronic liver disease or alcohol use in excess of two drinks per day for males or one per females, alternative conventional DMARDs such as sulfasalazine or hydroxychloroquine should be used in monotherapy. Early in the course of disease, NSAIDs and low-dose corticosteroids can be used for rapid control of inflammation in combination with DMARDs.

In cases of methotrexate failure or inadequate response with continued moderate to high disease activity, the subsequent choice of conventional and biologic DMARDs is not standardized and is instead based on clinical factors such as route of administration, side effects and risks of adverse events, cost, and patient and physician preference. Often combination therapy of multiple DMARDs is used for RA treatment. For patients with mild RA, hydroxychloroquine or sulfasalazine, or both, may be used as first-line drugs. Triple therapy, the combination of methotrexate, hydroxychloroquine, and sulfasalazine, was shown in two randomized, controlled trials to be noninferior to biologic TNF-α inhibitors. Tofacitinib and baricitinib are a new class of synthetic DMARDS that inhibit Janus kinase (JAK)s and reduce cytokine levels. JAK inhibitors are the one class of synthetic DMARDS that should not be used in combination with biologic DMARDS due to increased risk of infections.

Biologic DMARDs

Biologic DMARDs are targeted, immune-based therapies that were introduced in the 1990s with the initiation of cytokine-directed TNF-α inhibitors. Biologics are produced by living cells using recombinant DNA technology (Table 2.5). TNF-α inhibitors were the first of 10 biologic DMARDs approved by the U.S. Food and Drug Administration (FDA) for the treatment of RA (see Table 2.5). Five TNF-α–directed therapies are available. The TNF-α inhibitors are the most widely used biologic agents because of the rapid improvement they produce in patients resistant to methotrexate therapy. They are one class of the biologics recommended in addition to methotrexate after methotrexate failure.

Most biologic DMARDs are given by intravenous or subcutaneous injection and are quite expensive but very effective treatments. Biosimilars are biologic medications with a similar molecular structure to a sister biologic medication and that have no clinically meaningful differences from FDA-approved biologic DMARDs. Multiple biosimilars are available and more are in development as cheaper alternatives to

表 2.4	传统 DMARD
传统药物	毒性
硫唑嘌呤	感染、恶心、骨髓抑制、发热、胰腺炎
巴瑞替尼，托法替布（靶向合成口服 DMARD）	感染发生率与生物 DMARD 相似；骨髓和肝毒性、高脂血症；应用生物 DMARD 时禁用
羟氯喹	视网膜毒性，需要眼科监测
来氟米特	骨髓和肝毒性；若有毒性，用消胆胺洗脱；妊娠期禁用
甲氨蝶呤 a	口腔溃疡、恶心、骨髓抑制、肺炎；妊娠期及合并严重肺部疾病时禁用；肝毒性
柳氮磺吡啶	恶心、骨髓抑制

DMARD：改善病情抗风湿药。
a 中重度 RA 首选的 DMARD。

表 2.5	生物 DMARD
生物制剂	靶标
阿达木单抗、赛妥珠单抗、依那西普、戈利木单抗、英夫利昔单抗	靶向细胞因子，抗 -TNF-α
阿那白滞素	靶向细胞因子，抗 -IL-1
沙利鲁单抗、托珠单抗	靶向细胞因子，抗 -IL-6
阿巴西普	靶向 T 细胞，共刺激因子抑制剂
利妥昔单抗	靶向 B 细胞，抗 CD20

DMARD：改善病情抗风湿药；IL：白细胞介素；TNF：肿瘤坏死因子。

药物治疗

研究表明，早期启动改善病情抗风湿药（DMARD）治疗比延迟治疗可更有效地减缓 RA 疾病进展。目前，早期 RA 定义为诊断后 6 个月内，而确诊超过 6 个月者则定义为明确诊断的 RA。应根据 RA 疾病活动程度采取个体化治疗方案，以最大程度地减轻关节炎症。即使在长病程 RA 中，有效的 DMARD 治疗也能改善症状、体征及放射学进展。应尽可能全面、快速且持续地控制 RA 的炎症。传统 DMARD 和生物 DMARD 可防止疾病进展和致残。

疾病活动度

RA 的确诊有助于临床医生制订治疗方案，并为患者提供未来疾病进程、治疗需求和预后方面的咨询。治疗强度取决于疾病活动度。如前所述，RA 通常累及运动关节，但关节受累的具体形式因患者而异。受累关节越多，病情越严重，且与疾病的不良预后相关。衡量疾病活动度可以通过多种工具进行，这些工具综合考虑了体格检查结果（如肿胀和压痛关节数量）、患者对 RA 整体活动度的评估（不仅仅是疼痛）以及反映炎症的实验室指标（最常使用 ESR 和 CRP）。治疗的目标是消除关节炎症。一旦确诊，患者应与风湿病医生协商后接受治疗。如果条件允许，使用特定的工具进行评估，以减轻关节炎症，从而达到缓解或低疾病活动度的目标。这些疾病活动度评估工具包括 DAS28（28 个关节的疾病活动度评分）、ESR/CRP、CDAI（临床疾病活动度评分）、SDAI（简易疾病活动度评分）、RAPID3（由简短问卷得出的疾病活动度评分）和 PASDAS（包含 7 个内容的加权指数的 PAS 疾病活动度评分）。

传统 DMARD

许多 DMARD 可用于 RA 的治疗。所有传统 DMARD 均起效缓慢，需要 1～6 个月才能完全起效，并且需要密切监测其毒性（表 2.4）。一旦确诊为 RA，应立即启动 DMARD 治疗。

甲氨蝶呤因其明确的疗效和已知的毒性特征（来自多项随机对照试验的证据）而被广泛应用于早期 RA 患者的初始 DMARD 治疗。它可通过每周一次口服或肠外途径给药。需要监测的已知副作用包括口腔溃疡、恶心、肝毒性、血细胞减少和肺炎。如果存在甲氨蝶呤禁忌证，如慢性肝病或过度饮酒（男性每天饮酒超过两杯，女性每天饮酒超过一杯）的患者，则应在单药治疗中使用替代性传统 DMARD，如柳氮磺吡啶或羟氯喹。在疾病早期，非甾体抗炎药（NSAID）和低剂量皮质类固醇可与 DMARD 联合使用，以迅速控制关节炎症。

在甲氨蝶呤治疗失败或应答不足的疾病活动持续处于中高度的 RA 患者中，后续传统和生物 DMARD 的选择尚未标准化，而是基于诸如给药途径、副作用和不良事件风险、成本以及患者和医生偏好等临床因素综合决定。多种 DMARD 联合常被用于 RA 的治疗。对于轻症 RA 患者，羟氯喹或柳氮磺吡啶，或两者均可作为一线药物。在两项随机对照试验中，甲氨蝶呤、羟氯喹和柳氮磺吡啶的三联疗法的疗效被证明并不劣于生物制剂 TNF-α 抑制剂的疗效。托法替布和巴瑞替尼是一类新型的合成 DMARD，可抑制 Janus 激酶（JAK）并降低细胞因子水平。由于感染风险增加，JAK 抑制剂是合成 DMARD 中不应与生物 DMARD 联合使用的一类药物。

生物 DMARD

生物 DMARD 是基于免疫原理的靶向治疗，在 20 世纪 90 年代随着针对细胞因子 TNF-α 的抑制剂诞生而推出。生物制剂是利用重组 DNA 技术由活细胞产生的（表 2.5）。美国食品药品监督管理局（FDA）批准了 10 种生物 DMARD 用于 RA（表 2.5）治疗，TNF-α 抑制剂是第一种。目前有五种靶向 TNF-α 的治疗可供选择。由于 TNF-α 抑制剂可使甲氨蝶呤耐药的患者迅速改善病情，因此是目前使用最为广泛的生物制剂。在甲氨蝶呤治疗失败后，TNF-α 抑制剂推荐在甲氨蝶呤基础上加用。

大多数生物 DMARD 通过静脉注射或皮下注射给药，价格昂贵但疗效显著。生物类似药是与原研生物药分子结构相似的生物制剂，与 FDA 批准的生物 DAMRD 没有临床意义上的不同。多种生物类似药已经上市，还有很多正在研发中，可作为生物 DMARD

biologic DMARDs. Most biologics have an increased risk of infection, including risk of reactivation of tuberculosis. Other cytokine-directed therapies include the IL-6 receptor antagonists sarilumab and tocilizumab and the IL-1 receptor antagonist anakinra. Biologic DMARDs also include an inhibitor of T-cell co-stimulation, abatacept; and a B-cell–depleting agent, rituximab. All patients should be screened for tuberculosis within 12 months prior to starting the first biologic DMARD. Biologic DMARDs should not be used in combination with other biologics because of increased risk of atypical infections.

❖ For a deeper discussion of these topics, please see Chapter 33, "Biologic Agents and Signaling Inhibitors," in *Goldman-Cecil Medicine*, 26th Edition.

Symptomatic Control and Bridging Therapy

DMARDs often take up to 1 to 6 months to produce low disease activity or remission. Consequently, nonsteroidal anti-inflammatory drugs (NSAIDs), which are not disease modifying, are frequently used early in the disease process for symptomatic control. NSAIDs can have significant side effects, including renal toxicity and increased risk of gastrointestinal bleeding; NSAIDs should be used with caution in patients with multiple medical comorbidities but are a standby for many patients with chronic disease.

Glucocorticoids remain important in the treatment of RA, especially for acute exacerbations of disease. These agents are used for RA in low to medium doses. Glucocorticoids are useful for brief exacerbations and decrease bone erosions, but the long-term side effects of glucocorticoids can be substantial; they should be used primarily in episodes of RA flares or high disease activity as bridging therapy for further DMARD effects. Side effects include osteoporosis, avascular necrosis of bone, obesity, hypertension, and glucose intolerance. Screening, prevention, and treatment for osteoporosis should be considered for all patients who receive long-term glucocorticoid therapy for prevention of glucocorticoid-induced osteoporosis. Intra-articular glucocorticoids are extremely effective treatment for exacerbations involving only a few joints.

❖ For a deeper discussion of these topics, please see Chapter 230, "Osteoporosis," in *Goldman-Cecil Medicine*, 26th Edition.

Medical Care Specialized for Rheumatoid Arthritis

RA is a chronic disease that requires focused care for comorbidities. DMARDs themselves require frequent laboratory monitoring for toxicities, including bone marrow suppression, hepatotoxicity, and renal dysfunction.

Infection

All patients should be tested for hepatitis B and C prior to starting a DMARD or biologic. Patients should be tested for latent tuberculosis within the previous 12 months by either a purified protein derivative (PPD) or interferon-γ release assay (IGRA) before starting a biologic DMARD. Opportunistic infections can occur in patients receiving DMARDs and biologic therapies and should be considered in the clinical care if chronic cytopenias or respiratory disease. In the setting of acute infection, DMARDs and biologic therapies should be withheld.

Vaccinations

Vaccination status should be assessed by primary care and rheumatology in caring for patients with RA. Ideally, vaccinations should occur during quiescent disease and also prior to starting immunosuppressive therapy. Killed vaccines can be given to patients while on all immunosuppressive conventional and biologic therapy, but live vaccines should be avoided in patients on biologic therapy. Prophylactically, all RA patients should be vaccinated for pneumococcal, influenza, and hepatitis B infection if increased risk. Herpes zoster vaccine to prevent shingles should be given to patients greater than 50 years old. If the live vaccine is used, this should be used prior to starting or while off biologic agents.

Osteoporosis

RA itself is a risk factor for osteoporosis, and combined with glucocorticoid use, it can lead to severe osteoporosis and subsequent morbidity. In every RA patient, bone health should be addressed to prevent development of osteoporosis. Bone health can be evaluated by periodic dual-energy x-ray absorptiometry (DXA), a risk assessment tool including coexistent tobacco use, family history of fractures, and ensuring adequate vitamin D supplementation. Routine strength training and aerobic exercise in moderation is recommended to improve bone health and ensure joint stabilization.

Cardiovascular

RA is a risk factor for cardiovascular disease due to chronic inflammation and should be monitored and managed. Lipid treatment recommendations do not currently differ from the routine non-RA patient populations. Hypertension, exacerbated by both pain and coexistent medications such as NSAIDs and glucocorticoids, should be monitored and treated according to current guidelines.

Perioperative

Caution should be taken preoperatively when the RA patient is being anesthetized to avoid C1-C2 subluxation and spinal cord compression. Flexion and extension radiographs of the cervical spine should be considered preoperatively for general anesthesia to assess for atlanto-occipital joint instability. Joint replacement surgery plays an important role for patients who have had severe, destructive joint disease, particularly in the knees and hips. Medications should be evaluated preoperatively with biologic DMARDs held one treatment cycle prior to starting. Methotrexate and conventional DMARDs can be continued through joint replacement surgery with improvement in both surgical and RA outcomes.

CONCLUSION AND PROGNOSIS

Although the underlying cause of RA is unknown, advances in cell biology, immunology, and molecular biology have led to dramatic therapeutic advancements for this disease. Conventional and biologic DMARDs improve short- and long-term outcomes. Bone erosions can occur within 1 to 2 years of disease onset, and early initiation of DMARDs is essential to prevent further morbidity.

RF and/or CCP positivity and extra-articular features are characteristic of severe disease. Tobacco use is the most significant environmental risk factor for RA and smoking cessation should be recommended to patients at risk for and with RA. The incidence of lymphoma and other malignancies is increased among patients with RA, and the overall mortality rate is increased by coexisting cardiovascular disease and infection.

更为便宜的替代药。大多数生物制剂会增加感染风险，包括结核病复发风险。其他靶向细胞因子疗法包括白细胞介素-6受体拮抗剂沙利鲁单抗（sarilumab）和托珠单抗（tocilizumab）、白细胞介素-1受体拮抗剂阿那白滞素（anakinra）。生物DMARD还包括T细胞共刺激因子抑制剂阿巴西普（abatacept）以及B细胞清除剂利妥昔单抗（rituximab）。所有患者在开始使用第一种生物DMARD前的12个月内都应进行结核病筛查。由于非典型感染的风险增加，生物DMARD不应与其他生物制剂联合使用。

❖ 有关此专题的深入讨论，请参阅 *Goldman-Cecil Medicine* 第26版第33章"生物制剂和信号抑制剂"。

症状控制与桥接治疗

DMARD通常需要应用1~6个月才能使RA患者达到低疾病活动度或缓解。因此，在病程早期，非甾体抗炎药（NSAID）这种不具有疾病改善作用的药物常被用于控制症状。然而，NSAID可能会带来显著的副作用，包括肾毒性和胃肠道出血风险增加；对于有多种合并症的患者，需慎用NSAID。尽管如此，对于许多慢性病患者来说，NSAID仍然是一种备选药物。

糖皮质激素在RA的治疗中仍然具有重要地位，尤其是在疾病急性发作期。这些药物用于RA治疗的剂量通常为低至中等剂量。虽然糖皮质激素对急性发作的患者有效并能降低骨侵蚀，但长期使用可能会带来较大的副作用；因此主要应用于RA发作期或高疾病活动度下DMARD起效前的桥接治疗。糖皮质激素的副作用包括骨质疏松、骨缺血性坏死、肥胖、高血压和糖耐量异常。对于所有接受长期糖皮质激素治疗的患者，应考虑进行骨质疏松的筛查、预防和治疗，以预防糖皮质激素诱导的骨质疏松。对个别关节炎症活动的患者来说，关节内注射糖皮质激素是很有效的治疗方法。

❖ 有关此专题的深入讨论，请参阅 *Goldman-Cecil Medicine* 第26版第230章"骨质疏松症"。

RA的专科护理

RA是一种慢性疾病，需重点关注其并发症。由于DMARD具有骨髓抑制、肝毒性和肾功能障碍等毒副作用，应用DMARD本身需要密切监测实验室指标。

感染

在开始使用DMARD或生物制剂之前，所有患者均应接受乙型肝炎和丙型肝炎检测。在开始使用生物DMARD前，患者应在用药前12个月内通过纯化蛋白衍生物（PPD）或γ-干扰素释放试验（IGRA）筛查潜伏结核。接受DMARD和生物制剂的患者可能发生机会性感染，存在慢性血细胞减少症或呼吸系统疾病者，在临床护理中应予以重点关注。在急性感染情况下，应暂停使用DMARD和生物制剂。

疫苗

在RA管理过程中，初级保健和风湿病专家应评估患者疫苗接种情况。理想状态下，接种疫苗应在疾病稳定期进行，且应在开始免疫抑制治疗之前进行。所有传统和生物免疫抑制治疗期间，可予患者接种灭活疫苗，接受生物制剂治疗的患者应避免接种活疫苗。感染风险增加的情况下，所有RA患者都应预防性接种肺炎球菌、流感和乙型肝炎疫苗。对于50岁以上的患者，应接种带状疱疹疫苗以预防带状疱疹。如果使用活疫苗，应在开始使用生物制剂之前或停用生物制剂期间使用。

骨质疏松

RA本身就是骨质疏松的危险因素，再加上糖皮质激素的使用，可能会导致严重的骨质疏松及并发症。对于每一位RA患者，都应关注骨骼健康，以预防骨质疏松的发展。骨骼健康可以通过定期的双能X线吸收测定法（DXA）进行评估，风险评估指标包括吸烟情况、有无骨折家族史以及维生素D是否补充充足。建议进行适度常规力量训练和有氧运动，以改善骨骼健康并维持关节稳定。

心血管

由于慢性炎症的作用，RA是心血管疾病的一个危险因素，应当进行监测和管理。目前，RA患者血脂管理的推荐意见与非RA人群并无不同。疼痛以及诸如NSAID、糖皮质激素等药物的应用可加重高血压，应根据当前指南进行监测和治疗。

围术期

RA患者术前麻醉时，应注意避免C1~C2半脱位和脊髓受压情况的发生。在进行全身麻醉前，应考虑对颈椎进行屈伸位X线片检查，以评估寰枕关节的稳定性。对于严重破坏性关节病变患者，尤其是膝关节和髋关节受累的患者，关节置换手术有重要作用。术前应评估用药情况，生物DMARD应在术前停用一个治疗周期。甲氨蝶呤和传统DMARD在关节置换手术期间可以继续使用，有助于改善手术效果和RA的病情。

结论和预后

虽然RA的潜在病因尚不清楚，但细胞生物学、免疫学和分子生物学的进展已使该病的治疗取得了巨大进步。传统和生物DMARD能改善RA的短期和长期预后。骨侵蚀可能在起病后的1~2年内发生，早期启用DMARD对于防止病情进一步恶化至关重要。

RF和（或）抗CCP抗体阳性以及关节外表现是RA病情严重的特征。吸烟是RA最重要的环境风险因素，应建议有RA风险者和RA患者戒烟。RA患者中淋巴瘤和其他恶性肿瘤的发病率增加，合并心血管疾病和感染使总体死亡率升高。

Although up to 15% of patients can go into drug-free remission, long-term disability is still significant for most patients. Fifty percent of patients with RA are not working in their original occupation after 10 years, approximately 10 times the rate in the normal population. Most patients fall between these disease extremes with various levels of functional impairment. Some have a waxing and waning course over a period of years, with acute episodes of single- or multiple-joint exacerbations.

Future developments in RA therapy will include guidelines about when to institute and withdraw biologic DMARDS, novel targeted biologic agents, when to use biosimilars, and personalized approaches based on an understanding of individual disease pathogenesis and disease activity.

SUGGESTED READINGS

Aletaha D, Neogi T, Silman AJ, et al: 2010 Rheumatoid arthritis classification criteria: an American College of Rheumatology/European League Against Rheumatism collaborative initiative, Arthritis Rheum 62:2569–2581, 2010.

Furer V, Rondaan C, Heijstek MW, et al: 2019 update of the ULAR recommendations for vaccination in adult patients with autoimmune inflammatory rheumatic diseases, Ann Rheum Dis 0:1–14, 2019.

Karlson EW, Ding B, Keenan BT, et al: Association of environmental and genetic factors and gene-environment interactions with risk of developing rheumatoid arthritis, Arthritis Care Res 65:1147–1156, 2013.

Kim K, Band SY, Lee HS, Bae SC: Update on the genetic architecture of rheumatoid arthritis, Nat Rev Rheumatol 13:13–24, 2017.

McInnes IB, Schett G: The pathogenesis of rheumatoid arthritis, N Engl J Med 365:22052219, 2011.

Minichiello E, Semerano L, Boissier MC: Time trends in the incidence, prevalence, and severity of rheumatoid arthritis: a systematic literature review, Joint Bone Spine 83:625–630, 2016.

Moreland LW, O'Dell JR, Paulus HE, et al: A randomized comparative effectiveness study of oral triple therapy versus etanercept plus methotrexate in early aggressive rheumatoid arthritis: the treatment of Early Aggressive Rheumatoid Arthritis Trial, Arthritis Rheum 64:2824–2835, 2012.

O'Dell JR, Mikuls TR, Taylor TH, et al: Therapies for active rheumatoid arthritis after methotrexate failure, N Engl J Med 369:307–318, 2013.

Okada Y, Wu D, Trynka G, et al: Genetics of rheumatoid arthritis contributes to biology and drug discovery, Nature 506:376–381, 2014.

Singh JA, Saag KG, Bridges Jr SL, et al: 2015 American College of Rheumatology Guideline for the Treatment of Rheumatoid Arthritis, Arthritis Care Res 68:1–26, 2016.

Smolen JS, Aletaha D, Mcinnes IB: Rheumatoid arthritis, Lancet 388:2023–2038, 2016.

Smolen JS, Landwe B, et al: EULAR recommendations for the management of rheumatoid arthritis with synthetic and biological disease-modifying antirheumatic drugs: 2016 update, Ann Rheum Dis 17:960–977, 2017.

Sparks JA: Rheumatoid arthritis, Ann Intern Med 170:ITC1–ITC16, 2019.

van der Woude D, van der Helm-van Mil HM: Update on the epidemiology, risk factors, and disease outcomes of rheumatoid arthritis, Best Pract Res Clin Rheumatol 32:174–187, 2018.

15% 的患者可达到无药缓解，但对大多数患者来说，长期功能障碍仍然常见。RA 患者中有 50% 在发病 10 年后无法从事原来的工作，这一比例大约为正常人群的 10 倍。大多数 RA 患者伴有不同程度的功能障碍。有些患者在数年间病情起伏不定，可出现单个或多个关节急性加重的情况。

RA 治疗的未来发展方向包括制定生物 DMARD 启用和停用的指南、开发新的靶向生物制剂、明确生物类似药的使用时机，以及基于疾病发病机制和疾病活动度的个体化治疗方法。

推荐阅读

Aletaha D, Neogi T, Silman AJ, et al: 2010 Rheumatoid arthritis classification criteria: an American College of Rheumatology/European League Against Rheumatism collaborative initiative, Arthritis Rheum 62:2569–2581, 2010.

Furer V, Rondaan C, Heijstek MW, et al: 2019 update of the ULAR recommendations for vaccination in adult patients with autoimmune inflammatory rheumatic diseases, Ann Rheum Dis 0:1–14, 2019.

Karlson EW, Ding B, Keenan BT, et al: Association of environmental and genetic factors and gene-environment interactions with risk of developing rheumatoid arthritis, Arthritis Care Res 65:1147–1156, 2013.

Kim K, Band SY, Lee HS, Bae SC: Update on the genetic architecture of rheumatoid arthritis, Nat Rev Rheumatol 13:13–24, 2017.

McInnes IB, Schett G: The pathogenesis of rheumatoid arthritis, N Engl J Med 365:22052219, 2011.

Minichiello E, Semerano L, Boissier MC: Time trends in the incidence, prevalence, and severity of rheumatoid arthritis: a systematic literature review, Joint Bone Spine 83:625–630, 2016.

Moreland LW, O'Dell JR, Paulus HE, et al: A randomized comparative effectiveness study of oral triple therapy versus etanercept plus methotrexate in early aggressive rheumatoid arthritis: the treatment of Early Aggressive Rheumatoid Arthritis Trial, Arthritis Rheum 64:2824–2835, 2012.

O'Dell JR, Mikuls TR, Taylor TH, et al: Therapies for active rheumatoid arthritis after methotrexate failure, N Engl J Med 369:307–318, 2013.

Okada Y, Wu D, Trynka G, et al: Genetics of rheumatoid arthritis contributes to biology and drug discovery, Nature 506:376–381, 2014.

Singh JA, Saag KG, Bridges Jr SL, et al: 2015 American College of Rheumatology Guideline for the Treatment of Rheumatoid Arthritis, Arthritis Care Res 68:1–26, 2016.

Smolen JS, Aletaha D, Mcinnes IB: Rheumatoid arthritis, Lancet 388:2023–2038, 2016.

Smolen JS, Landwe B, et al: EULAR recommendations for the management of rheumatoid arthritis with synthetic and biological disease-modifying antirheumatic drugs: 2016 update, Ann Rheum Dis 17:960–977, 2017.

Sparks JA: Rheumatoid arthritis, Ann Intern Med 170:ITC1–ITC16, 2019.

van der Woude D, van der Helm-van Mil HM: Update on the epidemiology, risk factors, and disease outcomes of rheumatoid arthritis, Best Pract Res Clin Rheumatol 32:174–187, 2018.

3

Spondyloarthritis

Douglas W. Lienesch

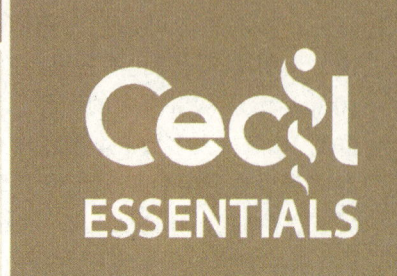

DEFINITION

Spondyloarthritis is a form of inflammatory joint disease characterized by inflammation of the axial skeleton (spine and sacroiliac joints) and/or the peripheral joints, often associated with inflammation of the eye, gastrointestinal tract, genitourinary system, and skin. *Axial spondyloarthritis* is the term used when the spine is the site of inflammation, and *peripheral spondyloarthritis* indicates inflammation of the joints and periarticular tissues in the extremities.

The cardinal clinical feature of spondyloarthritis is inflammation of the sacroiliac joints (i.e., sacroiliitis) and the spine (i.e., spondylitis). Inflammation of tendon insertion sites (i.e., enthesitis), inflammation of entire digits (i.e., dactylitis), and inflammation of one to four lower extremity joints (i.e., oligoarthritis) are extraspinal skeletal findings. A positive family history, eye inflammation (i.e., anterior uveitis or conjunctivitis), and the absence of rheumatoid factor and subcutaneous nodules are common.

Spondyloarthritis may be further subcategorized based on other clinical features. Patients with axial spondyloarthritis with typical radiographic features including sacroiliac joint erosions, spinal syndesmophytes, and ankylosis of the joints have *ankylosing spondylitis*. In the absence of these radiographic changes, *nonradiographic axial spondyloarthritis* may be present if there are typical symptoms accompanied by magnetic resonance imaging inflammatory signs at the sacroiliac joint or spine. Axial or peripheral inflammatory joint disease in the setting of psoriasis or inflammatory bowel disease (IBD) is termed *psoriatic arthritis* or *IBD-related spondyloarthritis*, respectively. *Reactive arthritis* refers to spondyloarthritis with onset within a few weeks of certain types of infection.

Spondyloarthritis is strongly associated with human leukocyte antigen B27 (HLA-27), a specific allele of the B locus of the HLA-encoding class I major histocompatibility complex genes. The frequency of HLA-B27 among white individuals is approximately 8%. However, up to 90% of white patients with ankylosing spondylitis and 80% of white patients with reactive arthritis or juvenile spondyloarthritis are HLA-B27 positive, and these percentages are even higher among patients with uveitis. The rate of HLA-B27 positivity among patients with inflammatory bowel disease or psoriasis with peripheral arthritis is not markedly increased unless they have spondylitis, in which case the frequency of HLA-B27 is 50%. The frequency of HLA-B27 varies widely among other ethnic groups and accounts for the broad variation of the prevalence of ankylosing spondylitis in different populations.

Ankylosing spondylitis is much more common among adolescent boys and young men, but this finding may reflect underdiagnosis in women, in whom disease manifestations may be milder than they are in men. Reactive arthritis is more common among men when it follows genitourinary *Chlamydia trachomatis* infection, but the sex distribution is even among patients after dysentery. Inflammatory arthritis including spondylitis affects approximately 5% to 8% of patients with psoriasis and 10% to 25% of patients with ulcerative colitis or Crohn's disease. Men and women are affected equally. The prevalence of spondyloarthritis, particularly psoriatic and reactive arthritis, is increased in populations with high human immunodeficiency virus (HIV) infection rates.

PATHOLOGY

Although the strong association of HLA-B27 with spondyloarthritis is well established, a specific role in the pathogenesis of these disorders has not been elucidated. Animal models in which rodents transgenic for HLA-B27 develop inflammatory abnormalities strikingly similar to those seen in HLA-B27–associated human diseases provide compelling indirect evidence for a pathogenic role. When raised in a germ-free environment, these animals remain disease free, suggesting a key additional environmental factor.

In addition to the strong genetic links for the risk of spondyloarthritis, important associations exist between specific bacterial agents and disease pathogenesis. Genitourinary infection with *C. trachomatis* or diarrheal illness with *Shigella*, *Salmonella*, *Campylobacter*, and *Yersinia* species can induce reactive arthritis. Several additional infectious agents are less commonly implicated. They appear to trigger an inflammatory response, possibly as a result of persistence of bacterial antigens, or cause an aberrant immunologic response to infection that results in misfolding of HLA-B27 molecules in antigen-presenting cells, generating a persistent inflammatory reaction.

No one theory of pathogenesis of spondyloarthritis explains the clinical spectrum of these disorders, and more research is clearly needed to solidify an understanding of their origin. The complex role of the immune system in spondyloarthritis is highlighted by the observation that patients infected with HIV appear more likely to have severe disease, especially psoriatic arthritis. When HIV infection is treated with antiviral agents, the incidence of spondyloarthritis declines.

Although many of the cellular and molecular mechanisms of inflammatory joint disease have been elucidated, the pathophysiology of spondyloarthritis remains incompletely understood. Inflammation of the sacroiliac joints, spine, and entheses is a unique feature of these disorders. Pathophysiologic studies show that the inflammation originates at the interface of bone and cartilage in the sacroiliac joint and bone and fibrocartilage in the enthesis. Macrophages and $CD4^+$ and $CD8^+$ T cells are present, and Th17 appears to play a critical role in the inflammatory process. Proinflammatory cytokines interleukin-17 (IL-17), interleukin-23 (IL-23), and tumor necrosis factor-α (TNF-α) and are abundant.

Synovial tissue becomes inflamed, and osteoclasts are activated, leading to bone resorption, reminiscent of rheumatoid arthritis joint

脊柱关节炎

罗贵 译　赵征 薛静 审校　李梦涛 通审

定义

脊柱关节炎是一种以中轴骨骼（脊柱和骶髂关节）和（或）外周关节的炎症为特征的炎症性关节病，常伴有眼部、胃肠道、泌尿生殖系统和皮肤的炎症。中轴脊柱关节炎是指以脊柱为炎症部位的疾病，而外周脊柱关节炎则是指四肢关节和周围组织的炎症。

脊柱关节炎的主要临床特征是骶髂关节炎症（即骶髂关节炎）和脊柱炎症（即脊柱炎）。肌腱插入部位的炎症（即附着点炎）、整个手指/足趾的炎症（即指/趾炎）以及1~4个下肢关节的炎症（即寡关节炎）是其脊柱外的骨骼症状。阳性家族史、眼部炎症（即前葡萄膜炎或结膜炎）、类风湿因子阴性且无皮下结节也是其常见临床表现。

脊柱关节炎还可根据其他临床特征进一步分类。具有典型放射学特征（包括骶髂关节侵蚀、脊柱韧带骨赘和关节强直）的中轴脊柱关节炎患者可归为强直性脊柱炎。在没有这些放射学改变的情况下，如果出现典型的症状并伴有骶髂关节或脊柱磁共振成像炎症改变者，则可归为非放射学中轴脊柱关节炎。银屑病或炎症性肠病（IBD）引起的中轴或外周炎症性关节病，分别称为银屑病关节炎或IBD相关脊柱关节炎。反应性关节炎是指在某些类型的感染后几周内发病的脊柱关节炎。

脊柱关节炎与人类白细胞抗原B27（HLA-B27）密切相关，HLA-B27是HLA编码的Ⅰ类主要组织相容性复合体基因B位点的特异等位基因。在白种人中，HLA-B27的阳性率约为8%。然而高达90%的强直性脊柱炎白人患者及80%的反应性关节炎或幼年脊柱关节炎白人患者HLA-B27为阳性，这一比例在葡萄膜炎患者中甚至更高。伴有外周关节炎的炎症性肠病或银屑病患者的HLA-B27阳性率并没有明显升高，除非他们出现脊柱炎，在这种情况下，HLA-B27阳性率为50%。HLA-B27在其他种族群体中的阳性率差异很大，这也是强直性脊柱炎在不同人群中患病率差异很大的原因。

强直性脊柱炎在青春期男孩和青年男性中更为常见，但这一发现可能反映了女性诊断不足，主要是由于她们的临床表现可能比男性轻微。在泌尿生殖系统沙眼衣原体感染后，反应性关节炎在男性中更为常见，但在痢疾感染后，其性别分布是均匀的。包括脊柱炎在内的炎症性关节炎影响着大约5%~8%的银屑病患者及10%~25%的溃疡性结肠炎或克罗恩病患者，男女性别差异较小。在人类免疫缺陷病毒（HIV）感染率较高的人群中，脊柱关节炎（尤其是银屑病关节炎和反应性关节炎）的患病率会有所升高。

病理学

虽然HLA-B27与脊柱关节炎的密切关系已得到证实，但其在这些疾病发病机制中的具体作用尚未得到阐明。在动物模型中，转基因HLA-B27的啮齿类动物出现的炎症异常与HLA-B27相关人类疾病中出现的炎症异常惊人地相似，这为HLA-B27的致病作用提供了令人信服的间接证据。当在无菌环境中饲养时，这些动物不会发病，这表明还有一个关键的环境致病因素。

脊柱关节炎发病机制除了与遗传因素密切相关以外，与特定细菌病原体之间也存在重要联系。泌尿生殖系统感染沙眼衣原体或感染志贺菌、沙门菌、弯曲杆菌及耶尔森菌出现腹泻时均可诱发反应性关节炎。其他感染性病原体则不太常见。它们似乎会触发炎症反应，这可能是细菌抗原持续存在的结果；或者导致对感染的异常免疫反应，使得抗原提呈细胞中的HLA-B27分子错误折叠，从而产生持续的炎症反应。

目前尚无有关脊柱关节炎发病机制的理论能解释这类疾病的临床表现，亟需更多研究来确认对其起源的认知。感染HIV的患者更容易罹患严重疾病，尤其是银屑病关节炎，这突显了免疫系统在脊柱关节炎中的复杂作用。当使用抗病毒药物治疗HIV感染时，脊柱关节炎的发病呈现下降趋势。

虽然炎症性关节病的许多细胞和分子机制已被阐明，但人们对脊柱关节炎的病理生理学仍不完全了解。骶髂关节、脊柱和附着点炎症是这类疾病的独特特征。病理生理学研究表明，炎症起源于骶髂关节的骨与软骨界面以及附着点的骨与纤维软骨界面。这些部位存在巨噬细胞、$CD4^+$和$CD8^+$ T细胞，而Th17细胞似乎在炎症过程中起关键作用。白细胞介素-17（IL-17）、白细胞介素-23（IL-23）和肿瘤坏死因子-α（TNF-α）等促炎细胞因子含量丰富。

滑膜组织出现炎症，破骨细胞被激活，导致骨

TABLE 3.1 Comparison of the Spondyloarthritis

Features	Ankylosing Spondylitis	Posturethral Reactive Arthritis	Postdysenteric Reactive Arthritis	Enteropathic Arthritis	Psoriatic Arthritis
Sacroiliitis	+++++	+++	++	+	++
Spondylitis	++++	+++	++	++	++
Peripheral arthritis	+	++++	++++	+++	++++
Articular course	Chronic	Acute or chronic	Acute or chronic	Acute or chronic	Chronic
HLA-B27	95%	60%	30%	20%	20%
Enthesopathy	++	++++	+++	++	++
Extra-articular manifestations	Eye, heart	Eye, GU, oral and/or GI, heart	GU, eye	GI, eye	Skin, eye
Other names	Bekhterev arthritis, Marie-Strümpell disease	Reactive arthritis, SARA, NGU, chlamydial arthritis	Reactive arthritis	Crohn's disease, ulcerative colitis	

GI, Gastrointestinal tract; *GU*, genitourinary tract; *HLA*, human leukocyte antigen; *NGU*, nongonococcal urethritis; *SARA*, sexually acquired reactive arthritis; *+*, relative prevalence of a specific feature.
Data from Cush JJ, Lipsky PE: The spondyloarthropathies. In Goldman L, Bennett JC, editors: *Cecil textbook of medicine,* ed 21, Philadelphia, 2000, Saunders, pp 1499-1507.

inflammation. Unlike in rheumatoid arthritis, early bone resorption is followed by a secondary phase during which osteoblast activity predominates, leading to new bone formation in periarticular bone (i.e., hyperostosis) and around joints (i.e., osteophytosis) or vertebral bodies (i.e., syndesmophytes). Ultimately, bony fusion of joints (ankylosis) occurs. The relationship between these paradoxical phases of bone resorption and proliferation is an area of active investigation.

CLINICAL PRESENTATION

Common Clinical Features of Spondyloarthritis

All forms of spondyloarthritis have considerable clinical overlap with one another and are most easily considered as a group of related disorders. Table 3.1 outlines the clinical features of these disorders. The cardinal clinical features common to all of them are inflammatory spine pain and an asymmetrical, predominantly lower extremity inflammatory joint or tendon disease. Inflammatory spine pain should be suspected in young patients (<40 years) who have an insidious onset of chronic low back pain or buttock pain associated with prolonged morning stiffness and relieved by exercise.

The characteristic peripheral joint disease involves one to four joints, usually in the lower extremities, and may be associated with tendon insertion inflammation (i.e., enthesitis) or sausage digits (i.e., dactylitis). Symmetrical polyarthropathy involving the upper extremities and clinically similar to rheumatoid arthritis is seen in some forms of psoriatic or inflammatory bowel disease–related spondyloarthritis. Anterior uveitis, enthesitis, dactylitis, psoriatic skin or nail changes, inflammatory bowel disease, a family history of spondyloarthritis, or a history of preceding gastrointestinal or genitourinary infection suggests spondyloarthritis. Subcutaneous nodules, rheumatoid factor, and antinuclear antibodies are usually absent.

In a given patient, the clinical features of these disorders may accumulate over a prolonged period. Some patients do not initially demonstrate the typical findings of a specific disorder. They are considered to have undifferentiated spondyloarthritis. Early disease can be subcategorized as predominately axial spondyloarthritis or predominately peripheral spondyloarthritis, depending on the site of the dominant symptoms. Many patients later have clinical findings consistent with a specific subtype of spondyloarthritis.

Inflammatory spine pain is the cardinal feature of axial disease and results from inflammation in the sacroiliac joints and spinal elements. Uncontrolled disease may lead to ankylosis (i.e., bony fusion) at sacroiliac joints and throughout the vertebral column, culminating in loss of spinal and costovertebral motion, deformity, and restrictive extrapulmonary physiology.

Enthesitis can occur in many different anatomic locations. They include spinous processes, costosternal junctions, ischial tuberosities, plantar aponeuroses, and Achilles tendons.

When peripheral arthritis of spondyloarthritis occurs, it frequently begins as an episodic, asymmetrical, oligoarticular process that often involves the lower extremities. The arthritis can progress and may become chronic and disabling. A unique feature of spondyloarthritis is the appearance of fusiform swelling of an entire finger or toe, referred to as *dactylitis* or *sausage digits*.

Anterior uveitis, or inflammation of the anterior chamber of the eye, is a common extra-articular manifestation of spondyloarthritis, especially among HLA-B27–positive patients. Acute bouts of uveitis are usually monocular, painful, and accompanied by eye redness and blurred vision. Recurrent attacks are common and can lead to blindness. Scleritis, episcleritis, and conjunctivitis are less commonly associated phenomena.

Spondyloarthritis may occasionally involve other organ systems and may cause significant morbidity and mortality. Aortitis, especially occurring in the ascending segment, can result in aortic insufficiency from aortic root dilation, aortic dissection, and cardiac conduction system abnormalities. Pulmonary fibrosis of the apical regions can occur, often in an insidious fashion. Spinal cord compression can result from atlantoaxial joint subluxation, cauda equina syndrome, or vertebral fractures. In rare cases, long-standing spondyloarthritis is associated with secondary amyloidosis.

Specific Clinical Features of Spondyloarthritis
Ankylosing Spondylitis

The cardinal clinical feature of ankylosing spondylitis is inflammatory spine pain. Over time, spine involvement ascends from the sacroiliac joints to involve all levels of the spine. Progressive loss of motion results from ankylosis of the vertebral column and apophyseal joints. Costovertebral involvement leads to decreased chest expansion and restrictive lung physiology.

Loss of mobility and secondary osteoporosis of the vertebral bodies increase the risk of traumatic spine fracture. Axial involvement of the shoulders and hips is common and associated with a worse prognosis.

表 3.1 脊柱关节炎的比较

特征	强直性脊柱炎	尿道感染后反应性关节炎	痢疾感染后反应性关节炎	肠病性关节炎	银屑病关节炎
骶髂关节炎	+++++	+++	++	+	++
脊柱炎	+++++	+++	++	++	++
外周关节炎	+	++++	++++	+++	++++
关节病程	慢性	急性或慢性	急性或慢性	急性或慢性	慢性
HLA-B27	95%	60%	30%	20%	20%
附着点病变	++	++++	+++	++	++
关节外表现	眼睛，心脏	眼睛，GU，口腔和（或）GI，心脏	GU，眼睛	GI，眼睛	皮肤，眼睛
其他名称	Bekhterev 关节炎，Marie Strümpell 病	反应性关节炎，SARA，NGU，衣原体关节炎	反应性关节炎	克罗恩病，溃疡性结肠炎	

GI，胃肠道；GU，泌尿生殖道；HLA，人类白细胞抗原；NGU，非淋球菌性尿道炎；SARA，性行为获得性反应性关节炎；+，某一特征的相对发生率。

引自 Cush JJ，Lipsky PE：The spondyloarthropathies. In Goldman L，Bennett JC，editors：Cecil textbook of medicine, ed 21，Philadelphia，2000，Saunders，pp 1499-1507.

吸收，使人联想到类风湿关节炎的关节炎症。与类风湿关节炎不同的是，脊柱关节炎在早期骨吸收后会有一个继发阶段，在这一阶段中，成骨细胞的活性占主导地位，导致关节周围骨（即骨质增生）和关节周围（即骨赘形成）或椎体（即韧带骨赘）新骨形成。最终，关节发生骨性融合（强直）。目前，骨吸收和骨增殖阶段之间的矛盾关系是研究的热点领域。

临床表现

脊柱关节炎的常见临床特征

所有形式的脊柱关节炎在临床表现上都有相当多重叠，因此最容易被视为一组相关疾病。表 3.1 概述了这些疾病的临床特征。它们共同的主要临床特征是炎性脊柱疼痛和不对称的、下肢为主的炎性关节或肌腱疾病。如果年轻患者（小于 40 岁）隐匿性地出现慢性腰背痛或臀区疼痛，并伴有长时间的晨僵，且运动后可缓解，则应怀疑炎性脊柱疼痛。

特征性的外周关节疾病涉及 1~4 个关节，通常发生在下肢，可能与肌腱插入部位炎症（即附着点炎）或腊肠指/趾（即指/趾炎）有关。累及上肢的对称性多关节病，临床表现与类风湿关节炎相似，可见于某些形式的银屑病或炎症性肠病相关的脊柱关节炎。前葡萄膜炎、附着点炎、指/趾炎、银屑病性皮肤或指甲病变、炎症性肠病、脊柱关节炎家族史、前驱胃肠道或泌尿生殖系统感染病史均提示脊柱关节炎。通常不会出现皮下结节，而类风湿因子和抗核抗体也常为阴性。

在特定患者身上，这些疾病的临床特征可能会长期逐步累加。有些患者最初并没有表现出某种特定疾病的典型症状。此时认为他们患有未分化脊柱关节炎。根据主要症状的部位，早期疾病可分为以中轴脊柱关节炎为主和以外周脊柱关节炎为主两类。许多患者后来的临床表现与脊柱关节炎的特定亚型一致。

炎性脊柱疼痛是中轴疾病的主要特征，由骶髂关节和脊柱的炎症引起。如果病情得不到控制，可能会导致骶髂关节和整个脊柱椎体发生强直（即骨融合），最终导致脊柱和肋椎关节运动功能丧失、畸形和肺扩张度下降导致的肺功能受限。

附着点炎可发生在不同的解剖位置，包括棘突、胸肋关节、坐骨结节、足底腱膜和跟腱。

当脊柱关节炎出现外周关节炎时，初期通常表现为发作性、非对称性、寡关节炎，常累及下肢。关节炎会逐渐进展，并可能发展为慢性、致残性关节炎。脊柱关节炎的一个特征性表现是整个手指或脚趾纺锤形肿胀，称为指/趾炎或腊肠指/趾。

前葡萄膜炎或眼前房炎症是脊柱关节炎常见的关节外表现，尤其是在 HLA-B27 阳性患者中。葡萄膜炎急性发作通常表现为单眼、疼痛、伴有眼红和视物模糊。反复发作很常见，可导致失明。巩膜炎、巩膜外层炎和结膜炎是较少见的相关表现。

脊柱关节炎偶尔会累及其他器官系统，并可能导致严重的并发症和死亡率升高。主动脉炎（尤其是发生在升主动脉段的主动脉炎）会因主动脉根部扩张、主动脉夹层和心脏传导系统异常而导致主动脉瓣关闭不全。肺尖部可能发生肺纤维化，通常是隐匿性的。寰枢关节脱位、马尾综合征或脊椎骨折可能导致脊髓压迫。在极少数情况下，长期的脊柱关节炎会伴有继发性淀粉样变性。

脊柱关节炎的特异性临床特征
强直性脊柱炎

强直性脊柱炎的主要临床特征为炎性脊柱疼痛。随着时间推移，脊柱受累会从骶髂关节发展至脊柱各个节段。椎体及关节突关节的强直会导致运动能力逐渐丧失。肋椎关节受累会导致胸廓扩张度下降和肺生理功能受限。

椎体活动度的丧失和继发性骨质疏松会增加脊柱外伤性骨折的风险。属于中轴部位的肩关节及髋关节受累很常见，预后较差。外周寡关节炎、附着点炎和

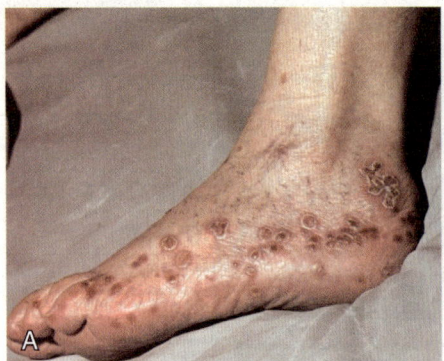 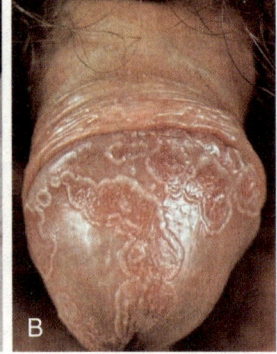 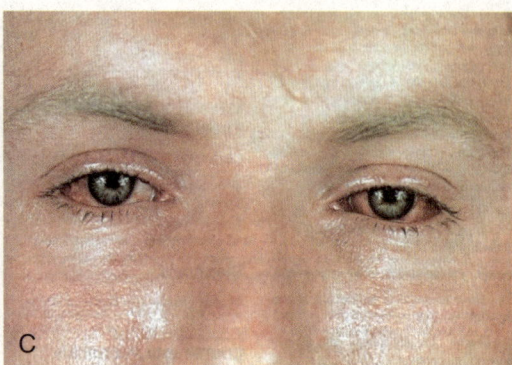

Fig. 3.1 Reactive arthritis. (A) Keratoderma blennorrhagicum. Red to brown papules, vesicles, and pustules with central erosion show characteristic crusting and peripheral scaling on the dorsolateral and plantar foot. (B) Balanitis circinata. Moist, well-demarcated erosions with a slightly raised micropustular circinate border on the glans penis. (C) Bilateral conjunctivitis associated with anterior uveitis. (From Fitzpatrick TB, Johnson RA, Wolff K, et al: *Color atlas and synopsis of clinical dermatology*, ed 3, New York, 1983, McGraw-Hill, pp 393, 395.)

Peripheral oligoarthritis, enthesitis, and dactylitis are more common in females. Diagnosis requires demonstration of radiographic sacroiliitis (i.e., sacroiliac joint erosions, sclerosis, and ankylosis). Anterior uveitis is common. Aortitis, upper lobe pulmonary fibrosis, cauda equina syndrome, and amyloidosis are less common and seen in late disease.

Reactive Arthritis (Posturethral/Postdysenteric)

Among the unique clinical features of reactive arthritis are urethritis, conjunctivitis, and certain dermatologic problems (Fig. 3.1). The urethritis may result from the chlamydial infection that triggers the disease, or it may be a sterile inflammatory discharge seen in diarrhea-associated disease. Conjunctivitis may be mild in reactive arthritis and is distinct from uveitis.

Keratoderma blennorrhagicum is a distinct papulosquamous rash usually found on the palms or soles. Circinate balanitis is a rash that may appear on the penile glans or shaft of men with reactive arthritis. Nonpitting nail thickening and oral ulcers may also occur in patients with reactive arthritis. These lesions can be confused with similar findings in patients with psoriasis and inflammatory bowel disease, respectively.

Most cases are self-limited. Chronic or relapsing arthritis and chronic spondylitis are associated with HLA-B27 and *Chlamydia* infection.

Psoriatic Arthritis

Five identifiable clinical patterns of psoriatic arthritis are recognized: distal interphalangeal joint involvement with nail pitting; asymmetrical oligoarthropathy of large and small joints; arthritis mutilans, a severe, destructive arthritis; symmetrical polyarthritis, which is identical to rheumatoid arthritis; and predominately axial disease. These patterns are not exclusive, and clinical overlap is significant.

Spondylitis or sacroiliitis may occur along with any of the other patterns. The prevalence of HLA-B27 is increased among the patients with spondylitis or sacroiliitis but not among patients with the other patterns. Psoriatic skin or nail disease predates arthritis in most cases, but both may occur concomitantly, or joint disease may precede skin involvement. Rarely, joint disease is indistinguishable from psoriatic arthritis, which can occur in patients with a family history but no personal history of psoriatic skin disease.

Enteropathic Arthritis: Inflammatory Bowel Disease

Crohn's disease and ulcerative colitis (see Chapter 38) are frequently associated with inflammatory spine disease and peripheral arthritis. The peripheral arthritis is typically nonerosive, oligoarticular, and episodic, and the degree of joint involvement fluctuates with gut activity. A more chronic, symmetrical polyarthritis may occur in patients with Crohn's disease.

DIAGNOSIS AND DIFFERENTIAL DIAGNOSIS

The diagnosis of spondyloarthritis remains a clinical diagnosis made by identifying typical history and physical examination phenomena, analyzing selected laboratory tests, and using musculoskeletal imaging. The diagnosis is suggested by inflammatory spine pain or chronic lower extremity asymmetric inflammatory oligoarthritis in two to four joints. In this setting, features that increase the probability of spondyloarthritis include uveitis, psoriasis, enthesitis, dactylitis, inflammatory bowel disease, family history of spondylarthropathy, elevated C-reactive protein (CRP) level, HLA-B27, preceding gastrointestinal or genitourinary infection, and sacroiliitis on radiography, computed tomography (CT), or magnetic resonance imaging MRI).

Differentiating spondyloarthritis from other inflammatory or degenerative joint or spine diseases can be challenging. Crystalline arthropathies can manifest with peripheral oligoarthritis, often in the lower extremities. However, the spine is rarely involved, and intracellular crystals can be demonstrated in the synovial fluid. Rheumatoid arthritis and other systemic autoimmune diseases usually manifest with symmetrical polyarthritis of the upper and lower extremities associated with abnormal serologies such as rheumatoid factors, anti–cyclic citrullinated peptide (CCP) antibodies, or antinuclear antibodies. Predominately axial spondyloarthritis must be differentiated from indolent infections of the sacroiliac joints, vertebrae, or intravertebral disks; degenerative disease of the spine and disks (i.e., spondylosis); and diffuse idiopathic skeletal hyperostosis (DISH).

The radiographic features of the spondyloarthritis are highly specific and, in the correct clinical setting, greatly increase the certainty of the diagnosis. Sacroiliitis is usually the earliest radiographic sign of spine disease and results in sclerosis and erosions of the sacroiliac joints with eventual bony fusion (Fig. 3.2A). Many radiographic changes result from chronic spondylitis, including ossification of the annulus fibrosus, calcification of spinal ligaments, bony sclerosis and squaring of vertebral bodies, and ankylosis of apophyseal joints. These changes can lead to vertebral fusion and a bamboo spine appearance (see Fig. 3.2B).

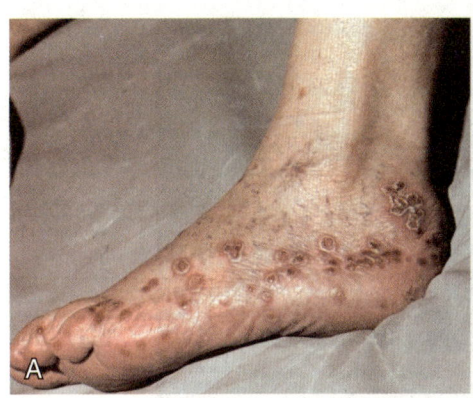 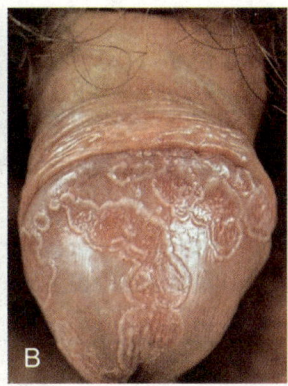 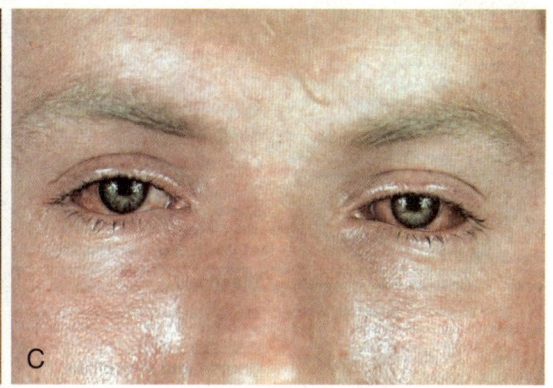

图 3.1 反应性关节炎。（A）脓溢性皮肤角化病。足背外侧和足底出现红色至棕色丘疹、水疱和脓疱，中央有糜烂，呈特征性结痂和周围脱屑。（B）环状龟头炎。龟头上有湿润、分界清楚的糜烂，微脓疱环状边界略微隆起。（C）双眼结膜炎伴前葡萄膜炎（引自 Fitzpatrick TB, Johnson RA, Wolff K, et al: Color atlas and synopsis of clinical dermatology, ed 3, New York, 1983, McGraw-Hill, pp 393, 395.）

指/趾炎在女性患者中更为常见。诊断需要骶髂关节炎的放射学表现（即骶髂关节侵蚀、硬化和强直）。前葡萄膜炎很常见。主动脉炎、肺上叶纤维化、马尾综合征和淀粉样变性较少见，且多出现于疾病晚期。

反应性关节炎（尿道感染后/痢疾感染后）

反应性关节炎的独特临床特征包括尿道炎、结膜炎和某些皮肤表现（图 3.1）。疾病的触发因素可能是衣原体感染所致的尿道炎或者是腹泻相关疾病产生的无菌性炎性分泌物。反应性关节炎患者的结膜炎一般比较轻微，这有别于葡萄膜炎。

脓溢性皮肤角化病是一种独特的丘疹鳞屑性皮疹，通常出现在手掌或足底。环状龟头炎是一种可能出现于男性反应性关节炎患者的阴茎龟头或阴茎体上的皮疹。反应性关节炎患者也可能出现非凹陷性指甲增厚和口腔溃疡。这些病变可能与银屑病和炎症性肠病患者的类似症状相混淆。

大多数病例都是自限性的。慢性或复发性关节炎和慢性脊柱炎与 HLA-B27 及衣原体感染有关。

银屑病关节炎

银屑病关节炎有 5 种临床类型：远端指间关节受累伴有指甲顶针样凹陷；大小关节均受累的非对称性寡关节炎；毁损型关节炎，一种严重的破坏性关节炎；对称性多关节炎，与类风湿关节炎相似；以及中轴受累为主型。这些类型之间并不矛盾，临床上经常相互重叠。

脊柱炎或骶髂关节炎可与任何其他类型同时出现。HLA-B27 的阳性率在脊柱炎或骶髂关节炎患者中会升高，而其他类型的患者则不会。在大多数情况下，银屑病的皮肤或指甲病变要早于关节炎，但两者也可能同时发生，或者关节病变先于皮肤受累。在极少数情况下，关节疾病与银屑病关节炎难以区分，这可能发生在有银屑病家族史但没有银屑病皮肤表现病史的患者身上。

肠病性关节炎：炎症性肠病

克罗恩病和溃疡性结肠炎（见第 38 章）常伴有炎症性脊柱疾病和外周关节炎。外周关节炎通常是非侵蚀性、寡关节性和发作性的，关节受累程度随肠道病情活动而波动。克罗恩病患者可能会出现慢性、对称性多关节炎。

诊断和鉴别诊断

脊柱关节炎的诊断仍然是一种临床诊断，通过确切典型的病史和体格检查、分析选定的实验室检查以及肌肉骨骼影像学检查来进行。脊柱炎症性疼痛或 2～4 个关节受累的慢性下肢非对称性炎性寡关节炎可提示该疾病的诊断。在这种情况下，提高脊柱关节炎诊断可能性的特征包括葡萄膜炎、银屑病、附着点炎、指/趾炎、炎症性肠病、脊柱关节炎家族史、C 反应蛋白（CRP）水平升高、HLA-B27、前驱胃肠道或泌尿生殖系统感染以及 X 线、计算机断层成像（CT）或磁共振成像（MRI）显示的骶髂关节炎。

将脊柱关节炎与其他炎症性或退行性关节或脊柱疾病区分开来具有一定挑战性。晶体性关节病可表现为外周寡关节炎，通常发生在下肢。但脊柱很少受累，且滑液中可检测出细胞内结晶。类风湿关节炎和其他系统性自身免疫性疾病通常表现为上下肢对称性多关节炎，并伴有血清学异常，如类风湿因子、抗环瓜氨酸肽（CCP）抗体或抗核抗体。以中轴受累为主的脊柱关节炎必须与骶髂关节、椎体或椎间盘内的惰性感染，脊柱和椎间盘的退行性疾病（即脊柱病）以及弥漫性特发性骨肥厚（DISH）相鉴别。

脊柱关节炎的放射学特征具有高度特异性，在正确的临床背景下，可大大提高诊断准确度。骶髂关节炎通常是脊柱病变最早的影像学表现，会导致骶髂关节硬化和侵蚀，最终骨性融合（图 3.2A）。慢性脊柱炎会导致许多影像学改变，包括纤维环骨化、脊柱韧带钙化、椎体骨质硬化和方形变以及关节突关节强直。这些变化可导致椎体融合和竹节状脊柱（图 3.2B）。

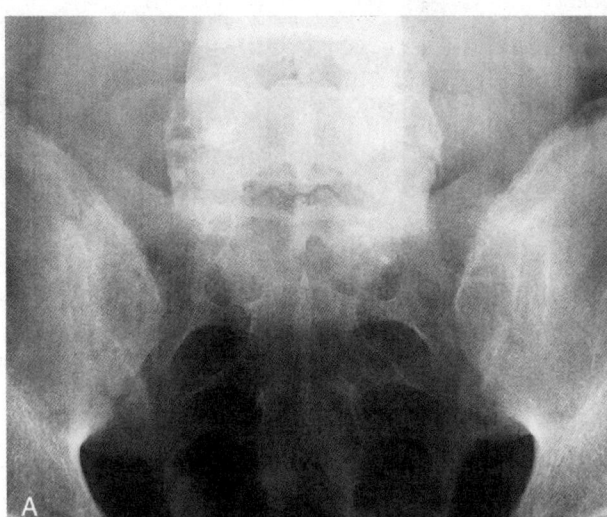
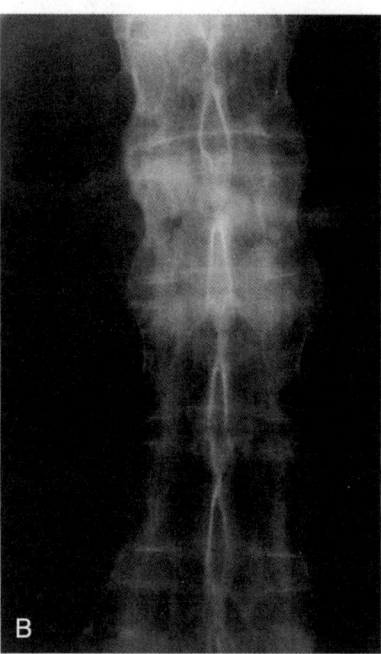

Fig. 3.2 (A) Bilaterally symmetrical sacroiliitis in ankylosing spondylitis. (B) Lumbar spondylitis in ankylosing spondylitis with symmetrical, marginal bridging syndesmophytes and calcification of the spinal ligament. (From Cush JJ, Lipsky PE: The spondyloarthropathies. In Goldman L, Bennett JC, editors: Cecil textbook of medicine, ed 21, Philadelphia, 2000, Saunders, pp 1499-1507.)

Radiographic findings progress over many years of illness and may not be apparent in early disease. However, during this preradiographic period, MRI demonstrates bone inflammation (i.e., osteitis) and erosion at the sacroiliac joints and vertebral bodies, and CT shows bony sclerosis and joint erosions.

Bone erosions, sclerosis, and new bone formation may occur at sites of enthesitis. Erosions at bone-cartilage interface (i.e., subchondral erosions), sclerosis, and bone proliferation are hallmarks of spondyloarthritis involving peripheral joints. In severe cases such as the arthritis mutilans form of psoriatic arthritis, total or subtotal bone resorption (i.e., osteolysis) of a phalange may occur.

TREATMENT

No cure has been found for any form of spondyloarthritis, but effective treatment for many of the manifestations is available. Patient education regarding the disease is essential and allows identification of affected family members and early detection of urgent clinical features such as uveitis. Physical therapy, including a daily stretching program, postural adjustments, and strengthening, helps to maintain proper bony alignment, reduce deformities, and maximize function, particularly for those with axial disease. Selective use of orthopedic surgery may be highly effective in correcting significant spinal deformities or instability.

Nonsteroidal anti-inflammatory drugs (NSAIDs) can provide significant relief of spinal pain and stiffness, and many patients take these drugs continually for years. No clear evidence indicates that systemic glucocorticoids benefit patients with spondyloarthritis, and these agents are usually avoided. Intra-articular glucocorticoid injection into the sacroiliac or other involved joints may provide temporary relief. Similarly, the role and efficacy of older immunosuppressive agents in the treatment of axial spondyloarthritis have not been established. In contrast, clinical trials have shown that the peripheral manifestations of spondylarthritis improve with sulfasalazine and methotrexate. Apremilast, a phosphodiesterase-4 inhibitor, has shown efficacy in peripheral joint inflammation in patients with psoriatic arthritis.

TNF-α blockers (i.e., infliximab, etanercept, adalimumab, certolizumab, and golimumab) represent a substantial breakthrough in the treatment of spondyloarthritis. The efficacy of these agents is well established for patients with axial inflammation who do not satisfactorily or fully respond to NSAIDs and physical therapy. TNF-α blockers can significantly reduce pain, improve function, and improve quality of life. They may also prevent or slow disease progression and structural damage. The drugs are effective in psoriatic arthritis, suppress the skin and nail disease of psoriasis, and retard radiographic progression in the peripheral joints. Infliximab and adalimumab reduce gut inflammation in ulcerative colitis and Crohn's disease, with concomitant reduction in symptoms of joint and spine inflammation. Ustekinumab, an inhibitor of IL-23, has demonstrated efficacy in psoriasis and psoriatic arthritis, as well as the intestinal manifestations of IBD. Secukinumab and ixekizumab, IL-17 inhibitors, have clinical efficacy in psoriasis, peripheral and axial spondyloarthritis.

Flares of uveitis require care by an ophthalmologist experienced in treating inflammatory eye diseases. Topical or intraocular glucocorticoids may suffice, but systemic therapy with glucocorticoids or immunosuppressive medications may be necessary to control the inflammation and prevent permanent visual loss. Methotrexate is frequently employed and the TNF-α inhibitor adalimumab has proven efficacy.

Reactive arthritis is usually self-limited, and joint symptoms are managed with NSAIDs or intra-articular corticosteroid injections. When chronic arthritis or spondylitis develops, interventions are similar to those employed for other forms of spondyloarthritis. Evaluation and treatment of *C. trachomatis* and associated sexually transmitted diseases in patients with reactive arthritis and their sex partners are essential. Early treatment reduces the frequency of reactive arthritis.

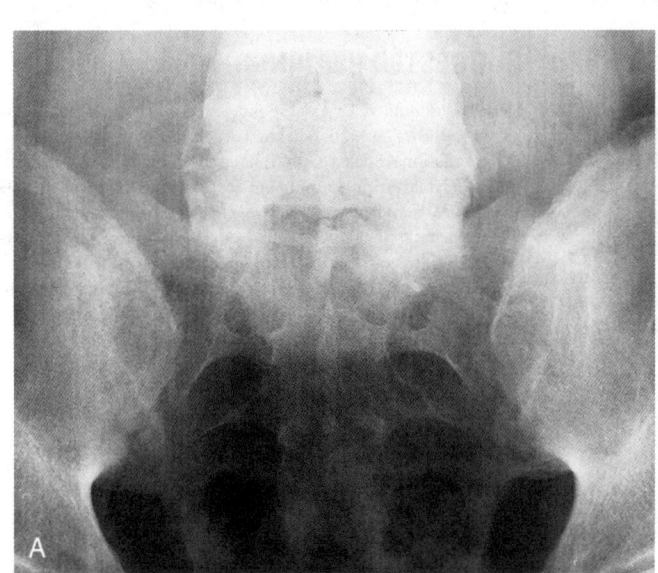
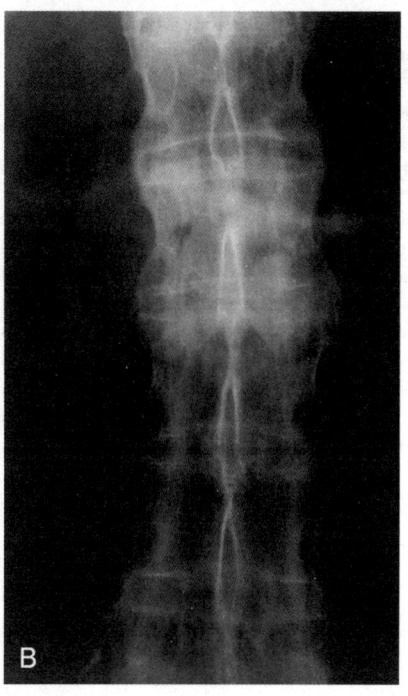

图 3.2 （A）强直性脊柱炎双侧对称性骶髂关节炎。（B）强直性脊柱炎的腰椎炎，表现为对称性边缘骨桥形成和脊柱韧带钙化（引自 Cush JJ, Lipsky PE: The spondyloarthropathies. In Goldman L, Bennett JC, editors: Cecil textbook of medicine, ed 21, Philadelphia, 2000, Saunders, pp 1499-1507.）

放射学改变在患病多年后才会出现，疾病早期可能并不明显。不过，在放射学改变前这一阶段，MRI可显示骶髂关节及椎体的骨骼炎症（即骨炎）和侵蚀，CT可显示骨质硬化和关节侵蚀。

骨侵蚀、硬化和新骨形成可发生在附着点炎部位。骨-软骨界面的侵蚀（即软骨下侵蚀）、硬化和骨质增生是脊柱关节炎累及外周关节的特征。在严重的病例中，例如银屑病关节炎中的毁损型关节炎，可能会出现趾骨全部或部分骨质吸收（即骨溶解）。

治疗

脊柱关节炎目前尚无根治方法，但许多临床症状都可以得到有效治疗。对患者进行疾病教育至关重要，这样可以识别受影响的家庭成员并及早发现葡萄膜炎等紧急临床症状。物理疗法包括日常伸展计划、姿势调整和力量训练，有助于保持正确的骨骼姿态、减少畸形，并最大限度地改善功能，对中轴受累的患者尤为重要。有选择性地进行矫形外科手术可以非常有效地矫正严重的脊柱畸形或不稳定。

非甾体抗炎药（NSAID）可以明显缓解脊柱疼痛及僵硬，许多患者多年持续服用这类药物。没有明确证据表明全身使用糖皮质激素对脊柱关节炎患者有益，因此通常避免使用这类药物。在骶髂关节或其他受累关节内注射糖皮质激素可暂时缓解症状。同样，传统免疫抑制剂在治疗中轴脊柱关节炎中的作用和疗效也尚未确定。但是，临床试验表明柳氮磺吡啶和甲氨蝶呤可改善脊柱关节炎的外周表现。磷酸二酯酶-4抑制剂阿普斯特对银屑病关节炎患者的外周关节炎有效。

TNF-α阻滞剂（即英夫利昔单抗、依那西普、阿达木单抗、培塞利珠单抗和戈利木单抗）在治疗脊柱关节炎方面取得了重大突破。对于NSAID和物理疗法效果不佳或完全无效的中轴炎症患者，这些药物的疗效已得到充分肯定。TNF-α阻滞剂可明显减轻疼痛、改善功能、提高生活质量，还能预防或减缓疾病的进展和结构性损害。这些药物对银屑病关节炎有效，能同时抑制银屑病的皮肤和指甲病变，并能延缓外周关节的影像学进展。英夫利昔单抗和阿达木单抗能减轻溃疡性结肠炎和克罗恩病的肠道炎症，同时减轻关节和脊柱的炎症症状。IL-23抑制剂乌司奴单抗对银屑病和银屑病关节炎以及IBD的肠道表现均有效。IL-17抑制剂司库奇尤单抗和依奇珠单抗对银屑病、外周和中轴脊柱关节炎均有临床疗效。

葡萄膜炎发作时需要由治疗炎症性眼病经验丰富的眼科医生进行治疗。局部或眼内使用糖皮质激素可能就足以缓解症状，但可能需要全身使用糖皮质激素或免疫抑制剂进行治疗，以控制炎症并防止永久性视力丧失。甲氨蝶呤是常用药物，TNF-α抑制剂阿达木单抗的疗效也已得到证实。

反应性关节炎通常是自限性的，关节症状可通过NSAID或关节内注射糖皮质激素得到控制。当出现慢性关节炎或脊柱炎时，干预措施与其他形式的脊柱关节炎类似。对反应性关节炎患者及其性伴侣进行沙眼衣原体及相关性传播疾病的评估和治疗至关重要。早

Long-term antibiotics are ineffective for gastroenteritis-associated reactive arthritis. Clinical trials of long-term antibiotics for reactive arthritis after *C. trachomatis* infection have had mixed results, and this practice requires further study before it can be adopted.

SUMMARY

Disability due to spondyloarthritis varies according to the subtype and severity of the specific syndrome. Historically, patients with spondyloarthritis usually experienced a lesser degree of disability compared with those with rheumatoid arthritis. Some patients with reactive arthritis experience self-limited disease with no long-term sequelae. Alternatively, those with more severe disease can have deformation and destruction of the axial and peripheral joints, leading to severe disability. Serious and potentially fatal extraskeletal manifestations can manifest.

With the advent of effective immunosuppressant medications such as methotrexate and biologic agents (i.e., TNF-α, IL-17 and IL-23 inhibitors), patients with more severe manifestations have markedly improved symptom control and quality of life.

SUGGESTED READINGS

Sieper J, Poddubnyy D: Axial spondyloarthritis, Lancet, 390:73–84, 2017.

Sieper J, Rudwaleit M, Baraliakos X, et al: The Assessment of Spondyloarthritis international Society (ASAS) handbook: a guide to assess spondyloarthritis, Ann Rheum Dis 68(Suppl lII):ii1–ii44, 2009.

Ward MW, Deodhar A, Gensler LS, et al: 2019 update of the American College of Rheumatology/Spondylitis Association of America/Spondylitis Research and Treatment Network recommendations for the treatment of ankylosing spondylitis and nonradiographic axial spondyloarthritis, Arthritis Rheumatol vol. 71(No. 10):1599–1613, 2019.

期治疗可降低反应性关节炎的发作频次。长期使用抗生素对胃肠炎相关反应性关节炎无效，而其治疗沙眼衣原体感染后反应性关节炎的临床试验结果不一，因此这种治疗方法的应用有待进一步研究。

总结

脊柱关节炎导致的残疾因具体亚型和严重程度而异。目前来看，脊柱关节炎患者的残疾程度通常低于类风湿关节炎患者。部分反应性关节炎患者的病情具有自限性，不会留下长期后遗症。而病情较重的患者会出现中轴和外周关节的变形和破坏，导致严重残疾。该疾病还可能出现严重的可能致命的骨骼外表现。

随着甲氨蝶呤等有效免疫抑制剂和生物制剂（即TNF-α、IL-17和IL-23抑制剂）的出现，病情较重患者的症状控制和生活质量都得到了明显提升。

推荐阅读

Sieper J, Poddubnyy D: Axial spondyloarthritis, Lancet, 390:73–84, 2017.

Sieper J, Rudwaleit M, Baraliakos X, et al: The Assessment of Spondyloarthritis international Society (ASAS) handbook: a guide to assess spondyloarthritis, Ann Rheum Dis 68(Suppl lII):ii1–ii44, 2009.

Ward MW, Deodhar A, Gensler LS, et al: 2019 update of the American College of Rheumatology/Spondylitis Association of America/Spondylitis Research and Treatment Network recommendations for the treatment of ankylosing spondylitis and nonradiographic axial spondyloarthritis, Arthritis Rheumatol vol. 71(No. 10):1599–1613, 2019.

Systemic Lupus Erythematosus

Sonia Manocha, Tanmayee Bichile, Susan Manzi

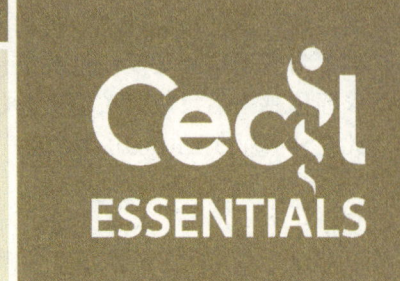

DEFINITION AND EPIDEMIOLOGY

Systemic lupus erythematosus (SLE) is a chronic multisystem autoimmune disease characterized by autoantibody production and immune complex deposition that can lead to organ inflammation and, if left untreated, organ damage. The cause of SLE is largely unknown. Clinical manifestations are heterogeneous, ranging from milder non-organ-threatening symptoms of fatigue or oral ulcerations to life-threatening organ involvement with nephritis and neurologic disease. Diagnosing SLE is often challenging due to its varied clinical presentation, and it can take up to several years and seeing multiple health care providers to accurately come to a diagnosis.

Incidence and Prevalence

New data regarding the incidence and prevalence of SLE in the United States have been derived from several lupus registries including Michigan, Georgia, California Lupus Surveillance Project (CLSP), Manhattan Lupus Surveillance Program (MLSP), CDC funded population-based registry, Minnesota, and a large national managed-care claims database. These lupus registries allowed for a comprehensive estimation of incidence and prevalence across various ethnicities, including African American, Caucasian, Alaskan Native/American Indian, Hispanic, and Asian populations.

There remains a female predominance in both incidence and prevalence of SLE. Overall, the incidence and prevalence of SLE ranges from 5.2 to 7.4 cases per 100,000 person years and 72.8 to 178 cases per 100,000 person years, respectively. There remains ethnic diversity with a higher incidence of SLE among non-white ethnic populations, with African Americans having the highest incidence and prevalence followed by Hispanic and Asian individuals.

During childbearing years, the female-to-male ratio of SLE prevalence is 10:1 to 15:1. This gender discrepancy also exists but is less distinct (2:1) in young children and older individuals, suggesting hormonal influences.

Mortality

Mortality rates due to SLE have waxed and waned over time. Initially, there was a decrease in mortality from 1968 to 1975 followed by a steady increase from 1975 to 1999. This increase was followed by a steady decrease in mortality after 1999. However, despite this sustained decrease, SLE mortality remains high compared with those without SLE. SLE mortality has a bimodal distribution, with infection and disease activity typically increasing mortality earlier in the course of disease and cardiovascular and renal disease increasing mortality later in the course of disease. Furthermore, a study of all-cause mortality utilizing Medicaid data found ethnic variability in SLE-related mortality showing Asians and Hispanics having lower mortality as compared with African Americans, Caucasians or Native Americans.

PATHOLOGY

Although SLE pathogenesis remains poorly understood, individuals who develop SLE likely have a genetic predisposition in the setting of immune system dysregulation, environmental triggers, and altered hormonal milieu. The genetic contribution to SLE is emphasized by the high concordance rate for monozygotic twins (>20%) and a lower concordance rate among other siblings (<5%). The search for genes involved in SLE pathogenesis is an active area of research. Genes coding for certain human leukocyte antigens, complement system components, immunoglobulin receptors, and various other proteins are being considered as candidate genes for SLE.

The many immune abnormalities in SLE implicate dysregulation of the humoral and cellular immune systems in the pathogenesis of the disease. Dysregulation leads to loss of self-tolerance and autoimmune destruction of healthy tissues, hallmarked by the production of autoantibodies and immune complexes. The heterogeneity of clinical manifestations of lupus and response to treatment is likely a result of the different genetic and molecular profiles of individual patients. This has led to the notion of lupus as a spectrum disorder that includes distinct phenotypes that require customized management strategies.

Various environmental triggers, including microorganisms and ultraviolet light exposure, may influence the development of SLE and lupus activity. The striking differences in SLE prevalence between genders and the effect of pregnancy on disease activity suggest a role for hormones in SLE pathogenesis.

CLINICAL PRESENTATION

SLE can affect virtually any organ system. Typically, patients experience fluctuating periods of increased disease activity, known as flares, alternating with periods of clinical quiescence. The frequency, intensity, and duration of flares are highly variable among patients, and when left untreated, may lead to irreversible organ damage.

A challenge with establishing a diagnosis of SLE has been to accurately estimate the onset of disease. Patients with SLE often have antibody positivity for many years prior to the onset of clinical symptoms. The type and severity of chief complaint in SLE depends on underlying organ involvement at the time of presentation, varying from vague constitutional symptoms to specific organ involvement such as seizures, glomerulonephritis, serositis, and thrombosis. In one study by Cervera and colleagues, most manifestations of SLE occurred in the first 5 years. Long-term prognosis in SLE varies greatly depending on whether patients are diagnosed early or late.

Constitutional Symptoms

Constitutional symptoms of SLE include fever, lymphadenopathy, weight loss, malaise, and fatigue. These are nonspecific and can be

系统性红斑狼疮

黄璨 赵萌萌 译 赵久良 杨娉婷 审校 李梦涛 通审

定义和流行病学

系统性红斑狼疮（SLE）是一种以自身抗体产生及免疫复合物沉积并导致脏器炎症反应为主要特征的慢性多系统受累的自身免疫性疾病，如不及时治疗，可造成器官损害。其临床表现多种多样，轻症患者可仅表现为疲劳或口腔溃疡，重症患者可出现肾炎或中枢神经系统病变等危及生命的器官受累。SLE 的诊断具有挑战性，可能需要几年或多次诊疗才能做出准确判断。

发病率和患病率

有关美国 SLE 发病率和患病率的新数据主要来自多个 SLE 登记注册研究队列，包括密歇根州、佐治亚州、加利福尼亚州 SLE 监测项目（CLSP）、曼哈顿 SLE 监测项目（MLSP）、美国疾病预防控制中心（CDC）资助的基于人群的登记注册研究队列，明尼苏达州以及全国医疗索赔数据库。通过这些 SLE 登记注册研究，可以全面估算不同种族中 SLE 的发病率和患病率，包括非裔美国人、高加索人、阿拉斯加原住民/美洲印第安人、西班牙裔和亚裔人群。

SLE 的发病率和患病率中，女性占主导地位。总体而言，SLE 的发病率和患病率分别为每 10 万人年 5.2～7.4 例，和每 10 万人年 72.8～178 例。在非白色人种中，SLE 的发病率较高，非裔美国人的发病率和患病率最高，其次是西班牙裔和亚裔。

育龄期 SLE 发病率的女男比例为 10∶1 到 15∶1，尽管这种性别差异在幼儿和老年人中也存在，但没有如此明显（2∶1），这表明性激素可能影响 SLE 发病。

死亡率

SLE 死亡率随时代而变迁。1968—1975 年间死亡率有所下降，1975—1999 年间持续上升，1999 年后持续下降，但 SLE 患者的死亡率仍高于非 SLE 患者。SLE 的死亡呈双峰分布，感染和疾病活动在病程早期增加死亡率，心血管疾病和肾脏疾病在病程晚期增加死亡率。此外，一项利用医疗补助系统（Medicaid）数据进行的全因死亡率研究发现，SLE 死亡率存在种族差异，相比于非裔美国人、高加索人或美国原住民，亚裔和西班牙裔的死亡率更低。

病理学

尽管对 SLE 发病机制仍知之甚少，但除了免疫系统失调、环境诱因和性激素水平改变等因素外，SLE 还具有遗传易感性。单卵双生子的 SLE 发病一致性较高（>20%），而其他同胞兄弟姐妹的一致性较低（<5%），进一步证实了 SLE 的遗传性。近年来，探讨与 SLE 发病机制有关基因的研究非常活跃。SLE 的候选基因包括编码某些人类白细胞抗原、补体系统成分、免疫球蛋白受体和其他相关蛋白的候选基因等。

SLE 许多免疫异常现象表明，体液免疫和细胞免疫系统的失调与发病有关。免疫失调会导致自身耐受性的丧失和健康组织的自身免疫性破坏，最终产生自身抗体和免疫复合物。SLE 临床表现和治疗反应具有明显的异质性，很可能由于不同 SLE 患者的基因和分子特征各不相同。

微生物和紫外线照射等各种环境诱因也会参与 SLE 发病和复发。不同性别间 SLE 发病率的显著差异以及妊娠对疾病活动性的影响，都表明性激素在 SLE 发病机制中的作用。

临床表现

SLE 可累及全身各器官。患者会经历疾病活动期（称为复发）与临床静止期的交替。SLE 复发的频率、强度和持续时间差异很大，如不及时治疗可导致不可逆转的器官损伤。

准确估计 SLE 发病时间一直是诊断 SLE 的一个难题。SLE 患者往往在出现临床症状前多年已出现自身抗体。SLE 主诉的类型和严重程度取决于发病时潜在的器官受累情况，从非特异的全身症状，到特定的器官受累，如癫痫发作、肾小球肾炎、浆膜炎和血栓形成。在 Cervera 及其同事的一项研究中显示，大多数 SLE 的表现发生在起病的前 5 年。SLE 长期预后因确诊早晚而有很大差异。

全身症状

SLE 全身症状包括发热、淋巴结肿大、体重减轻、乏力和疲劳。这些症状都是非特异的，可能与其他病

related to other etiologies, and it is therefore imperative to be cognizant of infection in a patient with SLE presenting with fever. One way to distinguish a fever caused by infection versus a fever from SLE would be to evaluate serologic activity from lupus, especially complement levels, which are often elevated in the setting of infection because they are acute-phase reactants and decreased in the setting of active lupus.

Lymphadenopathy in lupus is often cervical and axillary and generally painful, soft, and mobile. Weight loss in SLE indicates an ongoing inflammatory state. Malaise and fatigue are among the most common but often difficult to treat presentations of SLE.

Mucocutaneous Manifestations

Skin manifestations of SLE are wide ranging and divided into categories including acute cutaneous lupus, subacute cutaneous lupus, and chronic cutaneous lupus. Acute cutaneous lupus includes a wide range of presentations. Many patients will present with a malar rash described as a butterfly rash with erythema and crusting that spares the nasolabial folds. Other presentations may include maculopapular rash, urticaria, bullous lupus and a toxic epidermal necrolysis (TEN)-like rash.

Subacute cutaneous lupus erythematosus (SCLE) typically presents as a psoriasiform or annular, polycyclic rash.

Chronic cutaneous lupus can cause disfiguration and scarring, with the most common form being discoid lupus. Other forms include lupus panniculitis (which is an inflammatory involvement of the subcutis and fat), tumid lupus, chilblains, lichen planus overlap, and mucosal lesions (oral, nasal, genital).

The majority of these rashes are photosensitive, which is an exaggerated response to ultraviolet (UV) light leading to symptoms of redness, itching or burning. Typically, skin manifestations of SLE occur within 24 to 48 hours after UV exposure.

Oral ulcerations occur in approximately 45% of SLE patients. Those involving the hard palate and buccal mucosa are more commonly associated with SLE. It is important to keep in mind that oral ulcers may also be seen in multiple other comorbid conditions such as acid reflux as well as herpetic infections.

Nonscarring alopecia involving the temporal area or diffuse thinning is another common cutaneous manifestation.

Musculoskeletal Manifestations

Arthritis is common in SLE. Usually this is an inflammatory, nonerosive arthritis. Some patients may develop deformities referred to as Jaccoud arthropathy. The hand in a patient with Jaccoud arthropathy looks similar to someone with rheumatoid arthritis except that the deformities are reducible (manually corrected) as opposed to fixed and imaging demonstrates absence of erosions.

Myalgia is another common manifestation of SLE, especially during periods of flares. Muscle weakness along with elevated CPK levels should raise suspicion of an underlying myopathy/myositis.

Hematologic Manifestations

Leukopenia (defined as white blood cell [WBC] count <4000 cells/mL), primarily lymphopenia, anemia, and thrombocytopenia, is common in SLE. Coombs positive autoimmune hemolytic anemia (AIHA) is one of the criteria for classification of SLE. Thrombocytopenia, which is an immune-mediated peripheral destruction disorder, may also be seen. Evans syndrome is rare in SLE and defined as AIHA and autoimmune thrombocytopenia. Thrombotic thrombocytopenic purpura (TTP) is also reported in SLE.

Cardiopulmonary Manifestations

Cardiac involvement in SLE is manifold. SLE can affect all parts of the cardiac system including the endocardium, myocardium, pericardium, valves, conduction pathways, and the coronary arteries. Pericarditis is the most common of cardiac manifestations in SLE. Myocarditis is rare but can be fatal. Libman-Sacks endocarditis is valvular involvement in SLE described as sterile verrucous lesions typically seen on the left-sided heart valves. Cardiovascular disease in SLE is discussed separately.

Pulmonary manifestations in SLE can involve the pleura, parenchyma, and pulmonary vessels. Pleural involvement typically occurs with pleurisy and pleural effusions. Parenchymal involvement can present as acute lupus pneumonitis, interstitial lung disease, diffuse alveolar hemorrhage, and shrinking lung syndrome. Pulmonary vessel involvement typically presents as a pulmonary embolus often in the presence of antiphospholipid antibodies and pulmonary artery hypertension.

Gastrointestinal and Hepatic Manifestations

Gastrointestinal (GI) manifestations may be seen in about 50% of patients with SLE and are often difficult to diagnose. GI manifestations are often mild but may be life-threatening. Although acute abdominal pain in SLE is more commonly attributed to non-SLE etiologies, SLE-related causes of acute abdominal pain include pancreatitis, serositis, mesenteric vasculitis, and renal vein thrombosis. Lupus hepatitis is a controversial diagnosis. This has been described in the literature in SLE patients presenting with constitutional symptoms and elevated liver enzymes five times or greater the upper limit of normal. SLE patients with persistent elevations of LFTs without other symptoms should be further evaluated for autoimmune hepatitis (AIH) because this may be seen in association.

Renal Manifestations

Nephritis, which manifests with hematuria and proteinuria, is a major cause of morbidity and mortality for SLE patients. The International Society of Nephrology/Renal Pathology Society (ISN/RPS) revisited the 1982 World Health Organization classification of lupus nephritis (classes I through VI). ISN/RPS class IV (i.e., diffuse, proliferative) lupus nephritis is the most common form and has the worst prognosis, but it is also the most amenable to aggressive immunosuppressive therapy. See Table 4.1 for more details.

Neuropsychiatric Manifestations

Neuropsychiatric manifestations of systemic lupus erythematosus (NPSLE) can vary from mild to severe and may be difficult to diagnose. NPSLE may involve any area of the nervous system with diffuse or focal involvement of the central nervous system (CNS) as well as involvement of the peripheral nervous system (PNS). Diffuse involvement may manifest as cognitive dysfunction, acute confusional state, headache, aseptic meningitis, and mood disorders. Focal involvement may present as cerebrovascular disease, myelopathy, movement disorders, demyelinating syndromes, and seizures.

Vascular Manifestations

More than 40% of SLE patients have Raynaud's phenomenon. This is typically described as cold sensitivity followed by biphasic or triphasic color changes with white discoloration followed by cyanosis and reactive hyperemia in the digits of hands and feet. Other areas affected by Raynaud's phenomenon include nose, earlobes, lips, and nipples.

Livedo reticularis is a netlike discoloration over arms or legs commonly seen in SLE. Livedo racemosa, which is a more severe form of livedo reticularis, can be seen in patients with SLE and Sneddon syndrome (ischemic cerebrovascular disease along with antiphospholipid antibodies [APLs]).

因有关。SLE 患者出现发热必须警惕感染。区分感染性发热和 SLE 发热的一种方法是评估血清学活动性，尤其是补体水平，由于补体是急性期反应物，在感染时通常会升高，而 SLE 活动时会降低。

SLE 淋巴结肿大常累及颈部和腋窝淋巴结，常疼痛、质软、可移动。体重下降表明炎症状态仍在持续。乏力和疲倦是 SLE 最常见的症状，但治疗往往困难。

皮肤黏膜受累

SLE 皮肤表现多种多样，分为急性皮肤狼疮、亚急性皮肤狼疮和慢性皮肤狼疮。急性皮肤狼疮（ACLE）有多种表现。其中蝶形红斑表现为横跨鼻梁、覆盖双颊，而不累及鼻唇沟的蝶形皮疹，伴有红斑和结痂。其他表现还包括斑丘疹、荨麻疹、大疱性狼疮和中毒性表皮坏死松解（TEN）样皮疹。

亚急性皮肤型红斑狼疮（SCLE）通常表现为丘疹鳞屑性或环形、多环形皮疹。

慢性皮肤狼疮（CCLE）可导致瘢痕形成，最常见的是盘状红斑。其他表现还包括狼疮性脂膜炎（皮下组织和脂肪的炎症）、肿胀性红斑狼疮、冻疮样皮疹、苔藓样皮肤型重叠综合征和黏膜病变（口腔、鼻腔、生殖器）。

这些皮疹大多是光敏性的，是一种对紫外线（UV）的过敏反应，导致发红、瘙痒或灼痛等症状。SLE 皮肤表现一般会在紫外线照射后 24～48 h 内出现。

大约 45% 的 SLE 患者会出现口腔溃疡。硬腭和颊黏膜溃疡更常见。但口腔溃疡也可见于多种其他合并症，如胃酸反流和疱疹病毒感染。

累及颞部的非瘢痕性脱发或弥漫性头发稀疏是另一种常见的皮肤表现。

骨骼肌肉受累

关节炎在 SLE 中很常见，通常是炎性、非侵蚀性关节炎。有些患者会出现 Jaccoud 关节病，表现为手部关节畸形，看似类风湿关节炎，但其畸形可手动复位而非固定，在影像学上没有骨侵蚀。

肌痛是 SLE 另一种常见表现，尤其是病情活动期。对存在肌无力和肌酸激酶水平升高的患者，应警惕潜在肌病/肌炎。

血液系统受累

白细胞减少［定义为白细胞（WBC）计数小于 4000/ml］，主要是淋巴细胞减少，贫血和血小板减少，在 SLE 中很常见。Coombs 试验阳性的自身免疫性溶血性贫血（AIHA）是 SLE 的分类标准之一；也可见血小板减少，是由于免疫介导的外周破坏。伊文思（Evans）综合征在 SLE 中很罕见，即 AIHA 合并自身免疫性血小板减少。在 SLE 中也有血栓性血小板减少性紫癜（TTP）的报道。

呼吸心脏受累

SLE 可影响心脏系统的所有部位，包括心内膜、心肌、心包、瓣膜、传导系统和冠状动脉。心包炎是 SLE 最常见的心脏表现。心肌炎很少见却致命。利布曼-塞克斯（Libman-Sacks）心内膜炎是 SLE 相关瓣膜损害，表现为无菌性疣状病变，通常见于左心瓣膜。SLE 的心血管疾病将单独讨论。

SLE 肺部受累部位包括胸膜、肺实质和肺血管。胸膜受累通常表现为胸膜炎和胸腔积液。肺实质受累可表现为急性狼疮性肺炎、间质性肺病、弥漫性肺泡出血和萎缩肺综合征。肺血管受累通常表现为肺栓塞［常与抗磷脂抗体（APL）阳性相关］和肺动脉高压。

消化系统受累

大约 50% 的 SLE 患者会出现胃肠道（GI）受累，但通常诊断困难。胃肠道受累通常较轻，但也可能危及生命。与 SLE 相关的急性腹痛病因包括胰腺炎、腹膜炎、肠系膜血管炎和肾静脉血栓形成，但 SLE 患者的急性腹痛更常见于非 SLE 病因，需注意排查。狼疮性肝炎是一种存在争议的诊断。文献中描述过 SLE 患者出现全身症状合并正常上限 5 倍以上的肝酶升高。如 SLE 患者肝酶持续升高而无其他表现，则应进一步评估合并自身免疫性肝炎（AIH）的可能性。

肾受累

肾炎表现为血尿和蛋白尿，是 SLE 患者致残和致死的主要原因。国际肾脏病学会/肾脏病理学学会（ISN/RPS）修订了 1982 年世界卫生组织对狼疮性肾炎的分类（Ⅰ至Ⅵ型）。ISN/RPS Ⅳ型（即弥漫增生性）狼疮性肾炎是最常见的类型，预后最差，常需要最积极的免疫抑制治疗，详见表 4.1。

神经精神系统受累

SLE 神经精神表现（NPSLE）有轻有重，有时诊断困难。NPSLE 可累及神经系统的任何部位，中枢神经系统（CNS）受累可出现弥漫性或局灶性病变，周围神经系统（PNS）也可受累。弥漫性病变可表现为认知障碍、急性意识混乱状态、头痛、无菌性脑膜炎和情绪障碍。局灶性病变可表现为脑血管疾病、脊髓病、运动障碍、脱髓鞘性疾病和癫痫发作。

血管受累

40% 以上 SLE 患者有雷诺现象，指寒冷刺激后的指/趾端颜色变化，经典表现为先变白，再变紫，然后转为红色。其他易受累的部位还包括鼻子、耳垂、嘴唇和乳头。

网状青斑是 SLE 患者手臂或腿部常见皮肤表现。葡萄状青斑是一种更严重的网状青斑，可见于 SLE 和 Sneddon 综合征［伴有抗磷脂抗体（APL）阳性的缺血性脑血管疾病］患者。

TABLE 4.1 International Society of Nephrology/Renal Pathology Society (ISN/RPS) 2003 Classification of Lupus Nephritis

Class I	**Minimal mesangial lupus nephritis**
	Normal glomeruli by light microscopy, but mesangial immune deposits by immunofluorescence
Class II	**Mesangial proliferative lupus nephritis**
	Purely mesangial hypercellularity of any degree or mesangial matrix expansion by light microscopy, with mesangial immune deposits
	May be a few isolated subepithelial or subendothelial deposits visible by immunofluorescence or electron microscopy, but not by light microscopy
Class III	**Focal lupus nephritis**[a]
	Active or inactive focal, segmental or global endo- or extracapillary glomerulonephritis involving 50% of all glomeruli, typically with focal subendothelial immune deposits, with or without mesangial alterations
Class III (A)	Active lesions: focal proliferative lupus nephritis
Class III (A/C)	Active and chronic lesions: focal proliferative and sclerosing lupus nephritis
Class III (C)	Chronic inactive lesions with glomerular scars: focal sclerosing lupus nephritis
Class IV	**Diffuse lupus nephritis**[b]
	Active or inactive diffuse, segmental or global endo- or extracapillary glomerulonephritis involving 50% of all glomeruli, typically with diffuse subendothelial immune deposits, with or without mesangial alterations. This class is divided into diffuse segmental (IV-S) lupus nephritis when 50% of the involved glomeruli have segmental lesions, and diffuse global (IV-G) lupus nephritis when 50% of the involved glomeruli have global lesions. Segmental is defined as a glomerular lesion that involves less than half of the glomerular tuft. This class includes cases with diffuse wire loop deposits but with little or no glomerular proliferation.
Class IV-S (A)	Active lesions: diffuse segmental proliferative lupus nephritis
Class IV-G (A)	Active lesions: diffuse global proliferative lupus nephritis
Class IV-S (A/C)	Active and chronic lesions: diffuse segmental proliferative and sclerosing lupus nephritis
Class IV-G (A/C)	Active and chronic lesions: diffuse global proliferative and sclerosing lupus nephritis
Class IV-S (C)	Chronic inactive lesions with scars: diffuse segmental sclerosing lupus nephritis
Class IV-G (C)	Chronic inactive lesions with scars: diffuse global sclerosing lupus nephritis
Class V	**Membranous lupus nephritis**
	Global or segmental subepithelial immune deposits or their morphologic sequelae by light microscopy and by immunofluorescence or electron microscopy, with or without mesangial alterations
	Class V lupus nephritis may occur in combination with class III or IV in which case both will be diagnosed
	Class V lupus nephritis show advanced sclerosis
Class VI	**Advanced sclerosis lupus nephritis**
	90% of glomeruli globally sclerosed without residual activity

[a]Indicate the proportion of glomeruli with active and with sclerotic lesions.
[b]Indicate the proportion of glomeruli with fibrinoid necrosis and/or cellular crescents. Indicate and grade (mild, moderate, severe) tubular atrophy, interstitial inflammation and fibrosis, severity of arteriosclerosis or other vascular lesions.
Data from Wallace D, Hahn BH: Pathogenesis of Lupus Nephritis. In Dubois' lupus erythematosus and related syndromes, ed 9, Philadelphia, 2019, Elsevier, pp 273.

Venous clots (e.g., pulmonary emboli, deep vein thrombosis) and arterial clots typically are seen in association with APLs and antiphospholipid syndrome. Leg ulcers, gangrene, thrombophlebitis, nail fold infarcts, cutaneous necrosis, and necrotizing purpura may also occur. Small vessel vasculopathy or vasculitis can be seen in lupus and may be a life-threatening manifestation.

Ocular Manifestations

Keratoconjunctivitis sicca from secondary Sjögren's syndrome is the most common ocular manifestation of SLE. Episcleritis, scleritis, uveitis, optic neuropathy, and retinal vasculitis can occur but are less frequent.

DIAGNOSIS AND DIFFERENTIAL DIAGNOSIS

SLE is a clinical diagnosis; no single test or feature is definitively diagnostic of the disease. SLE is typically suspected in patients presenting with clinical symptoms and exam findings suggesting a multisystem disease. Serologic testing is utilized to confirm the suspected diagnosis. It is important to note that many clinical manifestations and serologic tests that help to diagnose SLE can be seen in other diseases. For example, arthralgias, myalgias, fevers, and rash are common presentations in many viral diseases that may also have a positive ANA. Anti-double-stranded DNA (anti-dsDNA) antibodies are reported in patients with hepatitis B and hepatitis C. Low complement levels could occur in patients with chronic liver disease or inherited complement deficiencies. Malignancy (lymphoma and other hematologic malignancies, solid organ cancer) is an important differential diagnosis to consider in an elderly patient with constitutional symptoms, lymphadenopathy, rash, arthralgias, myalgias and positive ANA.

Classification Criteria

Classification Criteria for SLE were designed to group similar patients for the purposes of research. There are several classification criteria currently used for SLE. The American College of Rheumatology (ACR) classification criteria for SLE were updated in 1997. Patients are considered to have SLE if they meet 4 of 11 criteria (Table 4.2).

The Systemic Lupus International Collaborating Clinics (SLICC) classification criteria were developed in 2012 to improve clinical relevance and incorporate new knowledge into the definition of SLE immunopathogenesis. Under the SLICC criteria, patients are classified to have lupus if they meet four criteria including at least one clinical and

表 4.1 国际肾脏病学会/肾脏病理学学会（ISN/RPS）2003年狼疮性肾炎（LN）分型	
Ⅰ型	**轻微系膜性 LN** 光镜正常，免疫荧光可见系膜区免疫复合物沉积
Ⅱ型	**系膜增生性 LN** 光镜下可见不同程度的单纯系膜细胞增生或系膜基质扩增，有系膜区免疫沉积 免疫荧光或电镜下可见内皮下或上皮下免疫复合物的散在沉积，但光镜下没有
Ⅲ型	**局灶性 LN**[a] 活动性或非活动性的局灶性、节段性或球性血管内皮或血管外肾小球肾炎，累及 <50% 的肾小球，通常伴有局灶性内皮下免疫沉积，伴或不伴系膜改变
Ⅲ（A）型	活动性：局灶节段性增生
Ⅲ（A/C）型	混合性：局灶节段性增生和局灶节段性硬化
Ⅲ（C）型	慢性非活动性伴肾小球瘢痕：局灶节段性硬化
Ⅳ型	**弥漫性 LN**[b] 活动性或非活动性的弥漫性的节段性或球性血管内皮或血管外肾小球肾炎，≥50% 的肾小球受累，通常伴有弥漫性内皮下免疫沉积，伴或不伴系膜改变。可进一步分为两个亚型，弥漫节段性 LN（Ⅳ-S）是指有 ≥50% 的小球存在节段性病变，弥漫球性 LN（Ⅳ-G）是指 ≥50% 的小球存在球性病变。节段性是指 <50% 的肾小球血管丛受累。此型包括弥漫性"金属圈"样沉积，而无或少有小球增生改变
Ⅳ-S（A）型	活动性：弥漫节段性增生
Ⅳ-G（A）型	活动性：弥漫球性增生
Ⅳ-S（A/C）型	混合性：弥漫节段性增生和弥漫节段性硬化
Ⅳ-G（A/C）型	混合性：弥漫球性增生和弥漫球性硬化
Ⅳ-S（C）型	慢性非活动性伴肾小球瘢痕：弥漫节段性硬化
Ⅳ-G（C）型	慢性非活动性伴肾小球瘢痕：弥漫球性硬化
Ⅴ型	**膜性 LN** 光镜及免疫荧光或电镜下可见球性或节段性上皮下免疫沉积，伴或不伴系膜改变 Ⅴ型 LN 可与Ⅲ或Ⅳ型合并存在，应分别诊断 Ⅴ型 LN 可有硬化表现
Ⅵ型	**晚期硬化性 LN** ≥90% 的肾小球表现为球性硬化，且不伴残余的活动性病变

[a] 应描述活动性病变和硬化性病变的肾小球占比。
[b] 应描述有纤维素坏死和（或）细胞新月体的肾小球比例。应描述并分级肾小管萎缩、间质炎症和纤维化、动脉硬化或其他血管病变的严重程度（轻、中、重度）。
引自 Wallace D, Hahn BH: Pathogenesis of Lupus Nephritis. In Dubois' lupus erythematosus and related syndromes, ed 9, Philadelphia, 2019, Elsevier, pp 273.

静脉血栓（如肺栓塞、深静脉血栓）和动脉血栓通常与抗磷脂抗体和抗磷脂综合征有关。SLE 还可能出现腿部溃疡、坏疽、血栓性静脉炎、甲周梗死、皮肤坏死和坏死性紫癜；也可以出现小血管病变或血管炎，严重者可危及生命。

眼部受累

继发性干燥综合征引起的干燥性角结膜炎（角结膜干燥症）是 SLE 最常见的眼部表现。巩膜外层炎、巩膜炎、葡萄膜炎、视神经病变和视网膜血管炎也会发生，但较少见。

诊断和鉴别诊断

SLE 是一种临床诊断，没有任何一种检查或特征可以明确诊断该疾病。如患者的临床症状和检查结果提示多系统受累，则需警惕 SLE，并建议进一步完善血清学检测以确诊。值得注意的是，许多有助于诊断 SLE 的临床表现和血清学检查亦可出现在其他疾病。例如，关节痛、肌痛、发热和皮疹是病毒感染的常见表现，并可能出现 ANA 阳性。研究显示，乙型肝炎和丙型肝炎患者体内可存在抗双链 DNA（dsDNA）抗体。补体减低可能出现在慢性肝炎或遗传性补体缺乏症患者中。对有全身症状、淋巴结肿大、皮疹、关节痛、肌痛和 ANA 阳性的老年患者，恶性肿瘤（淋巴瘤和其他血液系统恶性肿瘤，以及实体瘤）是重要的鉴别诊断。

分类标准

SLE 分类标准的设立旨在将患者进行分类研究。目前有几个 SLE 的分类标准。美国风湿病学会（ACR）SLE 分类标准于 1997 年更新。如患者符合 11 项标准中的 4 项，则被认为患有 SLE（表 4.2）。

系统性红斑狼疮国际临床协作组（SLICC）分类标准于 2012 年制定，强调了临床特征，并更新了 SLE 免疫学异常的定义。根据 SLICC 标准，如患者符合 4 项

TABLE 4.2 1997 American College of Rheumatology Criteria for Classification of Systemic Lupus Erythematosus[a]

Criteria	Definitions
Malar rash	Fixed, flat or raised erythema is observed over the malar eminences, tending to spare the nasolabial folds.
Discoid rash	Erythematous, raised patches develop with adherent keratotic scaling and follicular plugging; atrophic scarring may occur in older lesions.
Photosensitivity	Rash occurs as a result of unusual reaction to sunlight, determined by patient history or physician observation.
Oral ulcers	Oral or nasopharyngeal ulceration, usually painless, is observed by the physician.
Arthritis	Nonerosive arthritis involves two or more peripheral joints, characterized by tenderness, swelling, or effusion.
Serositis	a. Pleuritis: convincing history of pleuritic pain exists or rub is heard by a physician or pleural effusion is in evidence, or b. Pericarditis: documented by electrocardiogram or rub or evidence of pericardial effusion.
Renal disorder	a. Persistent proteinuria is >0.5 g/day or scored >3+ if quantitation is not performed, or b. Cellular casts: may be red cell, hemoglobin, granular, tubular, or mixed.
Neurologic disorder	a. Seizures: occurs in the absence of offending drugs or known metabolic derangements (e.g., uremia, ketoacidosis, or electrolyte imbalance), or b. Psychosis: occurs in the absence of offending drugs or known metabolic derangements (e.g., uremia, ketoacidosis, electrolyte imbalance)
Hematologic disorder	a. Hemolytic anemia: develops with reticulocytosis, or b. Leukopenia: <4000/mm^3 is documented on two or more occasions, or c. Lymphopenia: <1500/mm^3 is documented on two or more occasions, or d. Thrombocytopenia: <100,000/mm^3 develops in the absence of offending drugs.
Immunologic disorder	a. Anti–double-stranded DNA: antibody to native DNA in abnormal titer, or b. Anti-Smith: presence of antibody to Smith nuclear antigen, or c. Positive finding of antiphospholipid antibodies is based on (1) an abnormal serum level of IgG or IgM anticardiolipin antibodies, (2) a positive test result for lupus anticoagulant using a standard method, or (3) a false-positive serologic test for syphilis known to be positive for at least 6 months and confirmed by *Treponema pallidum* immobilization or fluorescent treponemal antibody absorption test.
ANA	An abnormal titer of antinuclear antibody is documented by immunofluorescence or an equivalent assay at any point in time and in the absence of drugs known to be associated with drug-induced lupus syndrome.

[a]This classification is based on 11 criteria. For the purpose of identifying patients in clinical studies, a patient is classified as having definite SLE if any 4 or more of the 11 criteria are present (cumulative) during any interval of observation.

one immunologic finding. SLICC criteria also allow classification of a patient with SLE with only renal-limited disease (biopsy proven) in the presence of a positive ANA (Table 4.3).

The newest criteria from 2019 are a result of collaboration between ACR and European League against Rheumatism (EULAR) (Table 4.4). There are seven clinical and three immunologic domains. Each domain has several criteria, which are weighted. Within each domain, only the highest weighted criterion is counted towards the total score. Patients are classified to have SLE if there is a positive ANA of 1:80 or greater, at least one clinical criteria and a score of 10 or greater. These classification criteria are unique in the sense that they are the first weighted criteria for SLE. These criteria are combined with a comprehensive examination to help guide a diagnosis of SLE.

The hallmark of SLE is the presence of various autoantibodies that at times may be detected before the initial clinical presentation of SLE. The prevalence of these autoantibodies varies across different SLE patient cohorts and ethnic groups; however, more than 95% of patients with SLE will have a positive ANA, often with titers 1:160 or greater. The HEP-2 indirect immunofluorescence ANA test is the preferred assay over direct ELISA testing. Indirect immunofluorescence is reported in titers and patterns, with the most common pattern reported in SLE being homogenous (diffuse). ANA is not specific for the diagnosis of SLE, particularly in the presence of low titers and can often be seen in patients with normal ageing, viral infections, malignancies, and other connective tissue diseases.

Anti-dsDNA and anti-Smith antibodies are more specific for SLE. Anti-Ro antibodies are commonly found in SLE and are associated with subacute cutaneous lupus. Anti-Ro antibodies have implications during pregnancy with increased risk of neonatal lupus. Anti-U1-RNP is associated with increased risk of pulmonary hypertension and is discussed further in the "Overlap Syndrome" section. Antihistone antibodies are generally associated with drug-induced lupus but can be seen in patients with idiopathic lupus (Table 4.5).

The complement system plays an integral role in immune activation in SLE. Low complements (low C3, C4, CH50) are often considered hallmarks of disease activity in SLE, in particular glomerular disease, making them a valuable tool for clinicians to monitor disease activity.

Drug-Induced Lupus

Many drugs have been associated with lupus-like symptoms and development of lupus-related antibodies. Drug-induced lupus generally affects older populations, and common causative medications include procainamide, isoniazid, hydralazine, propylthiouracil, TNF inhibitors, proton-pump inhibitors, minocycline, methyldopa, levodopa, and interferon-α.

Clinical symptoms generally manifest as musculoskeletal, cutaneous, serous, and hematologic. Rarely, there may be renal or CNS involvement. The typical gender inequality in SLE is not represented in drug-induced lupus, but rather there seems to be a higher incidence in older men. Serologies often present include ANA and antihistone antibodies. The presence of anti-dsDNA antibodies is rare and is more commonly found in patients that were exposed to TNF inhibitor medications versus other medications.

In most cases, removal of the offending drug leads to improvement in symptoms. Depending on the severity of manifestations, glucocorticoids may also be helpful.

Neonatal Lupus

Neonatal lupus is a rare autoimmune disorder that develops in utero in which maternal anti-SSA/Ro and/or SSB/La antibodies cross the placenta and affect the fetus. This was first described in 1957 by G.R. Hogg

表4.2　1997年美国风湿病学会（ACR）系统性红斑狼疮分类标准 [a]

蝶形红斑	在两颧突出部位分布的扁平或高起的固定红斑，通常不累及鼻唇
盘状红斑	高于皮肤的片状红斑，黏附有角质脱屑和毛囊栓，陈旧性病变可发生萎缩性瘢痕
光过敏	光照后出现皮疹，从病史中得知或医生观察到
口腔溃疡	经医生观察到的口腔和鼻咽部溃疡，一般为无痛性
关节炎	非侵蚀性关节炎，累及2个或更多外周关节，表现为压痛、肿胀或积液
浆膜炎	a. 胸膜炎：具有可信的胸膜痛病史或医生闻及摩擦音或具有胸腔积液的证据　或 b. 心包炎：经心电图或摩擦音记录的心包炎或具有心包积液的证据
肾脏病变	a. 持续性尿蛋白 > 0.5 g/d，或 > 3+（如果未进行定量）　或 b. 细胞管型：可以为红细胞、血红蛋白、颗粒、管状或混合
神经系统异常	a. 癫痫：除外药物或已知的代谢紊乱（如尿毒症、酮症酸中毒或电解质紊乱）　或 b. 精神病：除外药物或已知的代谢紊乱（如尿毒症、酮症酸中毒或电解质紊乱）
血液系统异常	a. 溶血性贫血：伴网织红细胞增多或 b. 白细胞减少：≥2次的白细胞计数 < 4000/mm³　或 c. 淋巴细胞减少：≥2次的淋巴细胞计数 < 1500/mm³　或 d. 血小板减少：血小板计数 < 100 000/mm³，除外药物所致
免疫学异常	a. 抗dsDNA抗体：天然DNA抗体滴度异常　或 b. 抗Sm抗体：存在抗Sm核原抗体　或 c. 下列情况下抗磷脂抗体阳性：①血清IgG或IgM型抗心磷脂抗体异常或②经标准方法检测，狼疮抗凝物结果呈阳性或③至少持续6个月的梅毒螺旋体制动试验或荧光梅毒螺旋体抗体吸收试验呈假阳性
抗核抗体阳性	在任何时候和未用药物诱发的情况下，通过免疫荧光法或等效试验测定抗核抗体滴度异常

[a] 分类标准包括11项标准。患者需满足其中至少4项标准（可累积）方可分类为SLE。

标准，包括至少1项临床标准和1项免疫学标准，则被归类为SLE。SLICC标准还允许在ANA阳性的情况下，将仅有肾脏病变（活检证实）的患者归类为SLE（表4.3）。

2019年的最新标准是ACR和欧洲抗风湿病联盟（EULAR）合作的成果（表4.4）。共有7个临床模块和3个免疫学模块，每个模块都有多条标准，具有不同的加权赋分。在每个模块内，权重最高的标准计入总分。当患者ANA≥1∶80，至少有1项临床模块积分，总分≥10分，可被归类为SLE。这是第一个SLE的加权评分分类标准，结合全面的系统评估，有助于指导SLE的诊断。

SLE的特征是存在多种自身抗体，有时可能早于临床发病。不同抗体在不同SLE队列和种族中的阳性率不同；但ANA的阳性率在95%以上，滴度通常≥1∶160。HEP-2间接免疫荧光法优于ELISA检测。间接免疫荧光可报告滴度和核型，SLE中最常见的是均质型（弥漫型）。ANA对于SLE的诊断并不具有特异性，尤其是在低滴度的情况下，因其可见于正常衰老、病毒感染、恶性肿瘤和其他结缔组织病的患者。

抗dsDNA抗体和抗Sm抗体对SLE更具特异性。抗Ro抗体常见于SLE，与亚急性皮肤狼疮有关。抗Ro抗体对妊娠有影响，会增加新生儿狼疮的风险。抗U1-RNP抗体与肺动脉高压的风险增加有关，将在"重叠综合征"部分进一步讨论。抗组蛋白抗体通常与药物诱发的狼疮有关，但也可见于特发性狼疮患者（表4.5）。

补体系统在SLE的免疫激活过程中发挥着重要作用。低补体（低C3、C4、CH50）通常被认为是SLE疾病活动的标志，尤其是肾小球疾病，是临床医生监测疾病活动的重要指标。

药物性狼疮

许多药物都与狼疮样症状或狼疮相关抗体的产生有关。药物诱发的狼疮通常多见于老年人群。常见的致病药物包括普鲁卡因胺、异烟肼、肼屈嗪、丙硫氧嘧啶、TNF拮抗剂、质子泵抑制剂、米诺环素、甲基多巴、左旋多巴和干扰素-α。

临床一般表现为肌肉骨骼、皮肤、浆膜和血液系统症状。肾脏或中枢神经系统受累的情况较为罕见。SLE典型的性别差异在药物性狼疮中并不存在。相反，老年男性的发病率似乎更高。血清学检查通常包括ANA和抗组蛋白抗体（AHA）。抗dsDNA抗体很少见，可见于使用TNF拮抗剂的患者。

在大多数情况下，停用相关药物会改善症状。根据严重程度，也可酌情使用糖皮质激素。

新生儿狼疮

新生儿狼疮是一种罕见的自身免疫性疾病，由于SLE母亲的抗SSA/Ro和（或）抗SSB/La抗体穿过胎盘影响胎儿。G.R. Hogg于1957年首次描述了这种疾病。

TABLE 4.3 Systemic Lupus International Collaborating Clinics (SLICC) Classification Criteria of Systemic Lupus Erythematosus

Clinical Criteria[a]	Examples
1. Acute cutaneous lupus	Bullous lupus
	Lupus malar rash (not malar discoid)
	Maculopapular lupus rash
	Photosensitive lupus rash (in the absence of dermatomyositis)
	Subacute cutaneous lupus
	Toxic epidermal necrolysis variant of SLE
2. Chronic cutaneous lupus	Classic discoid rash
	Localized (above the neck)
	Generalized (above and below the neck) Chilblains lupus
	Discoid lupus/lichen planus overlap
	Hypertrophic (verrucous) lupus
	Lupus erythematosus tumidus
	Lupus panniculitis (profundus)
	Mucosal lupus
3. Oral ulcers	Palate, buccal, tongue, or nasal ulcers (in the absence of other causes: vasculitis, Behçet's disease, infection, inflammatory bowel disease, reactive arthritis, and acidic foods)
4. Nonscarring alopecia	Diffuse thinning or hair fragility with visible broken hairs (in the absence of other causes: alopecia areata, drugs, iron deficiency, and androgenic alopecia)
5. Synovitis (≥2 joints)	Characterized by swelling or effusion or tenderness with ≥30 minutes of morning stiffness
6. Serositis	Typical pleurisy for >1 day or pleural effusions or pleural rub
	Typical pericardial pain for >1 day or pericardial effusion or pericardial rub or pericarditis by ECG (in the absence of other causes: infection, uremia, and Dressler pericarditis)
7. Renal	Urine protein/creatinine (or 24-hr protein) ≥500 mg of protein/24 hr or red blood cell casts
8. Neurologic	Acute confusional state (in the absence of other causes: toxic-metabolic, uremia, and drugs)
	Mononeuritis multiplex (in the absence of other known causes: primary vasculitis)
	Myelitis
	Peripheral or cranial neuropathy (in the absence of other known causes: primary vasculitis, infection, and diabetes mellitus)
	Psychosis
	Seizure
9. Hemolytic anemia	
10. Leukopenia	<4000 cells/mm^3 detected at least once (in the absence of other known causes: Felty syndrome, drugs, and portal hypertension)
11. or Lymphopenia	<1000 cells/mm^3 detected at least once (in the absence of other known causes: corticosteroids, drugs, and infection)
12. Thrombocytopenia	<100,000 cells/mm^3 detected at least once (in the absence of other known causes: drugs, portal hypertension, and thrombotic thrombocytopenic purpura)
Immunologic Criteria	
1. ANAs	Above laboratory reference range
2. Anti–double-stranded DNA	Above laboratory reference range, except ELISA: two times greater than laboratory reference range
3. Anti-Smith	
4. Antiphospholipid	Any of the following: lupus anticoagulant, false-positive RPR, medium- or high-titer anticardiolipin (IgA, IgG, or IgM), or anti-β_2 glycoprotein I (IgA, IgG, or IgM)
5. Low complement	Low C3
	Low C4
	Low CH50
6. Direct Coombs test	In the absence of hemolytic anemia

ANAs, Antinuclear antibodies; *ECG*, electrocardiogram; *ELISA*, enzyme-linked immunosorbent assay; *Ig*, immunoglobulin; *RPR*, rapid plasma reagin; *SLE*, systemic lupus erythematosus.

[a]Criteria are cumulative. A patient is classified as having SLE using lupus nephritis as a stand-alone criterion (in the setting of ANAs or anti-dsDNA antibodies) or four criteria (with at least one of the clinical criteria and one of the immunologic criteria).

Modified from Petri M, Orbai AM, Alarcon GS, et al: Derivation and validation of Systemic Lupus International Collaborating Clinics classification criteria for systemic lupus erythematosus, Arthritis Rheum 64:2677-2686, 2012.

表 4.3　系统性红斑狼疮国际临床协作组（SLICC）系统性红斑狼疮分类标准

临床标准 [a]	示例
1. 急性皮肤狼疮	大疱性狼疮 蝶形红斑（非颊部盘状红斑） 狼疮斑丘疹 光过敏（非皮肌炎皮疹） 亚急性皮肤狼疮 中毒性表皮坏死松解样皮疹
2. 慢性皮肤狼疮	典型盘状红斑 　　局灶（颈部以上） 　　弥漫（颈部以上及以下均可）冻疮样红斑狼疮 盘状红斑/扁平苔藓重叠 增殖性（疣状）狼疮 肿胀性红斑狼疮 狼疮性脂膜炎（深部红斑狼疮） 黏膜受累
3. 口腔溃疡	上颚、颊黏膜、舌、鼻腔溃疡（除外其他原因：血管炎、白塞病、感染、炎症性肠病、反应性关节炎、酸性物质等）
4. 非瘢痕性脱发	弥漫性头发变细、变脆、易折断（除外其他原因：斑秃、药物、缺铁、雄激素性脱发）
5. 关节炎（≥2 个关节）	肿胀、积液、疼痛伴晨僵≥30 min
6. 浆膜炎	典型胸膜炎＞1 天或胸腔积液或胸膜摩擦音，典型心包炎疼痛＞1 天或心包积液或心包摩擦音或心电图证实的心包炎（除外其他原因：感染、尿毒症、Dressler 心包炎）
7. 肾脏受累	24 h 尿蛋白（或尿蛋白肌酐比）≥500 mg 或红细胞管型
8. 神经系统受累	急性意识混乱状态（除外其他原因：中毒、代谢紊乱、尿毒症、药物） 多发性单神经病变（除外其他原因：原发血管炎） 脊髓炎 周围或脑神经病变（除外其他原因：原发血管炎、感染、糖尿病） 精神障碍 癫痫
9. 溶血性贫血	
10. 白细胞减少	至少一次＜4000/mm³（除外其他原因：Felty 综合征、药物、门脉高压）
11. 或淋巴细胞减少	至少一次＜1000/mm³（除外其他原因：糖皮质激素、药物、感染）
12. 血小板减少	至少一次＜100 000/mm³（除外其他原因：药物、门脉高压、血栓性血小板减少性紫癜）
免疫学标准	
1. 抗核抗体	超过检测上限
2. 抗 dsDNA 抗体	超过检测上限，ELISA 法需超过 2 倍检测上限
3. 抗 Sm 抗体	
4. 抗磷脂抗体	以下任一种阳性：狼疮抗凝物；梅毒快速血清反应素（RPR）试验假阳性；中高滴度的抗心磷脂抗体（IgA、IgG 或 IgM）；中高滴度的抗 β2 糖蛋白 I 抗体（IgA、IgG 或 IgM）
5. 低补体血症	低 C3 低 C4 低 CH50
6. 直接抗人球蛋白试验	无溶血性贫血

ELISA，酶联免疫吸附试验；Ig，免疫球蛋白；SLE，系统性红斑狼疮。

[a] 标准可累积。符合狼疮性肾炎（在抗核抗体或抗 dsDNA 抗体阳性时）或满足 4 条标准（至少有 1 条临床标准和 1 条免疫学标准），可归类为系统性红斑狼疮。

改编自 Petri M，Orbai AM，Alarcon GS，et al：Derivation and validation of Systemic Lupus International Collaborating Clinics classification criteria for systemic lupus erythematosus，Arthritis Rheum 64：2677-2686，2012.

TABLE 4.4 2019 EULAR/ACR Criteria for Classification of SLE

Entry Criterion
Antinuclear antibodies (ANA) at a titer of ≥1:80 on HEp-2 cells or an equivalent positive test (ever)
↓
If absent, do not classify as SLE
If present, apply additive criteria
↓

Additive Criteria
Do not count a criterion if there is a more likely explanation than SLE
Occurrence of a criterion on at least one occasion is sufficient
SLE classification requires at least one clinical criterion and ≥10 points
Criteria need not occur simultaneously
Within each domain, only the highest weighted criterion is counted toward the total score[a]

Clinical Domains and Criteria	Weight	Immunology Domains and Criteria	Weight
Constitutional		*Antiphospholipid antibodies*	
Fever	2	Anti-cardiolipin antibodies OR	
		Anti-β_2GPI antibodies OR	
		Lupus anticoagulant	2
Hematologic		*Complement proteins*	
Leukopenia	3	Low C3 OR low C4	3
Thrombocytopenia	4	Low C3 AND low C4	4
Autoimmune hemolysis	4		
Neuropsychiatric		*SLE-specific antibodies*	
Delirium	2	Anti-dsDNA antibody[b] OR	
Psychosis	3	Anti-Smith antibody	6
Seizure	5		
Mucocutaneous			
Non-scarring alopecia	2		
Oral ulcers	2		
Subacute cutaneous OR discoid lupus	4		
Acute cutaneous lupus	6		
Serosal			
Pleural or pericardial effusion	5		
Acute pericarditis	6		
Musculoskeletal			
Joint involvement	6		
Renal			
Proteinuria >0.5 g/24 h	4		
Renal biopsy Class II or V lupus nephritis	8		
Renal biopsy Class III or IV lupus nephritis	10		
Total Score:			

↓
Classify as Systemic Lupus Erythematosus with a score of ≥10 if entry criterion fulfilled.

Anti-β_2GPI, Anti-β_2-glycoprotein I; *anti-dsDNA*, anti–double-stranded DNA.
[a]Additional criteria within the same domain will not be counted.
[b]In an assay with 90% specificity against relevant disease controls.

in a full-term, 2-kg baby boy who had complete AV block and subendocardial fibrosis born to a mother with SLE. There is a 1% to 2% chance of having a child with neonatal lupus in mothers with anti-SSA/Ro or SSB/La antibodies. In women with a previous baby with neonatal lupus the risk of having a subsequent baby with cardiac involvement of neonatal lupus increases from 2% to 19%. The development of heart block is most common between 18 weeks' and 24 weeks' gestation in mothers with these antibodies; thus, screening with fetal heart tones and fetal echocardiography should begin at 16 weeks' gestation. If there are signs of heart block, the mother may be treated with fluorinated corticosteroids (i.e., dexamethasone or betamethasone). Many children with congenital heart block do not survive or have continued morbidities requiring pacemakers.

Other manifestations of neonatal SLE that are more common include rashes, cytopenias, and hepatosplenomegaly. These manifestations generally resolve after the baby begins to develop his or her own antibodies, at around 6 to 8 months. Although this is commonly a condition that is seen in children born to mothers with SLE, it may also be seen in other autoimmune conditions or in otherwise healthy mothers with SSA/Ro and/or SSB/La antibodies.

Overlap Syndrome

Some patients with clinical and laboratory features of two or more autoimmune diseases have an overlap syndrome. Mixed connective tissue disease is characterized by overlaps among SLE, scleroderma, and myositis with a high titer of anti–U1-RNP antibody levels. For

表 4.4　2019 EULAR/ACR 系统性红斑狼疮（SLE）分类标准

准入标准：
抗核抗体（ANA）滴度 ≥ 1∶80（HEp-2 细胞法）或（既往）等效的阳性检验结果

↓

如果不符合，不考虑 SLE 分类；
如果符合，应用附加标准。

↓

附加标准：
如果计分标准可以被其他比 SLE 更符合的疾病解释，则该项不计分；
满足标准至少一次即可；
SLE 分类标准要求：至少包括 1 条临床标准，且总分 ≥ 10 分；
不需要同时满足所有标准；
在每个模块中，只取最高权重分计入总分 [a]。

临床模块及标准	权重	免疫学模块及标准	权重
全身状况		抗磷脂抗体	
发热	2	抗心磷脂抗体或	
		抗 β₂GPⅠ抗体或	
		狼疮抗凝物	2
血液系统		补体	
白细胞减少	3	低 C3 或低 C4	3
血小板减少	4	低 C3 和低 C4	4
自身免疫性溶血	4		
神经精神系统		*SLE 特异性自身抗体*	
谵妄	2	抗 dsDNA 抗体 [b] 或	
精神错乱	3	抗 Smith 抗体	6
癫痫	5		
皮肤黏膜			
非瘢痕性脱发	2		
口腔溃疡	2		
亚急性皮肤狼疮或盘状狼疮	4		
急性皮肤狼疮	6		
浆膜			
胸膜或心包渗出液	5		
急性心包炎	6		
肌肉骨骼			
关节受累	6		
肾脏			
蛋白尿 > 0.5 g/24 h	4		
肾脏病理Ⅱ型或Ⅴ型狼疮性肾炎	8		
肾脏病理Ⅲ型或Ⅳ型狼疮性肾炎	10		
总分：			

↓

如果符合准入标准，且总分 ≥ 10 分，则分类为系统性红斑狼疮

抗 β₂GPⅠ抗体：抗 β₂ 糖蛋白Ⅰ抗体；抗 dsDNA 抗体：抗双链 DNA 抗体。
[a] 同一模块内的多项标准不予重复计分。
[b] 与对照组相比，该检验方法特异性达到 90%。

一例足月分娩男婴，出生体重 2000 g，患有完全性房室传导阻滞和心内膜下纤维化，其母亲为 SLE 患者。抗 SSA/Ro 或抗 SSB/La 抗体阳性的母亲中，有 1%～2% 的概率生出新生儿狼疮患儿。如果母亲曾生育过新生儿狼疮患儿，则再次妊娠时出现新生儿狼疮所致心脏受累患儿的风险，将从 2% 增加到 19%。在这些抗体阳性的母亲中，胎儿心脏传导阻滞最常出现于孕 18 周至孕 24 周之间。因此，建议从孕 16 周开始进行胎心监测和胎儿心脏超声检查。如果发现心脏传导阻滞的迹象，可以应用氟化皮质类固醇（如地塞米松或倍他米松）对母亲进行治疗。许多罹患先天性心脏传导阻滞的儿童无法存活，或因疾病需要安装心脏起搏器。

新生儿狼疮的其他常见表现包括皮疹、血细胞减少和肝脾肿大。在患儿开始产生自己的抗体，即出生后 6～8 个月时，这些表现通常可以消退。虽然这种情况通常见于患有 SLE 的母亲所生的儿童，但也可能见于患有其他自身免疫性疾病或携带抗 SSA/Ro 和（或）抗 SSB/La 抗体的健康母亲。

重叠综合征

一些患者具有两种或更多自身免疫性疾病的临床和实验室特征，称之为重叠综合征。混合性结缔组织病则可出现 SLE、系统性硬化症和肌炎的重叠表现，且伴有高滴度的抗 U1-RNP 抗体。对于那些具有多种

TABLE 4.5 Prevalence of Autoantibodies in Systemic Lupus Erythematosus	
Target Autoantigen	Positive (%)
Nuclear antigens	>95
Double-stranded DNA	30–60
Smith	10–44
Ribonucleoprotein (U1-RNP)	25–40
SSA/Ro	30–40
SSB/La	38
Phospholipids	16–60
Ribosomal P	5–10
Histone	21–90

Data from Wallace D, Hahn BH: Other Clinical laboratory tests in SLE. In Dubois' lupus erythematosus and related syndromes, ed 8, Philadelphia, 2013, Saunders, pp 526–531.

patients who have multiple autoimmune manifestations but do not meet the criteria of a specific autoimmune disease, the term *undifferentiated connective tissue disease* is used. In some instances, these patients may be early in their disease course and eventually develop a specific autoimmune disease.

TREATMENT

There is no known cure for SLE. Management can be challenging and is aimed at treating the underlying organ manifestations. Treatment is often multipronged with patient education; one or more medications including anti-inflammatories, antimalarials, glucocorticoids and immunosuppressive drugs; and management of other aspects such as fatigue, depression, and other psychosocial factors. General goals for treatment are to achieve low disease activity or remission and prevent flares with the least amount of glucocorticoid use possible. At this time, there are only four FDA-approved treatments for SLE: aspirin, glucocorticoids, hydroxychloroquine, and belimumab.

It is essential to establish the type of SLE and the extent of organ involvement prior to initiating treatment. This is important because prognosis of SLE varies based on the severity of disease at presentation.

Every patient with SLE should be educated on sun protection techniques and smoking cessation because both are important triggers of flares and ongoing disease activity. Sunscreen with at least SPF 30 and preferably one that blocks both UVA and UVB is recommended. Avoiding sun exposure during peak hours, typically midmorning to early evening, and use of long-sleeve shirts and wide-brimmed hats are advisable. Smoking not only increases all-cause mortality but also worsens SLE activity and may decrease efficacy of certain medications such as hydroxychloroquine.

Nonsteroidal anti-inflammatory drugs (NSAIDs) are commonly used to treat certain manifestations of SLE including musculoskeletal symptoms, pericarditis, pleurisy, and fever. Typically, NSAIDs are used as short-term therapies. One should be cognizant of renal involvement prior to initiation and continuation of NSAIDs. Aspirin is often used in SLE patients with other cardiac risk factors to mitigate the increased risk of cardiovascular events. Aspirin is often used in patients with SLE who have high titer antiphospholipid antibodies without a history of thrombosis and in most pregnant women.

Glucocorticoids remain a very effective treatment modality in SLE. They are fast acting and halt ongoing inflammation in many organ systems, making them valuable during initial treatment and as bridge therapy for flares. Doses of glucocorticoids vary widely from oral low-dose alternate-day regimen to very high doses of IV formulations. As a general rule, using the lowest effective dose for the shortest amount of time limits potential long-term side effects. Long-term use of moderate to high doses of glucocorticoids leads to a higher cumulative dose exposure over time and increased risk of toxicity. This includes obesity, diabetes mellitus, hypertension, hyperlipidemia, accelerated atherosclerosis, osteoporosis with increased risk of fracture, avascular necrosis, cataracts, glaucoma, and increased risk of infections. To avoid these toxicities, steroid-sparing immunomodulating or immunosuppressant agents are used.

Antimalarial agents are the cornerstone of therapy in SLE. Hydroxychloroquine is the most commonly used agent because it has less retinal toxicity compared to chloroquine. Quinacrine is an antimalarial agent with no retinal toxicity, but the oral formulation has to be compounded at a specialty pharmacy. Hydroxychloroquine is an immunomodulatory agent that is beneficial in treating cutaneous and musculoskeletal manifestations. It has also been shown to prevent organ flares, prevent organ damage, modulate risk factors for atherosclerosis and thrombosis, and prevent placental transfer of anti-Ro antibodies that cause congenital heart block and neonatal lupus. Newer guidelines for the screening and prevention of hydroxychloroquine retinopathy suggest use of 5 mg/kg/day or less and regular ophthalmologic monitoring. Ophthalmologic monitoring at baseline (within the first year) and then annually after 5 years (more frequent in high risk individuals) with a dilated eye exam, Humphrey visual field testing, and spectral domain optical coherence tomography (SD-OCT) is recommended to monitor for retinal toxicity. Risk for retinal toxicity is dose dependent and influenced by comorbidities.

Azathioprine (AZA), methotrexate (MTX), leflunomide (LEF), and mycophenolate mofetil (MMF) are immunosuppressive agents used in SLE. AZA is effective in treating a variety of manifestations including skin disease, musculoskeletal disease, and nephritis. It is safe during pregnancy and breast-feeding. Toxicity includes cytopenias, hepatoxicity with transaminitis, and increased risk for infections. MTX is effective in treating cutaneous, arthritis, and serositis manifestations. MTX is teratogenic and should be discontinued 3 to 6 months prior to conception. Toxicity is similar to AZA. LEF works well for cutaneous and musculoskeletal manifestations. LEF is teratogenic and contraindicated in pregnancy and lactation. MMF has been used for more than 20 years for the treatment of lupus nephritis, but it is also effective for skin disease and serositis. MMF toxicity is primarily related to gastrointestinal intolerance, cytopenias, and infectious complications. Mycophenolic acid, which is an active form of MMF, has less gastrointestinal intolerance. MMF is teratogenic and contraindicated in both pregnancy and lactation.

In organ- or life-threatening SLE, the alkylating agent cyclophosphamide (CTX) is used. Scenarios where CTX is utilized include rapidly progressive glomerulonephritis, lupus cerebritis, and diffuse alveolar hemorrhage. However, it is associated with significant toxicity, particularly bone marrow suppression, hemorrhagic cystitis, gonadal toxicity, increased risk of infections, and certain malignancies. The use of lower doses of intravenous CTX has resulted in equal efficacy and fewer side effects and has replaced many of the older regimens.

Great potential and optimism exist for biologic immunomodulating agents that focus on various aspects of the immune system, including B cells, interactions between B and T cells, and cytokines. The most promising agents are those that target B cells, which produce autoantibodies. In 2011, belimumab, a monoclonal antibody that inhibits B-lymphocyte stimulator, was the first therapeutic agent approved for the treatment of SLE in more than 50 years (Table 4.6). There are a number of other potential biologic therapies for lupus in the pipeline and currently being tested in clinical trials.

表 4.5 系统性红斑狼疮中自身抗体阳性率	
目标自身抗原	阳性率（%）
核抗原	>95
双链 DNA	30～60
Smith	10～44
核糖核蛋白（U1-RNP）	25～40
SSA/Ro	30～40
SSB/La	38
磷脂	16～60
核糖体 P	5～10
组蛋白	21～90

引自 Wallace D, Hahn BH: Other Clinical laboratory tests in SLE. In Dubois' lupus erythematosus and related syndromes, ed 8, Philadelphia, 2013, Saunders, pp 526-531.

自身免疫表现，但不符合某一特定的自身免疫性疾病标准的患者，则诊断为未分化结缔组织病。在某些情况下，这些患者可能处于疾病的早期阶段，并最终发展为某种特定的自身免疫性疾病。

治疗

目前 SLE 尚不能治愈。疾病管理具有挑战性，治疗目标为控制潜在的器官损害。治疗常包括多个方面：患者教育、药物治疗（如抗炎药、抗疟药、糖皮质激素、免疫抑制剂）、其他方面管理（如疲乏、抑郁以及社会心理因素等）。通常治疗的目标是达到低疾病活动度或疾病缓解，尽可能以最低剂量糖皮质激素预防疾病复发。目前仅有 4 种药物通过 FDA 批准用于 SLE 治疗：阿司匹林、糖皮质激素、硫酸羟氯喹以及贝利尤单抗。

在进行初始治疗之前，明确 SLE 类型和脏器受累程度非常重要。主要是由于 SLE 的预后取决于初始呈现的疾病严重程度。

应向所有 SLE 患者进行防晒及戒烟宣教，从而避免疾病复发和持续疾病活动的重要诱发因素。推荐防晒霜至少达到 SPF30，最好能够同时阻隔 UVA 和 UVB。避免暴露在阳光最强的时刻（一般为上午中段到傍晚），可以穿长袖衬衫和戴宽边遮阳帽。吸烟不仅提高全因死亡率，还会加重 SLE 病情活动，同时还可能会降低硫酸羟氯喹等药物的疗效。

非甾体抗炎药（NSAID）一般用于治疗 SLE 的以下临床表现：骨骼肌肉症状、心包炎、胸膜炎以及发热。通常 NSAID 用于短期治疗。在启动和持续应用 NSAID 之前，应注意识别有无肾脏受累。阿司匹林常用于 SLE 患者合并其他心脏风险因素，以降低心血管事件的高风险。阿司匹林也常用于具有高滴度抗磷脂抗体且无血栓事件的 SLE 患者的一级预防，以及大部分妊娠期 SLE 女性患者。

糖皮质激素仍然是非常有效的 SLE 治疗方法。糖皮质激素起效迅速并可以阻止多数器官系统的持续性炎症，在初始诱导治疗和复发时的桥接治疗中具有价值。糖皮质激素应用剂量具有较大的差异，从隔日低剂量口服到大剂量静脉冲击疗法。一般的原则是在最短的时间内应用最低的有效剂量，可以控制潜在的长期不良反应。长时间应用中、大剂量糖皮质激素会导致更高的累积暴露剂量并增加毒副作用，包括：肥胖、糖尿病、高血压、高脂血症、加速性动脉硬化、骨质疏松伴骨折高风险、骨缺血性坏死、白内障、青光眼以及增加感染风险。为避免上述毒副作用，需联合应用非类固醇的免疫调节剂或免疫抑制剂。

抗疟药是 SLE 治疗的基石。硫酸羟氯喹最为广泛应用，相较于氯喹具有更低的视网膜毒性。奎纳克林是一种无视网膜毒性的抗疟药，但其口服剂型需要在专业药房合成。硫酸羟氯喹作为一种免疫调节剂，适用于治疗皮肤和骨骼肌肉受累。硫酸羟氯喹还可以防止器官复发和损伤，调节动脉硬化及血栓的风险因素，预防引起先天性心脏传导阻滞和新生儿狼疮的抗 Ro 抗体的胎盘转运。筛查和预防硫酸羟氯喹相关视网膜病变的更新指南推荐应用每日 ≤ 5 mg/kg 的剂量，同时进行定期眼科监测。眼科监测需要在基线（1 年内）以及应用 5 年后每年进行（高风险人群可增加检查频次），推荐用于监测视网膜毒性的检查包括散瞳验光、汉弗莱（Humphrey）视野测验、频域光学相干断层成像（SD-OCT）。视网膜毒性发生风险具有剂量依赖性，合并症也会影响视网膜病变。

用于 SLE 治疗的免疫抑制剂包括硫唑嘌呤（AZA）、甲氨蝶呤（MTX）、来氟米特（LEF）及吗替麦考酚酯（MMF）。硫唑嘌呤在治疗皮肤、肌肉骨骼及肾炎等病变方面有效。在妊娠期及哺乳期安全性高。其不良反应包括血细胞减少、肝毒性（转氨酶升高）以及增加感染风险。甲氨蝶呤用于治疗皮疹、关节炎及浆膜炎。甲氨蝶呤具有致畸性，孕前应停药 3～6 个月。其不良反应与硫唑嘌呤类似。来氟米特在治疗皮疹及肌肉骨骼症状中发挥作用。来氟米特也具有致畸性，严禁应用于妊娠期及哺乳期。吗替麦考酚酯治疗狼疮性肾炎已经超过 20 年，在治疗皮肤病变及浆膜炎中亦有效。其不良反应主要有胃肠道不耐受、血细胞减少以及感染并发症。霉酚酸（mycophenolic acid）作为吗替麦考酚酯的活性形式，可以减轻胃肠道不耐受。吗替麦考酚酯也具有致畸性，禁止应用于妊娠期及哺乳期。

在器官受累或危重症 SLE 治疗中，常应用烷化剂环磷酰胺（CTX）。环磷酰胺一般应用于快速进展性肾小球肾炎、狼疮性脑病以及弥漫性肺泡出血。环磷酰胺的不良反应也十分显著，尤其是骨髓抑制、出血性膀胱炎、性腺毒性、增加感染以及某些恶性肿瘤风险。应用小剂量环磷酰胺静脉滴注具有同样的疗效，且不良反应较少，已经取代以往的使用方法。

针对免疫系统不同靶点的生物制剂具有很好的治疗前景，包括以 B 细胞、B 细胞与 T 细胞相互作用以及细胞因子等为靶点的生物制剂。目前，最具希望的生物制剂是以产生自身抗体的 B 细胞为靶点的药物。2011 年，抑制 B 淋巴细胞刺激因子（BLys）的单克隆抗体——贝利尤单抗，50 多年来首次被批准应用于治疗系统性红斑狼疮（表 4.6）。还有许多用于治疗狼疮的潜在生物疗法即将或正在进行临床试验。

TABLE 4.6 Treatment Options in Systemic Lupus Erythematosus

Medication	Mechanism of Action	Monitoring	Pregnancy Concern
NSAIDS	Inhibits cyclooxygenase, reducing prostaglandin and thromboxane synthesis	CBC and CMP, caution with renal disease	Caution in 1st trimester, avoid use in 3rd trimester
Glucocorticoids[a]	Inhibits multiple cytokines	Electrolytes, BP, blood sugar. Caution with comorbid diabetes mellitus	May be used. Increased risk of low birth weight and premature birth.
Hydroxychloroquine[a]	Exact mechanism unknown. Inhibits TLR and various enzymes.	Ophthalmologic exam at baseline (within 6 months of starting), in 5 years then annually. If there are increased risk factors, every 6 months or annually.	Safe in pregnancy and lactation. May decrease risk of neonatal lupus in mothers with anti-Ro or anti-La antibodies
Azathioprine	Inhibits T-lymphocytes	Check TPMT[b] prior to initiation. CBC and CMP	May be used in pregnancy
Methotrexate	Inhibits dihydrofolate reductase and inhibits lymphocyte proliferation	Pregnancy test, hepatitis B and C serologies and CXR at baseline. CBC and CMP. Caution with renal disease, hepatitis or alcohol use.	Teratogenic. Avoid use in both men and women considering pregnancy
Leflunomide	Inhibits pyrimidine synthesis via dihydroorotate dehydrogenase inhibition	Pregnancy test, TB test at baseline. CBC and CMP	Teratogenic
Mycophenolate mofetil	Inhibits B and T lymphocyte proliferation	Pregnancy test at baseline. CBC and CMP	Teratogenic
Belimumab[a]	Inhibits B lymphocyte stimulator (BLyS) binding to B cells which inhibits B-cell survival and decreased B-cell differentiation into immunoglobulin producing plasma cells	No routine testing	Avoid use during pregnancy and lactation. Not enough data available
Cyclophosphamide	Alkylates and cross-links DNA	Creatinine at baseline. CBC, UA and CMP. May need to adjust dose in renal impairment	May cause gonadal failure. Teratogenic. Avoid use in pregnancy as well as lactation

[a]Denotes medications that are FDA approved for the treatment of SLE.
[b]Testing for thiopurine methyltransferase deficiency.

PROGNOSIS

Prognosis in SLE has improved with early diagnosis and advances in treatment. In 1955, 5-year survival of SLE was 55%, which improved to 64% to 87% in the 1980s, and most recently, it was reported at 95%. Survival rates are influenced by geographic location and ethnicity.

With improved mortality from lupus disease activity, the focus has been on prevention and management of comorbid conditions. Premature atherosclerotic heart disease, malignancy, bone health, and psychosocial well-being may be secondary to the inflammatory state seen in lupus or as a result of treatment.

SPECIAL CONSIDERATIONS IN SYSTEMIC LUPUS ERYTHEMATOSUS

Pregnancy

Women with SLE have normal fertility but have higher rates of pregnancy loss (i.e., miscarriage and stillbirths) and preterm delivery (i.e., premature rupture of membranes, preeclampsia, and intrauterine growth restriction) than their healthy counterparts. Lupus activity preceding conception, especially nephritis, hypertension, and APS, are risk factors for pregnancy complications in SLE. Pregnancy itself may place women with SLE at a greater risk of a flare, particularly if the disease was active before conception.

With careful prenatal screening and planning, women with SLE can successfully have a healthy child. Prenatal monitoring of anti-SSA/Ro and anti-SSB/La antibodies and APLs and pre-pregnancy consultation with an obstetrician caring for high-risk pregnancies are critical. Ideally, women with SLE should have clinical quiescence for 6 months prior to a planned pregnancy.

Hormone Therapy

Contraception plays an important role in pregnancy planning for women with lupus. Often it is important to avoid unintended pregnancy during periods of severe disease activity and fetal exposure to potentially teratogenic drugs.

Because SLE is more prevalent in women of childbearing ages there has been consideration of a hormonal role in pathogenesis. There have been concerns raised that estrogen-containing compounds could induce a flare. In the past, estrogen-containing contraceptives were considered relatively contraindicated. However, randomized controlled trials evaluating the rate of disease flares in women with SLE on estrogen-containing contraceptives found no significant difference in rates of serious flares. Still, as a general rule, women with SLE who have APLs should avoid contraception with estrogen-containing compounds due to increased risk of thrombotic events. More recently, intrauterine devices are becoming a recommended alternative, given the efficacy and safety profile.

The use of postmenopausal hormone replacement therapy for treating vasomotor symptoms in SLE should be restricted to patients with negative APLs and at the lowest dose and shortest duration.

表 4.6 系统性红斑狼疮治疗方案

药物	作用机制	监测指标	妊娠关注
非甾体抗炎药	抑制环氧化酶，减少前列腺素和凝血酶的合成	全血细胞计数、生化全项 注意肾脏病变	谨慎应用于妊娠早期，避免妊娠晚期应用。
糖皮质激素[a]	抑制多种细胞因子	电解质、血压、血糖 注意合并糖尿病	可以应用，会增加婴儿低体重及早产的风险。
硫酸羟氯喹[a]	确切机制尚不明确。抑制 Toll 样受体及多种酶	基线期（开始应用6个月内）及应用5年后每年进行眼科检查。如果合并高危因素，每6个月或每年进行检查。	妊娠期及哺乳期安全 对于抗 Ro 或抗 La 抗体阳性的母亲，可降低其新生儿狼疮的风险。
硫唑嘌呤	抑制 T 淋巴细胞	应用前进行 TPMT[b] 全血细胞计数、生化全项	妊娠期可以应用。
甲氨蝶呤	抑制二氢叶酸还原酶以及抑制淋巴细胞增殖	基线期进行妊娠试验、乙型肝炎、丙型肝炎血清学及胸部 X 线检查 全血细胞计数、生化全项 注意肾脏病变、肝炎及饮酒	有致畸性 若考虑妊娠，男性及女性均应该避免应用。
来氟米特	通过抑制二氢乳清酸脱氢酶，从而抑制嘧啶合成	基线期进行妊娠试验、结核筛查 全血细胞计数、生化全项	有致畸性
吗替麦考酚酯	抑制 B、T 淋巴细胞增殖	基线期进行妊娠试验 全血细胞计数、生化全项	有致畸性
贝利尤单抗[a]	抑制 B 淋巴细胞刺激因子（BLyS）与 B 细胞结合，抑制 B 细胞存活，降低 B 细胞分化为产生免疫球蛋白的浆细胞	无常规检测	避免妊娠期及哺乳期应用 尚无充分的临床数据
环磷酰胺	烷基化并交联 DNA	基线期检测肌酐 全血细胞计数、血尿酸、生化全项 肾功能不全时需要调整剂量	可能引起性腺早衰 有致畸性 避免妊娠期及哺乳期应用

[a] 标识药物均经 FDA 批准用于治疗 SLE。
[b] 硫嘌呤甲基转移酶缺乏症检测。

预后

SLE 的预后随着早期诊断和治疗进展而提高。1955 年，SLE 的 5 年生存率为 55%，到 1980 年代提高到 64%～87%，最近报道的则为 95%。生存率受地域和种族的影响。

随着狼疮疾病活动导致的死亡率下降，现在更为关注并发症的预防和管理。早发性动脉粥样硬化性心脏病、恶性肿瘤、骨骼健康和心理健康受损，既可能继发于狼疮炎症状态，也可能是治疗所致。

SLE 中的特殊注意事项

妊娠

患有 SLE 的女性具有正常的生育能力，但相比健康女性，她们的妊娠丢失（如流产和死胎）率以及早产（如胎膜早破、先兆子痫和胎儿宫内生长受限）率更高。在受孕前的狼疮活动，尤其是肾炎、高血压和抗磷脂综合征（APS），是 SLE 妊娠并发症的危险因素。妊娠本身可能会使患有 SLE 的女性面临病情复发风险增加，尤其是在受孕前已处于疾病活动期。

通过仔细的产前筛查和计划，患有 SLE 的女性可以成功生育健康的孩子。产前应监测抗 SSA/Ro、抗 SSB/La 抗体以及抗磷脂抗体，最重要的是向具有高危妊娠管理经验的产科医生进行孕前咨询。一般推荐，患有 SLE 的女性在计划妊娠前 6 个月应持续达到临床缓解状态。

激素治疗

避孕在狼疮女性的妊娠计划中十分重要。通常，在疾病高度活动和应用可能的致畸药物期间，应着重避免意外妊娠。

由于 SLE 在育龄期女性中发病率较高，因此激素被认为参与发病机制。含有雌激素的化合物也被认为可能会诱发疾病复发。过去，含雌激素的避孕药一般是相对禁忌的。然而，评估使用含雌激素避孕药的 SLE 女性患者疾病复发率的随机对照试验发现，严重复发率没有统计学差异。尽管如此，一般原则是，患有 SLE 且具有抗磷脂抗体的女性应避免使用含雌激素的避孕药，因其增加了血栓事件的风险。最近，鉴于宫内节育器的效果和安全性，宫内节育器正在成为推荐的替代方案。

SLE 患者使用绝经后雌激素替代疗法治疗血管舒缩性症状，应限于抗磷脂抗体阴性的患者，并应使用最低剂量和最短疗程。

TABLE 4.7 Revised Classification Criteria of Antiphospholipid Syndrome

Classification Criteria[a]	Definition
Clinical Criteria	
1. Vascular thrombosis	One or more clinical episodes of arterial, venous, or small vessel thrombosis in any tissue or organ
	Thrombosis must be confirmed by objective validated criteria (i.e., unequivocal findings of appropriate imaging studies or histopathology). For histopathologic confirmation, thrombosis should be present without significant evidence of inflammation in the vessel wall.
2. Pregnancy morbidity	a. One or more unexplained deaths of a morphologically normal fetus at or beyond 10 weeks' gestation, with normal fetal morphology documented by ultrasound or by direct examination of the fetus
	or
	b. One or more premature births of a morphologically normal neonate before 34 weeks' gestation because of (i) eclampsia or severe preeclampsia or (ii) recognized features of placental insufficiency
	or
	c. Three or more unexplained consecutive spontaneous abortions before 10 weeks' gestation, with maternal anatomic or hormonal abnormalities and paternal and maternal chromosomal causes excluded
Laboratory Criteria	
1. Lupus anticoagulant	LAC detected in plasma on two or more occasions at least 12 weeks apart
2. Anticardiolipin antibody	The ACA antibody of IgG and/or IgM isotype in serum or plasma in medium or high titer (i.e., >40 GPL units, or >the 99th percentile) on two or more occasions at least 12 weeks apart, measured by a standardized ELISA
3. Anti-β_2 glycoprotein I antibody	β_2GPI antibody of IgG and/or IgM isotype in serum or plasma (in titer >the 99th percentile), detected on two or more occasions at least 12 weeks apart, measured by a standardized ELISA

ACA, Anticardiolipin antibody; β_2GPI, anti-β_2 glycoprotein I antibody; *ELISA*, enzyme-linked immunosorbent assay; *Ig*, immunoglobulin; *LAC*, lupus anticoagulant.
[a]Antiphospholipid antibody syndrome is diagnosed if at least one clinical criterion and one laboratory criterion are met.
Modified from Miyakis S, Lockshin MD, Atsumi T, et al: International consensus statement on an update of the classification criteria for definite antiphospholipid syndrome (APS), J Thromb Haemost 4:295-306, 2006.

Bone Health

Women with SLE have an increased risk for osteoporosis due to multiple factors. Some of these factors are more specific to SLE, such as chronic inflammation, renal disease, photosensitivity and avoidance of sun exposure, medication use (especially glucocorticoids), and premature ovarian failure, which may be due to SLE or the use of CTX. In addition, there are still the typical risk factors for osteoporosis such as smoking, alcohol use, family history, and low BMI. One challenging aspect in treating osteoporosis in young women with SLE is the use of bisphosphonates as these medications are not safe in pregnancy and may be present for years after discontinuation.

Cardiovascular Health

As survival and therapies for SLE have improved, and patients are living longer, cardiovascular disease (CVD) has emerged as a leading cause of morbidity and mortality. SLE patients are 5 to 10 times more likely than healthy individuals to have a coronary event. More striking, premenopausal women between 35 and 44 years of age are 50 times more likely than healthy women to have a myocardial infarction.

Autopsy series reveal atherosclerotic heart disease as the underlying mechanism of CVD in SLE. The cause of premature atherosclerosis in SLE is multifactorial and likely includes inflammatory mediators, SLE-related factors (e.g., premature menopause, corticosteroid therapy, disease activity), and traditional cardiovascular risk factors.

Although no firm cardiovascular management guidelines exist for SLE patients, the 2011 updated guidelines from the American Heart Association for prevention of CVD in women included (for the first time) autoimmune diseases (i.e., SLE and rheumatoid arthritis) in the increased-risk category. Physicians should consider premature atherosclerotic CVD and aggressively evaluate SLE patients with typical and atypical cardiac symptoms, regardless of age and sex.

Secondary Antiphospholipid Syndrome

Antiphospholipid syndrome (APS) is a condition characterized by an increased risk of thrombosis and/or pregnancy loss in the setting of APLs. The term *lupus anticoagulant* is a misnomer because the in vitro anticoagulant effect reflects the prolonged activated partial thromboplastin time (aPTT), but the term does not indicate a diagnosis of SLE or an increased risk of bleeding. In fact, lupus anticoagulant is associated with an increased risk of thrombotic events.

If APS occurs in the absence of another autoimmune disease it is considered primary APS. When it occurs in the setting of SLE or another autoimmune disease it is considered secondary APS. Both primary and secondary APS have similar clinical manifestations and the treatment is also similar. Clinical manifestations of APS typically include increased risk for venous and arterial thrombosis, pregnancy complications, cerebrovascular and cardiovascular events, pulmonary hypertension, Libman-Sacks endocarditis, and neurologic complications.

Catastrophic APS (CAPS) is the most severe manifestation of APS, which affects multiple organs with microthromboses leading to rapid organ failure and potentially death. CAPS may be difficult to discern from sepsis or TTP.

For patients with presence of APS but no thrombotic events or pregnancy loss there is no indication for anticoagulation. If there is an episode of vascular thrombosis, treatment with lifelong anticoagulation is generally recommended. Warfarin remains the drug of choice for these patients despite the development of several other novel oral anticoagulants. Unfractionated and low-molecular-weight heparin are also effective anticoagulants for APS and are used for patients who suffer recurrent events while on warfarin therapy or patients who are or plan to become pregnant (Table 4.7).

表 4.7　修订的抗磷脂综合征分类标准

分类标准[a]	定义
临床标准	
1. 血栓形成	任何组织或器官的一次或多次动脉、静脉或小血管发生血栓。血栓形成必须通过客观有效的标准来证实（包括适当的影像学检查或组织病理学证实）。对于组织病理学证实，需要确保血栓形成存在，并且没有明显的血管壁炎症的证据。
2. 病理妊娠	a. ≥1次发生于妊娠10周或10周以上无法解释的形态学正常的胎儿死亡，经超声或直接检查证实胎儿形态正常。 或 b. ≥1次发生于妊娠34周之前，因以下原因所致的形态学正常的新生儿早产：（i）子痫或严重的先兆子痫；（ii）胎盘功能不全。 或 c. ≥3次发生于妊娠10周之前的无法解释的自发性流产，必须排除母体解剖或激素异常以及双亲染色体异常。
实验室标准	
1. 狼疮抗凝物（LAC）	血浆中出现LAC，至少2次阳性，每次间隔至少12周。
2. 抗心磷脂抗体（ACA）	用标准ELISA在血清或血浆中检测到中/高滴度的IgG和（或）IgM型ACA（>40 GPL，或滴度>99百分位数），至少检测2次，间隔至少12周。
3. 抗β$_2$糖蛋白I抗体（β$_2$GPI）	用标准ELISA在血清或血浆中检测到的IgG和（或）IgM型的抗β$_2$GPI抗体（滴度>99百分位数），至少检测2次，间隔至少12周。

ELISA：酶联免疫吸附试验；Ig：免疫球蛋白。
[a] 当符合至少1项临床标准和1项实验室标准，即可诊断为抗磷脂综合征。
改编自 Miyakis S, Lockshin MD, Atsumi T, et al: International consensus statement on an update of the classification criteria for definite antiphospholipid syndrome (APS), J Thromb Haemost 4：295-306，2006.

骨骼健康

由于多种因素，患有SLE的女性患骨质疏松的风险增加。其中一些因素为SLE特异性的，如慢性炎症、肾脏疾病、光敏感及避免日晒、药物使用（特别是糖皮质激素）和早发性卵巢衰竭（可能由于SLE或使用CTX引起）。此外，还有骨质疏松的典型危险因素，如吸烟、饮酒、家族史和低体重指数（BMI）。在治疗SLE年轻女性患者的骨质疏松时，谨慎应用双膦酸盐类药物，因为这些药物在妊娠期不安全，且停药后可能存在于体内数年。

心血管健康

随着SLE生存率的提高和治疗方法的改善，以及患者寿命的延长，心血管疾病（CVD）已成为致死和致残的主要原因。SLE患者发生冠状动脉事件的概率是健康人的5～10倍。更需注意的是，35～44岁的绝经前女性患者发生心肌梗死的概率是健康女性的50倍。

尸检系列报道的结果显示，动脉粥样硬化性心脏病是SLE中CVD的潜在机制。SLE中的早发性动脉粥样硬化的原因是多因素的，可能包括炎症介质、与SLE相关的因素（如早发性绝经、皮质类固醇治疗、疾病活动度）以及传统的心血管危险因素。

尽管目前还没有针对SLE患者明确的心血管管理指南，但美国心脏协会在2011年更新的女性CVD预防指南中，首次将自身免疫性疾病（即SLE和类风湿关节炎）纳入了高风险类别。医生应考虑早期动脉粥样硬化性CVD，并积极评估有典型和不典型心脏症状的SLE患者，无论其年龄和性别如何。

继发性抗磷脂综合征

抗磷脂综合征（APS）是一种以血栓形成和（或）妊娠失败风险增加，同时伴有APL（抗磷脂抗体）阳性为主要特征的疾病。"狼疮抗凝物"这个术语使用并不恰当，因为其仅仅反映了体外抗凝作用导致活化部分凝血活酶时间（aPTT）延长，并其不能直接提示SLE的诊断或出血风险的增加。实际上，狼疮抗凝物与血栓发生率增加有关。

APS在不伴其他自身免疫性疾病发生时，被称为原发性APS。而在伴有系统性红斑狼疮或其他自身免疫性疾病时，则被称为继发性APS。原发性或继发性APS的临床表现和治疗非常相似。通常，APS典型临床表现包括动静脉血栓事件、妊娠相关并发症、脑血管和心血管事件、肺动脉高压、利布曼-塞克斯（Libman-Sacks）心内膜炎、神经系统并发症。

灾难性抗磷脂综合征（CAPS）是APS最严重的临床表现，由于微血栓形成，影响多个器官并且伴随着器官迅速衰竭，甚至死亡。CAPS与感染中毒症或血栓性血小板减少性紫癜（TTP）很难区分。

对于患有APS但未出现血栓事件或病理妊娠的患者，没有抗凝治疗的指征。在发生血管栓塞的情况下，通常建议终身抗凝治疗。尽管已经有多种新型口服抗凝剂上市，但华法林仍是APS抗凝的首选药物。普通肝素和低分子量肝素也是治疗APS的有效抗凝剂，可用于在接受华法林治疗期间反复发生血栓的患者或已经怀孕或计划怀孕的患者（表4.7）。

Malignancy

Patients with SLE have an increased risk of solid organ cancers as well as lymphoma. A multicenter international cohort study by SLICC of more than 16,000 SLE patients reported an increased risk of malignancy compared with the general population. Most striking was a 4-fold increased risk of non-Hodgkin's lymphoma. Other hematologic, vulvar, lung, and thyroid cancers were also increased, whereas breast and endometrial cancers were observed less often in lupus. Malignancy risk appears to be highest early in the disease course, but risk remains elevated throughout a patient's lifespan. Although lymph node enlargement is a common manifestation of SLE, physicians must consider malignancy if the lymphadenopathy does not resolve with SLE treatment, is nontender or nonmobile, or if it occurs without other lupus symptoms.

Vaccines

Patients with SLE are at an increased risk of infection due to immune dysregulation in addition to the use of immunosuppressive medications. Vaccines play a vital role in prevention of infections. As a general rule, live attenuated vaccines are contraindicated in lupus patients on biologic therapy or high-dose immunosuppressive treatments with a few exceptions. Patients with SLE should receive pneumococcal vaccines (PCV 13 and 23) and annual influenza vaccine. Patients with SLE have a higher risk of HPV-related cancers, and younger individuals should receive the HPV vaccination to mitigate this risk. There is also an increased risk of latent varicella zoster reactivation. There is now an inactivated vaccine available for the use in immunocompromised individuals such as those with SLE. The long-term safety of this vaccine is still being evaluated.

Psychosocial Effects of Systemic Lupus Erythematosus

When deciding upon management of SLE one must take into consideration other factors that influence outcomes. There is an immune response to acute stress as well as physical and emotional trauma. Although commonly reported by patients, it has been difficult to demonstrate a causal relationship between stress and increased flares in clinical studies. Regardless, anxiety, depression, and social determinants of health can impact adherence to medications and treatment plans as well as overall quality of life and should be considered when caring for patients with lupus.

Fatigue

Fatigue is extremely common in SLE, affecting up to 80% of patients. The cause is often multifactorial, and it is essential to rule out reversible etiologies that may be contributing, such as thyroid disease, depression, non-restorative sleep, obstructive sleep apnea, deconditioning, poor nutrition, celiac disease and nutritional deficiencies, fibromyalgia, and medication side effects. It is often difficult to pinpoint the exact cause of fatigue, and this makes management challenging. Treatment requires addressing the underlying causes of fatigue as well as improving nutrition, sleep, and encouraging aerobic exercise.

Depression and Anxiety

Patients with SLE are at increased risk for depression and anxiety, which have been associated with worse outcomes and medication response. Management of depression and anxiety is essential to the overall treatment of patients with SLE. Along with pharmacologic modalities such as antidepressants and anxiolytics, nonpharmacologic interventions such as psychological counseling, biofeedback, and guided imagery should be incorporated into management of lupus when appropriate.

SUMMARY

Systemic lupus erythematosus is a chronic multisystem autoimmune disease characterized by periods of disease flares and quiescence, and when left untreated it can lead to permanent organ damage and increased mortality. Diagnosis of SLE can be difficult and relies on a combination of clinical and laboratory factors. The Classification Criteria serve as a helpful reminder of common manifestations to aid in diagnosis. The heterogeneity of clinical manifestations of lupus has raised the concept of lupus as a spectrum disorder with different genetic and molecular profiles that define distinct phenotypes requiring customized management strategies.

Antimalarials remain the cornerstone of SLE treatment and have benefits beyond managing lupus disease activity. Immunosuppressive and biologic agents are available for manifestations that are not controlled by antimalarials. It is crucial to recognize the increased risk of comorbidities in lupus, including cardiovascular disease, malignancy, and bone loss. Addressing social determinants of health should be a part of the overall treatment plan in lupus. There is a pipeline of new agents currently being tested to improve management, morbidity, and mortality of patients with SLE.

SUGGESTED READINGS

Arbuckle MR, et al: Development of autoantibodies before clinical onset of systemic lupus erythematosus, N Engl J Med 314:614–619, 1986.

Aringer M, Costenbader K, Daikh D, et al: 2019 European League Against Rheumatism/American College of Rheumatology Classification Criteria for Systemic Lupus Erythematosus, Arthritis Rheumatol 71(9):1400–1412, 2019.

Bernatsky S, Ramsey-Goldman R, Labrecque J: Cancer risk in systemic lupus: an updated international multi-center cohort study, J Autoimmun 42:130–135, 2013.

Borchers AT, Keen CL, Shoenfeld Y, Gershwin ME: Surviving the butterfly and the wolf: mortality trends in systemic lupus erythematosus, Autoimmun Rev 3(6):423–453, 2004.

Buyon JP: Updates on lupus and pregnancy, Bull NYU Hosp Jt Dis 67:271–275, 2009.

Cervera R, Khamashta MA, Font J, et al: Morbidity and mortality in systemic lupus erythematosus during a 10-year period. A comparison of early and late manifestations in a cohort of 1000 patients, Medicine (Baltimore) 82(5):299–308, 2003.

Churg J, Sobin LH: Renal disease: classification and atlas of glomerular disease, Tokyo, 1982, Igaku-Shoin.

Data from Wallace D, Hahn BH: Other clinical laboratory tests in SLE. In Dubois' lupus erythematosus and related syndromes, ed 8, Philadelphia, 2013, Saunders, pp 526–531.

Data modified from Gilliam classification scheme. Gilliam JN, Sontheimer RD: Distinctive cutaneous subsets in the spectrum of lupus erythematosus, J Am Acad Dermatol 4(4):471–475, 1981.

Fanouriakis A, Kostopoulou M, Alunno A, et al: 2019 update of the EULAR recommendations on the management of systemic lupus erythematosus, Ann Rheum Dis 78:736–745, 2019.

Gomez-Puerta J, Barbhaiya M, Guan H, et al: Racial/ethnic variation in all-cause mortality among U.S. medicaid recipients with, systemic lupus erythematosus: an hispanic and asian paradox, Arthritis Rheumatol 67(3):752–760, 2015.

Hochberg MC: Updating the American College of Rheumatology revised criteria for the classification of systemic lupus erythematosus, Arthritis Rheum 40:1725, 1997.

Hull D, Binns BA, Joyce D: Congenital heart block and widespread fibrosis due to maternal lupus erythematosus, Arch Dis Child 41:688–690, 1996.

Izmirly PM, Llanos C, Lee LA, et al: Cutaneous manifestations of neonatal lupus and risk of subsequent congenital heart block, Arthritis Rheumatol 62:1153–1157, 2010.

Llanos C, Izmirly PM, Katholi M, et al: Recurrence rates of cardiac manifestations associated with neonatal lupus and maternal/fetal risk factors, Arthritis Rheumatol 60:3091–3097, 2009.

Manzi S, Meilahn EN, Rairie JE, et al: Age-specific incidence rates of MI and angina in women with SLE: comparison with Framingham study, Am J Epidemiol 145(5):408–415, 1997.

恶性肿瘤

SLE 患者罹患实体器官癌症和淋巴瘤的风险较高。根据 SLICC 对 16 000 多名 SLE 患者进行的一项多中心国际队列研究显示，与普通人群相比，SLE 患者罹患恶性肿瘤的风险增加。其中非霍奇金淋巴瘤的风险甚至增加了 4 倍，而其他血液系统疾病、外阴癌、肺癌和甲状腺癌的发生率也有所增加，但乳腺癌和子宫内膜癌的发生率较低。恶性肿瘤的风险似乎在疾病病程初期最高，但在患者的整个生命周期内风险仍持续升高。淋巴结肿大是 SLE 的常见临床表现，但当淋巴结肿大在接受 SLE 治疗后仍不消退，无触痛或不移动，或者在出现淋巴结肿大时没有其他狼疮症状时，医生需考虑恶性肿瘤。

疫苗

除使用免疫抑制剂外，SLE 患者的免疫紊乱也增加了感染的风险。因此，疫苗在预防感染方面起着至关重要的作用。一般来说，接受生物制剂或大剂量免疫抑制剂治疗的狼疮患者禁用减毒活疫苗，但也有少数例外。对于 SLE 患者来说，应当接种肺炎球菌疫苗（PCV 13 和 23）和年度流感疫苗。SLE 患者患人乳头瘤病毒（HPV）相关癌症的风险较高，因此年轻患者应接种 HPV 疫苗以降低这种风险。同时潜伏性水痘-带状疱疹再活化的风险也增加。目前已有一种灭活水痘疫苗可用于狼疮等免疫妥协人群，但其长期安全性仍在评估中。

社会心理影响

在决定如何治疗 SLE 时，必须考虑影响治疗效果的其他因素。急性应激以及身体和精神创伤会引起免疫反应，尽管患者经常出现这类问题，但在临床研究中很难证明压力与复发增加之间存在因果关系。焦虑、抑郁及健康的社会决定因素会影响患者对药物和治疗计划的依从性以及整体生活质量，因此在护理狼疮患者时应考虑这些因素。

疲乏

疲乏在 SLE 中极为常见，多达 80% 的患者会出现疲乏。造成疲乏的原因通常是多方面的，需排除可能导致疲乏的可逆病因，如甲状腺疾病、抑郁、睡眠质量不佳、阻塞性睡眠呼吸暂停综合征、体力下降、营养不良、乳糜泻及营养缺乏、纤维肌痛以及药物不良作用等。一般很难确定导致疲乏的确切原因，这也给治疗带来了一定的挑战。治疗需要解决引起疲劳的根本原因，同时改善营养摄入、睡眠质量，并鼓励患者进行有氧运动。

抑郁和焦虑

SLE 患者抑郁和焦虑的风险更高，这与较差的预后和药物反应密切相关。因此，控制抑郁和焦虑对于 SLE 患者的整体治疗至关重要。除抗抑郁及抗焦虑药物治疗外，心理咨询、生物反馈和引导想象等合适的非药物干预也可改善患者的精神症状。

总结

系统性红斑狼疮是一种慢性多系统的自身免疫性疾病，其特点是疾病活动期和稳定期交替，如不及时治疗，可能导致永久性器官损伤和死亡率升高。SLE 的诊断比较困难，需要综合考虑临床和实验室因素。分类标准有助于提示常见的临床表现，并帮助进行诊断。由于狼疮临床表现的异质性，因此提出了该疾病是一种谱系疾病的概念。不同的基因和分子特征定义了不同的表型，需要制订个体化的管理策略。

抗疟药仍然是 SLE 治疗的基石，在控制狼疮的疾病活动同时还有其他受益。若抗疟药无法控制病情，可以考虑使用免疫抑制剂和生物制剂进行治疗。需要注意狼疮患者并发心血管疾病、恶性肿瘤和骨质疏松的风险增加。因此，在整体治疗计划中应纳入解决健康的社会决定因素问题。目前有一系列新药正在进行临床试验，以期改善 SLE 患者的疾病管理、发病率和死亡率。

推荐阅读

Arbuckle MR, et al: Development of autoantibodies before clinical onset of systemic lupus erythematosus, N Engl J Med 314:614–619, 1986.

Aringer M, Costenbader K, Daikh D, et al: 2019 European League Against Rheumatism/American College of Rheumatology Classification Criteria for Systemic Lupus Erythematosus, Arthritis Rheumatol 71(9):1400–1412, 2019.

Bernatsky S, Ramsey-Goldman R, Labrecque J: Cancer risk in systemic lupus: an updated international multi-center cohort study, J Autoimmun 42:130–135, 2013.

Borchers AT, Keen CL, Shoenfeld Y, Gershwin ME: Surviving the butterfly and the wolf: mortality trends in systemic lupus erythematosus, Autoimmun Rev 3(6):423–453, 2004.

Buyon JP: Updates on lupus and pregnancy, Bull NYU Hosp Jt Dis 67:271–275, 2009.

Cervera R, Khamashta MA, Font J, et al: Morbidity and mortality in systemic lupus erythematosus during a 10-year period. A comparison of early and late manifestations in a cohort of 1000 patients, Medicine (Baltimore) 82(5):299–308, 2003.

Churg J, Sobin LH: Renal disease: classification and atlas of glomerular disease, Tokyo, 1982, Igaku-Shoin.

Data from Wallace D, Hahn BH: Other clinical laboratory tests in SLE. In Dubois' lupus erythematosus and related syndromes, ed 8, Philadelphia, 2013, Saunders, pp 526–531.

Data modified from Gilliam classification scheme. Gilliam JN, Sontheimer RD: Distinctive cutaneous subsets in the spectrum of lupus erythematosus, J Am Acad Dermatol 4(4):471–475, 1981.

Fanouriakis A, Kostopoulou M, Alunno A, et al: 2019 update of the EULAR recommendations on the management of systemic lupus erythematosus, Ann Rheum Dis 78:736–745, 2019.

Gomez-Puerta J, Barbhaiya M, Guan H, et al: Racial/ethnic variation in all-cause mortality among U.S. medicaid recipients with, systemic lupus erythematosus: an hispanic and asian paradox, Arthritis Rheumatol 67(3):752–760, 2015.

Hochberg MC: Updating the American College of Rheumatology revised criteria for the classification of systemic lupus erythematosus, Arthritis Rheum 40:1725, 1997.

Hull D, Binns BA, Joyce D: Congenital heart block and widespread fibrosis due to maternal lupus erythematosus, Arch Dis Child 41:688–690, 1996.

Izmirly PM, Llanos C, Lee LA, et al: Cutaneous manifestations of neonatal lupus and risk of subsequent congenital heart block, Arthritis Rheumatol 62:1153–1157, 2010.

Llanos C, Izmirly PM, Katholi M, et al: Recurrence rates of cardiac manifestations associated with neonatal lupus and maternal/fetal risk factors, Arthritis Rheumatol 60:3091–3097, 2009.

Manzi S, Meilahn EN, Rairie JE, et al: Age-specific incidence rates of MI and angina in women with SLE: comparison with Framingham study, Am J Epidemiol 145(5):408–415, 1997.

Marmor MF, Kellner U, Lai TYY, et al: Recommendations on Screening for Chloroquine and Hydroxychloroquine Retinopathy (2016 Revision), Ophthalmology 123(6):1386–1394, 2016.

Merola JF, Bermas B, Lu B, et al: Clinical manifestations and survival among adults with SLE according to age of diagnosis, Lupus 23(8):778–784, 2014.

Merrell M, Shulman LE: Determination of prognosis in chronic disease, illustrated by systemic lupus erythematosus, J Chronic Dis 1(1):12–32, 1955.

Modified from Miyakis S, Lockshin MD, Atsumi T, et al: International consensus statement on an update of the classification criteria for definite antiphospholipid syndrome (APS), J Thromb Haemost 4:295-306, 2006.

Modified from Petri M, Orbai AM, Alarcón GS, et al: Derivation and validation of Systemic Lupus International Collaborating Clinics classification criteria for systemic lupus erythematosus, Arthritis Rheum 64: 2677–2686, 2012.

Mosca L, Benjamin EJ, Berra K, et al: Circulation 123(11):1243–1262, 2011.

Petri M, Kim MY, Kalunian KC, et al: Combined oral contraceptives in women with systemic lupus erythematosus, N Engl J Med 353(24):2550–2558, 2005.

Sánchez-Guerrero J, Uribe AG, Jiménez-Santana L, et al: A trial of contraceptive methods in women with systemic lupus erythematosus, N Engl J Med 353(24):2539–2549, 2005.

Stojan G, Petri M: Epidemiology of systemic lupus erythematosus: an update, Curr Opin Rheumatol 30(2):144–150, 2018.

Tan EM, Cohen AS, Fries, et al: The 1982 revised criteria of the classification of systemic lupus erythematosus, Arthritis Rheum 25:1271, 1982.

Tench CM, McCurdie I, White PD, D'Cruz DP: The prevalence and associations of fatigue in systemic lupus erythematosus, Rheumatology 39(11):1249–1254, 2000.

Weening JJ, D'Agati VD, Schwartz MM, et al: Classification of glomerulonephritis in systemic lupus erythematosus revisited, Kidney Int 65:521–530, 2004.

Marmor MF, Kellner U, Lai TYY, et al: Recommendations on Screening for Chloroquine and Hydroxychloroquine Retinopathy (2016 Revision), Ophthalmology 123(6):1386–1394, 2016.

Merola JF, Bermas B, Lu B, et al: Clinical manifestations and survival among adults with SLE according to age of diagnosis, Lupus 23(8):778–784, 2014.

Merrell M, Shulman LE: Determination of prognosis in chronic disease, illustrated by systemic lupus erythematosus, J Chronic Dis 1(1):12–32, 1955.

Modified from Miyakis S, Lockshin MD, Atsumi T, et al: International consensus statement on an update of the classification criteria for definite antiphospholipid syndrome (APS), J Thromb Haemost 4:295-306, 2006.

Modified from Petri M, Orbai AM, Alarcón GS, et al: Derivation and validation of Systemic Lupus International Collaborating Clinics classification criteria for systemic lupus erythematosus, Arthritis Rheum 64: 2677–2686, 2012.

Mosca L, Benjamin EJ, Berra K, et al: Circulation 123(11):1243–1262, 2011.

Petri M, Kim MY, Kalunian KC, et al: Combined oral contraceptives in women with systemic lupus erythematosus, N Engl J Med 353(24):2550–2558, 2005.

Sánchez-Guerrero J, Uribe AG, Jiménez-Santana L, et al: A trial of contraceptive methods in women with systemic lupus erythematosus, N Engl J Med 353(24):2539–2549, 2005.

Stojan G, Petri M: Epidemiology of systemic lupus erythematosus: an update, Curr Opin Rheumatol 30(2):144–150, 2018.

Tan EM, Cohen AS, Fries, et al: The 1982 revised criteria of the classification of systemic lupus erythematosus, Arthritis Rheum 25:1271, 1982.

Tench CM, McCurdie I, White PD, D'Cruz DP: The prevalence and associations of fatigue in systemic lupus erythematosus, Rheumatology 39(11):1249–1254, 2000.

Weening JJ, D'Agati VD, Schwartz MM, et al: Classification of glomerulonephritis in systemic lupus erythematosus revisited, Kidney Int 65:521–530, 2004.

Systemic Sclerosis

Anna Papazoglou, Robyn T. Domsic

INTRODUCTION

Systemic sclerosis (SSc) is a multisystem, autoimmune disease characterized by cutaneous and visceral fibrosis. The more common term for the disease, *scleroderma*, reflects this hallmark feature as it is derived from the Greek *scleros*, which means thick, and *derma*, which means skin. The pathology and damage from the disease reflects a complex interplay of vascular injury, immune system activation, and excessive fibrosis.

The disorder can range from a relatively benign condition to a rapidly progressive disease leading to significant morbidity or death. Although cutaneous manifestations are the most obvious features, visceral and vascular involvement can be severe and disabling. Monitoring for potential organ complications is essential in caring for SSc patients because early detection and treatment may minimize morbidity and mortality. There is ongoing research aiming to increase in-depth understanding of the complex mechanisms leading to SSc, which would facilitate the discovery of curative treatment.

EPIDEMIOLOGY

The annual US incidence of SSc is approximately 32 cases per million persons and the estimated prevalence is 254 cases per million persons. Incidence and prevalence vary somewhat throughout the world, and they typically are lower in Europe and Asia. SSc more commonly affects women, with a 3-5:1 female-to-male ratio. It occurs in individuals of all ages, from childhood to the elderly, but it most frequently affects those between the ages of 40 and 60 years. There are studies that indicate differences in the frequency and severity of SSc clinical manifestations as well as complications between men and women.

A familial pattern of inheritance is not as evident in SSc as in other connective tissue diseases, although first-degree relatives appear to be at somewhat increased risk. Twin studies have demonstrated only a 5% rate of concordance in monozygotic and dizygotic twins, implying that there are significant environmental contributions to its occurrence. Many patients with SSc, however, have family histories of other autoimmune diseases (e.g., thyroid disease, rheumatoid arthritis, systemic lupus erythematosus [SLE]). Genome-wide association studies have revealed a handful of genes associated with SSc that are shared with other diseases such as rheumatoid arthritis and SLE (e.g., major histocompatibility complex class I and II genes, *STAT4, IRF5, TNFSF4, IRF8*). These findings suggest a shared genetic predisposition to autoimmune conditions.

PATHOLOGY

The pathogenesis of SSc remains unclear. A combination of genetic and environmental factors results in complicated interaction of three clearly identified components, consisting of vascular abnormalities, immunologic abnormalities and extracellular membrane abnormalities leading to tissue fibrosis, the hallmark of SSc (Fig. 5.1).

The initial event is postulated to be tissue injury including endothelial damage with subsequent endothelial cell activation and chemokine production as well as vascular injury. Vascular damage is characterized by vascular obliteration, defective vasculogenesis, and tissue hypoxia. Vascular changes are seen in the skin and may also occur in the pulmonary, cardiac, and renal blood vessels, affecting arteries, arterioles, and capillaries. True vasculitis is conspicuously absent. Early vascular involvement consists of an imbalance between vasodilatory and vasoconstrictive factors, endothelial cell activation with resultant leukocyte migration and smooth muscle cell proliferation.

Immune system activation is evident in several respects. The secretion of multiple chemokines leads to perpetuating cycles of inflammation and autoimmunity. SSc-associated autoantibodies are detected in more than 95% of patients with SSc. All 10 of the recognized SSc-associated autoantibodies are directed against distinct nuclear antigens. They are helpful in classifying patients, but their pathogenic role has not been clarified. There is evidence of T-cell activation, with a T_H2-predominant cytokine profile. Elevated levels of interleukins (i.e., IL-1, IL-2, IL-2R, IL-4, IL-8, IL-13, and IL-17) and interferon have been reported. The role of T_H17 cells is not understood, but studies suggest that dysregulation of these proinflammatory T cells contributes to disease pathogenesis. In addition, there is increasing evidence of innate immune dysregulation in the setting of activated macrophages and altered expression and function of toll-like receptors.

The complex interplay between the chemokines produced by the inflammatory cells leads to activation of fibroblasts and presumed differentiation into myofibroblast. As such, there is overproduction of extracellular matrix, which results in progressively worsening fibrosis. Of note, fibroblasts are found in increased numbers in the skin and other tissues, and they develop an SSc phenotype when grown in vitro, producing an overabundance of collagen and living longer in tissue culture. Fibroblast persistence in culture suggests a perpetuated abnormality not requiring continued immune stimulation. Over the past decades, increasing evidence suggests that macrophages are important in the pathogenesis of systemic sclerosis through secretion of inflammatory cytokines; however, their exact role needs to be further clarified. Transforming growth factor β (TGF-β), specifically, is secreted by macrophages and has been found to have effect on the fibrotic mechanism through regulation of fibroblast function as well as various important processes in fibrosis.

CLINICAL PRESENTATION

Patients with SSc can have several clinical presentations, although Raynaud's phenomenon is the most common symptom (>95%). Distinctive phenotypes may manifest differently. SSc can have many

系统性硬化症

周佳鑫 译　徐东　田新平 审校　李梦涛 通审

引言

系统性硬化症（SSc）是一种多系统受累的自身免疫性疾病，其特征为皮肤和内脏纤维化。该病另一个更常用的名称，硬皮病（scleroderma），反映了疾病的特征，其源于希腊语scleros，意思是增厚的，以及derma，意思是皮肤。该病的病理学和损伤过程反映了血管损伤、免疫系统活化，以及过度纤维化之间一系列复杂的相互作用。

该病的表现可从相对较轻的状态，到快速进展性疾病导致严重合并症或死亡。虽然皮肤表现是本病最明显的临床特征，但该病也可出现严重的内脏和血管受累并导致功能障碍。由于早期发现并进行治疗可最大程度上降低发病率和死亡率，因此在诊治SSc患者时，监测可能的脏器合并症很重要。目前已有研究正在进行中，以期更深入地认识SSc复杂的发病机制，这也有助于发现更好的治疗方案。

流行病学

SSc在美国的年发病率约为32/100万人，预计的患病率为254/100万人。该病的发病率和患病率在世界的不同地区存在差异，在欧洲及亚洲更低。SSc更常影响女性，女：男的比率为（3～5）：1。该病各年龄阶段均可受累，从儿童到老年，但最常累及40～60岁之间的人群。有研究表明在男性和女性患者之间，SSc的临床表现的发生率和严重度存在差异。

尽管SSc患者的一级亲属发生SSc的风险有所增高，但和其他结缔组织病相比，SSc的家族遗传倾向相对较轻。针对双胞胎的研究表明在同卵和异卵双胞胎中仅有5%的可能同时患病，提示在该病的发生中环境因素起着重要的作用。然而，很多SSc患者具有其他自身免疫性疾病的家族史［如甲状腺疾病、类风湿关节炎、系统性红斑狼疮（SLE）］。全基因组关联研究发现SSc与其他疾病如类风湿关节炎和SLE享有少数相同的基因（如主要组织相容性复合体Ⅰ和Ⅱ基因，STAT4，IRF5，TNFSF4，IRF8）。这些发现表明自身免疫性疾病可能存在共有的遗传倾向。

病理学

SSc的发病机制目前尚不清楚。基因和环境因素共同导致了三种已知发病过程的复杂相互作用，包括血管异常、免疫学异常和细胞外膜异常导致组织纤维化，后者是SSc的特征性表现（图5.1）。

目前的假说认为最早发生的事件是组织损伤，包括内皮损伤并进一步导致内皮细胞活化，以及趋化因子产生和血管损伤。血管损伤的特征包括血管闭塞，血管生成缺陷和组织缺氧。血管病变可见于皮肤，也可发生于肺、心，以及肾脏的血管，影响动脉、小动脉，以及毛细血管。真性血管炎明显是不存在的。早期血管受累主要表现为血管舒张和血管收缩因素之间的失衡，内皮细胞活化及由此产生的白细胞迁移和平滑肌细胞增生。

免疫系统活化在某些方面明显。多种趋化因子的释放会导致炎症和自身免疫的持续存在。多于95%的SSc患者中可以检测出SSc相关的自身抗体。已知的10种SSc相关自身抗体均直接作用于特定的核抗原。这些抗体有助于患者分类，但是它们的病理机制尚不明确。患者体内存在T细胞活化的证据，及以TH2为主的细胞因子特征。已报告多种白介素（如IL-1、IL-2、IL-2R、IL-4、IL-8、IL-13和IL-17）以及干扰素水平增高。TH17细胞的作用尚不明确，但是研究表明这类促炎T细胞的失调参与了疾病的发生。此外，越来越多的证据表明在巨噬细胞活化和Toll样受体表达和功能改变的背景下存在固有免疫失调。

炎症细胞所分泌趋化因子之间复杂的相互作用导致成纤维细胞活化，并向肌成纤维细胞分化。同样地，细胞外基质过度生成，并导致进行性加重的纤维化。值得强调的是，在皮肤和其他组织中发现了增多的成纤维细胞，体外研究表明它们可向SSc的表型分化，分泌过量的胶原并能在组织培养中长期存活。体外培养中成纤维细胞的持续存活表明它们可永久存在而不需要持续的免疫刺激。在过去的数十年中，愈来愈多的证据表明巨噬细胞通过分泌炎症因子在系统性硬化症的发病机制中起着重要作用；然而，它们的具体作用还需进一步研究证实。需特别指出的是，转化生长因子-β（TGF-β）由巨噬细胞分泌，已发现可通过调节成纤维细胞功能以及纤维化的多个重要过程，在纤维化的发生中发挥作用。

临床表现

SSc患者最常见的症状为雷诺现象（>95%），此外也会有多种临床表现。不同的临床表型可能会有不

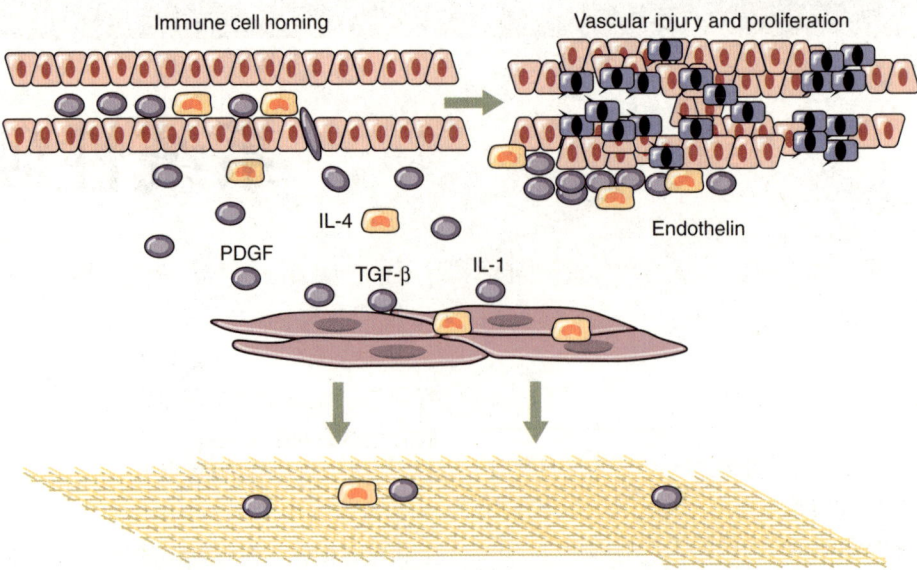

Fig. 5.1 Pathogenetic processes in systemic sclerosis. Vascular injury leads to intimal proliferation of endothelial cells *(red)* and smooth muscle cells *(blue with black nuclei)*. Immune cells consisting of T cells *(blue, small)* and monocyte/macrophages *(yellow with orange nuclei)* are activated and home to sites in the dermis. Fibroblasts are activated to deposit increased amounts of interstitial matrix. *IL,* Interleukin; *PDGF,* platelet-derived growth factor; *TGF-β,* transforming growth factor-β.

internal organ manifestations, producing various clinical presentations and requiring tailored work-up protocols.

Classification by Cutaneous Features

Historically, SSc has been separated into two major clinical subsets defined by the degree and extent of skin involvement: limited cutaneous (lc) and diffuse cutaneous (dc) disease. Patients with lcSSc experience skin thickening limited to the distal extremities (i.e., below the elbows and knees) as well as the face. The dcSSc patients have similar distal changes in addition to involvement of the upper arms, thighs, or trunk at some time during the disease course. Few patients (<1%) have no skin thickening but have one or more typical SSc visceral manifestations. The term *scleroderma sine scleroderma* has been used to describe patients with minimal or no skin involvement whose clinical course resembles that of individuals with lcSSc.

The distinct cutaneous patterns are important, because patients with dcSSc are more likely to develop internal organ complications (e.g., renal crisis, cardiac involvement) early in their illness, whereas those with lcSSc can develop internal organ involvement at any point throughout their disease, even decades after the initial symptoms. Several classification criteria have been suggested that do not particularly assist in diagnosis of SSc but are rather intended primarily to help classify SSc patients for studies (Table 5.1). These clinical characteristics are derived from a long-standing registry at the University of Pittsburgh. Some patients with lcSSc or dcSSc may have typical features of another connective tissue disease (most commonly polymyositis, SLE, or rheumatoid arthritis-like features), and they are considered to have *SSc in overlap*.

Of note, as an attempt for early identification of individuals at risk for future development of SSc, the Very Early Diagnosis of Systemic Sclerosis (VEDOSS) approach has been considered recently as a potentially useful tool for predicting SSc disease development. Its role in clinical and research work at this time still requires better understanding. This approach, which includes patients with manifestations of Raynaud's phenomenon, puffy fingers, certain positive SSc antibodies, and reported nailfold capillaroscopy changes, may be helpful in identifying those at risk for developing established disease over shorter-term follow-up.

Serologic Classification

Serologic classification refers to SSc-associated serum autoantibodies. Patients with the same autoantibody tend to have a similar cutaneous pattern, natural history of disease, and risk of internal organ involvement.

Serologic classification can augment the clinical classification described previously. For example, 95% of patients with anticentromere antibody have lcSSc and are at increased risk for pulmonary hypertension during the course of the disease. Individuals with anti–topoisomerase I (i.e., anti-SCL70) or anti–RNA polymerase III antibody are more likely to have dcSSc. Those with anti–RNA polymerase III antibody have an increased risk of renal crisis, and those with anti-SCL70 have a higher frequency of interstitial lung disease.

The primary internal organ risks and cutaneous associations are depicted in Fig. 5.2, which illustrates the combined clinical-serologic classification of SSc. It is uncommon for patients to have more than one SSc autoantibody.

Raynaud's Phenomenon and Peripheral Vascular Involvement

Nearly all patients with SSc experience Raynaud's phenomenon during their disease course, often as the initial symptom. Raynaud's phenomenon is a triphasic vasospastic response to cold consisting of pallor (i.e., blanching) with or without cyanosis (i.e., bluish discoloration followed by reactive hyperemia manifested by erythema) with a characteristic distinct line of demarcation on the digits separating the affected from unaffected areas.

The onset of Raynaud's phenomenon can precede the development of skin changes by years in some patients. Beyond Raynaud's phenomenon, SSc patients can develop progressive peripheral vasculopathy. This may lead to loss of digital tip tissue with resulting digital pitting scars, ulcers, or gangrene (rare) that can lead to autoamputation. Digital tip ulcers occur more frequently in patients who are anticentromere or

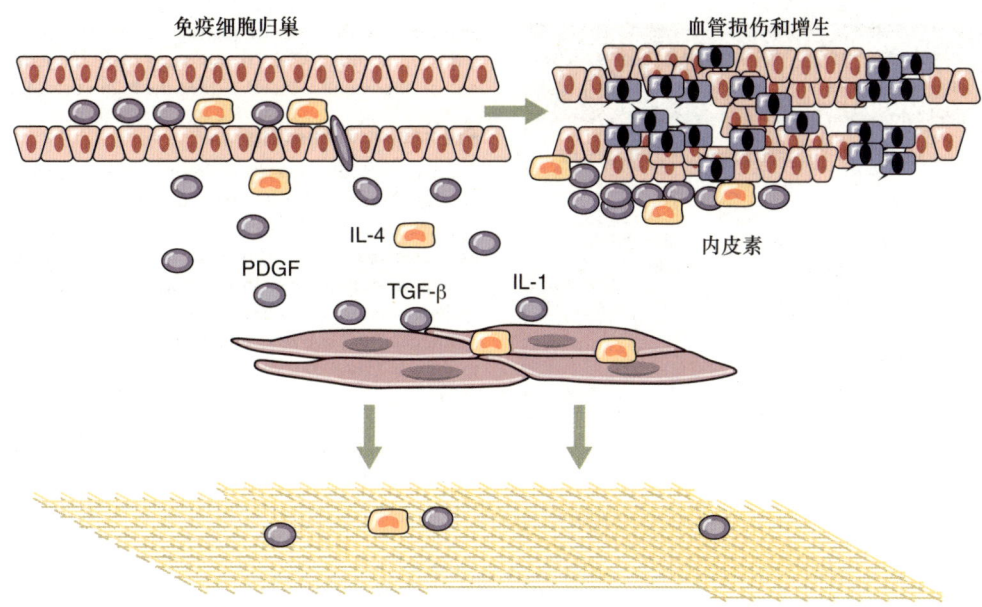

图 5.1 系统性硬化症的发病过程。血管损伤导致内皮细胞（红色）和平滑肌细胞（蓝色黑核）的内膜增生。由 T 细胞（蓝色，小）和单核细胞/巨噬细胞（黄色橙核）组成的免疫细胞被活化并归巢至真皮。成纤维细胞被活化使数量增多的间质基质沉积。IL，白介素；PDGF，血小板源性生长因子；TGF-β，转化生长因子-β

同的临床表现。SSc 患者可能会出现多个内脏受累，从而导致不同的临床表现，需要针对性的诊疗流程。

通过皮肤特征进行分类

长期以来，根据皮肤受累的程度和范围，SSc 被分为两种临床亚型，局限皮肤型（lc）和弥漫皮肤型（dc）疾病。lcSSc 患者的皮肤增厚局限于肢体远端（即，肘和膝的远端）以及面部。dcSSc 患者有类似的远端改变，在疾病发展过程中，可有上臂、大腿，以及躯干部位受累。极少数患者（＜1%）可没有皮肤增厚，但有一种或者更多的 SSc 典型的内脏受累表现。对于那些临床病程与 lcSSc 类似但是没有皮肤硬化或者仅有非常轻微皮肤硬化的患者，称为无硬皮的硬皮病。

上述皮肤分型具有重要意义，因为 dcSSc 患者更可能在疾病早期出现内脏受累（如肾危象、心脏受累），而 lcSSc 患者可在疾病的任何阶段出现内脏受累，甚至是在首发症状的数十年后。目前 SSc 有多种分类标准，但并非特意用来诊断 SSc，更多的是帮助对 SSc 患者进行分类来研究（表 5.1）。这些临床特征来源于匹兹堡大学的一个长期注册队列。部分 lcSSc 或者 dcSSc 患者可能会具有其他结缔组织病的典型表现（最常见的为多肌炎、SLE，或类风湿关节炎样的表现），他们被认为有 SSc 重叠综合征。

需要强调的是，为尝试早期发现将来可能发展为 SSc 的高危患者，近期提出的系统性硬化症极早期诊断（VEDOSS）模型可能会成为预测 SSc 发生的有力工具。该模型目前在临床和科研工作中的价值还需更深入的理解。该模型包括雷诺现象、手指肿胀、某种 SSc 抗体阳性，以及甲襞微循环异常，可能有助于确定在短期随访后具有发展为明确 SSc 风险的患者。

血清学分类

血清学分类主要是基于 SSc 相关的血清自身抗体。具有同种自身抗体的患者可能会有类似的皮肤表现、疾病自然病程，以及内脏受累的风险。

血清学分类可进一步强化上面提及的临床分型。例如，95% 的抗着丝点抗体阳性的患者表现为 lcSSc，在病程中出现肺动脉高压的风险增加。抗拓扑异构酶Ⅰ（即抗 -SCL70 抗体）或抗 -RNA 聚合酶Ⅲ抗体阳性的患者更有可能表现为 dcSSc。抗 -RNA 聚合酶Ⅲ抗体阳性患者出现肾危象的风险增加，而抗 -SCL70 抗体阳性的患者更有可能出现间质性肺病。

图 5.2 显示了主要内脏受累风险和皮肤受累的相关性，说明了 SSc 的临床 - 血清学联合分类。患者很少会出现一种以上 SSc 自身抗体。

雷诺现象和外周血管受累

几乎所有的 SSc 患者在病程中都会出现雷诺现象，且通常为首发症状。雷诺现象指遇冷后出现的三相程血管痉挛反应，包括苍白（即，指端变白），可伴或不伴发绀（即，变成青黑色，之后反应性充血而变红），同时在指端的受累部位和未受累部位间存在一条明确的分界线。

部分患者雷诺现象可以在皮肤病变出现数年之前发生。除雷诺现象之外，SSc 患者能出现进展性的周围血管病变。这可以引起指尖部位组织缺失产生指尖凹陷性瘢痕、溃疡或者坏疽（罕见）而导致截肢。指尖溃疡更多见于抗着丝点抗体或抗拓扑异构酶Ⅰ抗体阳

TABLE 5.1 Manifestations of Systemic Sclerosis by Clinical Classification in the Pittsburgh Scleroderma Center Database

Manifestations	Diffuse (N = 1646)	Limited (N = 2124)
Cutaneous		
Puffy fingers	83%	80%
Skin induration, thickening	Widespread: trunk, face, extremities	Face, below the elbow and knee
Telangiectasias	62%	65%
Calcinosis	10%	13%
Peripheral Vascular		
Raynaud's phenomenon	95%	98%
Digital ulcerations	41%	37%
Pulmonary		
Interstitial lung disease	38%	34%
Pulmonary arterial hypertension	6%	18%
Cardiac		
Arrhythmias	12%	10%
Diastolic dysfunction	7%	9%
Myocarditis	3%	1%
Pericarditis	3%	2%
Renal		
Renal crisis	16%	3%
Gastrointestinal		
Esophageal hypomotility, reflux	84%	83%
Small intestine dysmotility	11%	8%
Malabsorption	5%	4%
Incontinence	3%	4%
Joint and Musculoskeletal		
Tendon friction rubs	51%	6%
Joint contractures	87%	37%
Myositis	6%	7%

Data from the University of Pittsburgh Scleroderma Databank, 1980-2018.

anti–topoisomerase I autoantibody positive. Lower extremity ulcerations in SSc patients have been increasingly reported in recent years.

Interstitial Lung Disease

Interstitial lung disease (ILD) can be one of the most serious complications of SSc and should be monitored for routinely, because it plays a major role in mortality and morbidity. The initial presentation is often a nonproductive cough and a gradual onset of dyspnea on exertion over several months to years. However, the onset can be abrupt.

High-resolution chest computed tomography (CT) typically shows bibasilar fibrotic changes, which can be progressive. Pulmonary function tests reveal reduced forced vital capacity (FVC). On pathologic examination, the most frequently seen pattern is nonspecific interstitial pneumonitis (NSIP) or fibrosing NSIP. Patients with anti-SCL70 autoantibody and U11/U12 are at the highest risk for ILD.

Pulmonary Hypertension

SSc patients can develop pulmonary hypertension of three World Health Organization (WHO) classifications. Pulmonary arterial hypertension (PAH, WHO group 1) is the most common, with an estimated 10% to 15% of patients in cohort studies developing PAH. It occurs most commonly in those with lcSSc. The clinical presentation includes rapidly progressive dyspnea occurring over several months. Pulmonary function tests reveal a reduced diffusion capacity for carbon monoxide (D_{LCO}) out of proportion to any concomitant reduction in the FVC.

Less frequently, SSc patients develop pulmonary hypertension associated with ILD (WHO group 3) or pulmonary hypertension associated with left ventricular diastolic dysfunction from myocardial fibrosis or non–SSc-associated left ventricular disorders (WHO group 2). Screening for all types of pulmonary hypertension is performed by echocardiogram, and results should be confirmed by right heart cardiac catheterization.

Scleroderma Renal Crisis

Scleroderma renal crisis (SRC) manifests as the abrupt onset of accelerated arterial hypertension accompanied by a rise in serum creatinine levels and by microscopic hematuria and proteinuria on urinalysis. Microangiopathic hemolytic anemia and thrombocytopenia are common. Although once the major cause of mortality in SSc, SRC is now managed by aggressive blood pressure control with an angiotensin-converting enzyme (ACE) inhibitor, which should be maintained lifelong.

The typical setting for SRC is early dcSSc with a recent increase in skin thickening, palpable tendon friction rubs, and anti–RNA polymerase III antibody. During active, early dcSSc, patients should check their blood pressure once weekly and report a rise in systolic blood pressure of more than 20 mm Hg from baseline. Prednisone given at a dose of 15 mg daily or higher has been associated with the development of SRC and should be avoided in at-risk patients.

Cardiac Manifestations

In general, all cardiac structures may be affected with subsequent serious functional consequences. Underlying PAH contributes as well to cardiac manifestations of SSc. Patients with SSc have three primary types of cardiac involvement: pericarditis, myocarditis, and myocardial fibrosis. The latter can lead to congestive heart failure and arrhythmias due to fibrosis of the conduction system. These complications can be asymptomatic and underrecognized in SSc patients, but pathologic changes have been found in 70% of patients in older autopsy series. Later studies using cardiac magnetic resonance imaging (MRI) have supported the autopsy findings of subclinical cardiac involvement.

Diastolic dysfunction is becoming increasingly recognized as a complication of fibrosis and can be evaluated by echocardiogram during pulmonary hypertension screening. Many SSc deaths occur suddenly, possibly due to ventricular arrhythmias. It is prudent to obtain a resting electrocardiogram early in the disease course. Palpitations noticed by the patient should be addressed with a formal cardiac arrhythmia evaluation.

Gastrointestinal Tract Manifestations

At least one gastrointestinal manifestation will affect 80% or more of SSc patients, and all areas of the gastrointestinal tract may be affected. Gastrointestinal involvement is a significant cause of morbidity.

表 5.1　系统性硬化症临床分类表现——匹兹堡硬皮病中心数据库

临床表现	弥漫型（n = 1646）	局限型（n = 2124）
皮肤		
手指肿胀	83%	80%
皮肤硬化，增厚	弥漫分布：躯干，颜面，肢体	颜面、肘和膝部远端
毛细血管扩张	62%	65%
钙化	10%	13%
周围血管		
雷诺现象	95%	98%
指溃疡	41%	37%
肺		
间质性肺病	38%	34%
（动脉型）肺动脉高压	6%	18%
心脏		
心律失常	12%	10%
舒张功能障碍	7%	9%
心肌炎	3%	1%
心包炎	3%	2%
肾脏		
肾危象	16%	3%
胃肠道		
食管动力减低，反流	84%	83%
小肠动力障碍	11%	8%
吸收不良	5%	4%
大便失禁	3%	4%
关节和肌肉骨骼		
肌腱摩擦感	51%	6%
关节挛缩	87%	37%
肌炎	6%	7%

引自 the University of Pittsburgh Scleroderma Databank，1980-2018.

性的患者。近年来，SSc 患者合并下肢溃疡的报道也逐渐增加。

间质性肺病

间质性肺病（ILD）是 SSc 患者最严重的并发症之一，由于其在死亡率和发病率中扮演了重要的角色，因此需要常规监测。初始的表现常为干咳，在数月乃至数年后逐渐发生活动后气短。然而，该病也可以突然发生。

高分辨胸部 CT 的典型表现为双肺底部纤维化改变，可逐渐进展。肺功能检查表现为用力肺活量（FVC）下降。病理检查最常见的类型为非特异性间质性肺炎（NSIP）或者纤维化型 NSIP。抗-SCL70 抗体和抗-U11/U12 自身抗体阳性的患者出现 ILD 的风险最高。

肺动脉高压

SSc 患者可出现 3 种世界卫生组织（WHO）分类的肺动脉高压。动脉型肺动脉高压（PAH，WHO 1 组）是最常见的，队列研究中估计 10%～15% 的患者出现 PAH。其最常见于 lcSSc 患者。临床表现包括在数月内快速进展的气短。肺功能检查提示一氧化碳弥散量（D_{Lco}）减低，与共同发生的 FVC 的减低不成比例。

更少见的，SSc 患者出现与 ILD 相关的肺动脉高压（WHO 3 组）或心肌纤维化导致的左心舒张功能障碍或非 SSc 相关的左心室疾病相关肺动脉高压（WHO 2 组）。各种肺动脉高压的筛查主要依靠超声心动图，结果需要通过右心导管检查证实。

硬皮病肾危象

硬皮病肾危象（SRC）表现为突然开始的加速的动脉高血压，同时有血清肌酐水平升高，尿检镜下血尿和蛋白尿。微血管病性溶血性贫血和血小板减少常见。尽管 SRC 曾为 SSc 主要的死亡因素，目前可通过使用血管紧张素转换酶（ACE）抑制剂积极控制血压来处理，应终身维持。

典型的 SRC 多见于早期 dcSSc 患者，伴近期皮肤硬化明显进展，可触及肌腱摩擦感，以及抗-RNA 聚合酶Ⅲ抗体阳性。对于活动性的早期 dcSSc 患者，需要每周一次监测血压，当收缩压较基线上升大于 20 mmHg 时需报告。每天应用 15 mg 或更高剂量泼尼松与 SRC 的发生相关，在有风险的患者中应避免。

心脏表现

总体来说，所有的心脏结构均有可能受累并导致相应的严重功能受损。潜在的 PAH 也导致 SSc 心脏表现。SSc 患者有 3 种主要类型的心脏受累：心包炎、心肌炎和心肌纤维化。后者可导致充血性心力衰竭以及由于传导系统纤维化所引起的心律失常。在 SSc 患者中这些并发症可以是无症状和未被发现的，但在老年尸检系列中 70% 的患者已被发现有病理改变。后来的心脏磁共振成像（MRI）研究也支持了尸检发现的亚临床心脏受累。

舒张功能障碍作为心脏纤维化的并发症正被愈来愈多地认识，可在应用超声心动图筛查肺动脉高压的同时被评估。很多 SSc 患者的死亡是突然发生的，可能是由于室性心律失常。谨慎的做法是在疾病早期完善静息状态的心电图检查。若患者自觉心悸，应进行正规的心律失常评估。

胃肠道表现

80% 或以上的 SSc 患者会出现至少一种胃肠道表现，且胃肠道所有部位均可受累。胃肠道受累是发病的重要组成部分。

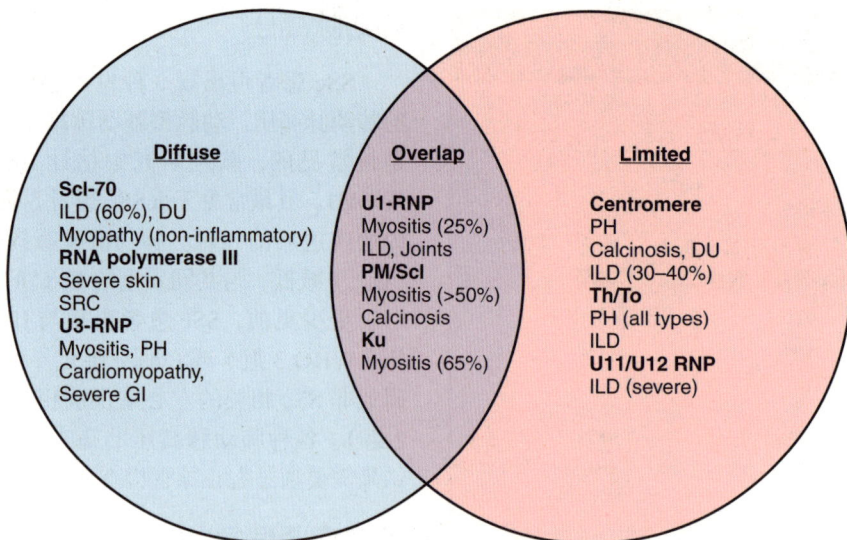

Fig. 5.2 Clinical-serologic classification of systemic sclerosis and antibody-associated internal organ manifestations. *Bold text* indicates an antibody; clinical manifestations listed below are associated with that antibody. *DU*, Digital ulcers; *ILD*, interstitial lung disease; *Ku*, 70/80-kD protein (XRCC6/XRCC5); *PH*, pulmonary hypertension; *PM*, polymyositis; *RNP*, ribonucleoprotein; *Scl*, sclerosis; *SRC*, scleroderma renal crisis.

When the esophagus is affected, patients experience heartburn and/or regurgitation due to a reduced lower esophageal sphincter pressure and distal dysphagia for solid foods due to esophageal dysmotility. The former can be determined by manometry. Less invasively, a barium swallow can reveal hypo- or aperistalsis to determine esophageal dysfunction. Neuropathic changes and fibrosis of the muscularis of the small intestine can lead to motor dysfunction and symptoms of postprandial abdominal distention. Small intestinal hypomotility may lead to bacterial overgrowth, causing bloating and diarrhea. When severe atony of the small intestine develops, patients occasionally develop a functional ileus or intestinal pseudo-obstruction. Parenteral nutrition may be necessary for severe malabsorption with accompanying weight loss and steatorrhea. Similar to the small bowel, the colon may develop impaired motor function leading to constipation and occasionally overflow diarrhea. Wide-mouthed diverticula on the antimesenteric border of the colon can be seen. The internal anal sphincter may become fibrotic, resulting in fecal incontinence.

Musculoskeletal Manifestations

Musculoskeletal manifestations are common. Tendons can become inflamed and fibrotic, particularly in early, diffuse disease. Palpable tendon or bursal friction rubs are virtually pathognomonic of SSc and often indicate progression to dcSSc before widespread skin thickening has occurred. Finger joint flexion contractures develop frequently within the first years of diffuse SSc. True arthritis with palpable synovitis should raise the question of an overlap condition or concomitant Sjögren's syndrome, because synovitis is not a typical feature of SSc.

Some patients develop a bland myopathy with nonprogressive, mild proximal muscle weakness and wasting. A few, particularly with features that overlap with other connective tissue diseases or mixed connective tissue disease, can develop true myositis, which can result in morbidity and disability.

DIAGNOSIS AND DIFFERENTIAL DIAGNOSIS

Raynaud's phenomenon is prominent in the differential diagnosis for SSc. Features that identify Raynaud's patients who have or may later develop SSc or another connective tissue disease are abnormal nail fold capillaries (i.e., megacapillaries, hemorrhages, neovascularization, and avascular areas), tissue loss at the tips of the fingers, and a positive antinuclear antibody (ANA) test result. None of these features is found in Raynaud's disease (i.e., primary Raynaud's phenomenon).

Mixed connective tissue disease (MCTD) is also on the differential for SSc. MCTD patients have features of two or more autoimmune diseases and are U1-RNP antibody positive. This most frequently includes SSc, polymyositis, and SLE. Patients with MCTD can develop any or all of the following SSc manifestations: Raynaud's phenomenon, puffy fingers, limited or diffuse skin thickening, myositis, ILD, PAH, and esophageal dysmotility.

Scleroderma mimics are sometimes difficult to distinguish from SSc (Table 5.2). They include eosinophilic fasciitis, the localized forms of scleroderma such as linear scleroderma (more frequently seen in children), and plaque or generalized morphea.

Nephrogenic systemic fibrosis is a complication of gadolinium administration for radiographic studies that occurs in the setting of renal failure. Nephrogenic systemic fibrosis manifests as symmetrical, bilateral, fibrotic, indurated papules, plaques, or subcutaneous nodules, which can be erythematosus and occur on the lower legs or hands. The lesions are often preceded by edema and may initially be misdiagnosed as cellulitis. This diagnosis should be considered in patients being evaluated for a fibrotic disorder who have renal failure, regardless of the cause of renal disease.

Scleromyxedema and scleredema are cutaneous fibrotic disorders in which excessive mucin accumulation is found on skin biopsy. Scleromyxedema can mimic dcSSc on the physical examination or can manifest with multiple, firm, nodular skin lesions (i.e., papular mucinosis). A frequent association is a monoclonal gammopathy (i.e., immunoglobulin [IgG] paraprotein). Scleredema typically involves the nape of the neck and shoulders, sparing the distal extremities. All SSc mimics lack Raynaud's phenomenon, characteristic SSc internal organ involvement, and SSc-associated serum antibodies.

TREATMENT

No single efficacious therapy has been demonstrated in a randomized, placebo-controlled phase III study for SSc. Thus, patients must

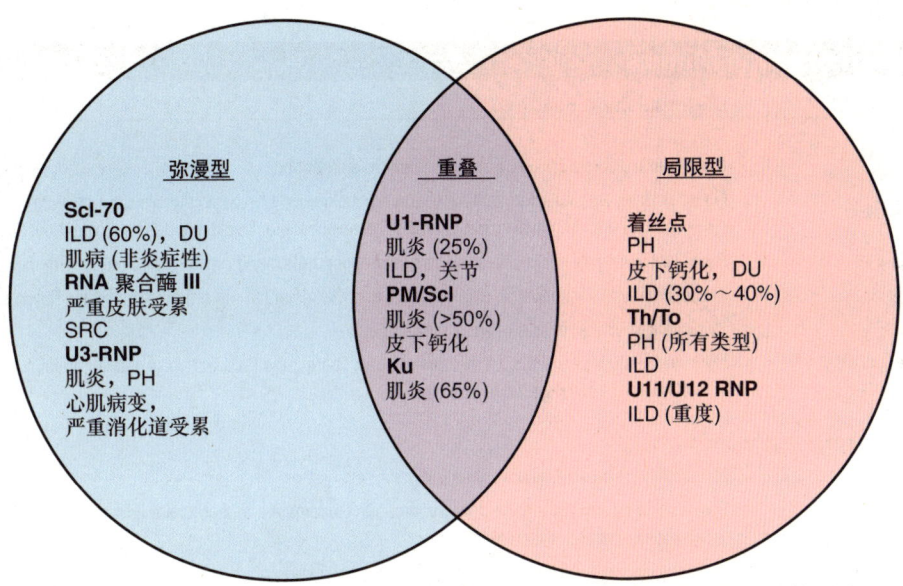

图 5.2　系统性硬化症的临床-血清学分类以及抗体相关的内脏受累表现。粗体字指某种自身抗体；其下列出的是与抗体相关的临床表现。DU，指端溃疡；ILD，间质性肺病；Ku，70/80-kD 蛋白（XRCC6/XRCC5）；PH，肺动脉高压；PM，多肌炎；RNP，核糖核蛋白；Scl，硬化；SRC，硬皮病肾危象

当食管受累时，患者可表现为由于下食管括约肌压力降低造成的烧心和（或）反流，以及由于食管运动障碍引起的对固体食物的远端吞咽困难。前者可通过食管测压确定。钡餐检查可发现蠕动低下或无运动，从而确定食管功能障碍。小肠肌层神经的改变和纤维化可导致运动障碍和餐后腹胀的症状。小肠动力减低可能会导致细菌过度增长，引起腹胀和腹泻。当小肠严重迟缓进一步发展时，患者偶尔出现功能性肠梗阻或者小肠假性肠梗阻。当患者出现严重吸收不良伴体重下降和脂肪泻时，需进行肠外营养。与小肠类似，结肠也有可能出现功能障碍并导致便秘，以及偶尔的溢流性腹泻。于结肠肠系膜游离部边缘可见宽口憩室。肛门内括约肌也可能纤维化，并导致大便失禁。

肌肉骨骼表现

肌肉骨骼症状常见。尤其在早期、弥漫型患者中，肌腱可出现炎症和纤维化。肌腱或者滑囊的摩擦感几乎是 SSc 的特征性表现，常在广泛皮肤硬化出现前就提示向 dcSSc 进展。指关节挛缩常发生于弥漫型 SSc 的第一年。由于滑膜炎并非 SSc 的典型表现，因此当 SSc 患者出现可触及滑膜炎的真正关节炎时应考虑是否重叠其他疾病或合并出现干燥综合征。

一些患者会出现轻度的肌病，表现为非进展性的、轻度的近端肌无力和消耗。少数患者，特别是有重叠其他结缔组织病或者混合性结缔组织病特征时，可出现明确的肌炎，其能导致合并症和致残。

诊断和鉴别诊断

雷诺现象在 SSc 的鉴别诊断中很重要。当雷诺现象的患者具有以下特征，包括异常的甲襞微循环（即巨大毛细血管、出血、新生血管和无血管区），指尖组织缺失，以及抗核抗体（ANA）阳性时，则提示其可能是或将来会发展为 SSc 或其他结缔组织病。在雷诺病（即原发雷诺现象）中这些特征不存在。

混合性结缔组织病（MCTD）也需要和 SSc 鉴别。MCTD 患者具有两种或更多的自身免疫性疾病特征以及抗 -U1-RNP 抗体阳性。最常见的自身免疫性疾病包括 SSc、多肌炎和 SLE。MCTD 患者能出现部分或者全部的下列 SSc 表现：雷诺现象、手指肿胀、局限或弥漫的皮肤增厚、肌炎、ILD、PAH 和食管运动障碍。

类硬皮病样疾病有时很难与 SSc 鉴别（表 5.2）。它们包括嗜酸细胞性筋膜炎，局灶型硬皮病如线状硬皮病（更常见于儿童），及斑块状或泛发性硬斑病。

肾源性系统性纤维化是一种在肾衰竭时使用钆造影剂进行影像学检查时所出现的并发症。肾源性系统性纤维化表现为对称性、双侧、纤维化样、硬节样的丘疹、斑块或皮下结节，可表现为红斑并发生于下肢或者手部。皮损常先表现为水肿，最初可能被误诊为蜂窝织炎。当肾衰竭患者出现纤维化样异常表现时，不管肾衰竭的病因如何，均应考虑是否存在该病。

硬化性黏液性水肿和硬肿病均为皮肤纤维化性疾病，在皮肤活检时均可见过量的黏蛋白沉积。硬化性黏液性水肿在查体时可像 dcSSc，或者表现为多发、质硬、结节样皮损（即，丘疹性黏蛋白病）。硬化性黏液性水肿经常同时存在单克隆丙种球蛋白病［即免疫球蛋白（IgG）异常蛋白］，后者可能是其原因。典型的硬肿病累及颈背部和肩部，不累及肢体远端。所有类 SSc 样疾病均缺乏雷诺现象、典型 SSc 的内脏受累以及 SSc 相关的血清抗体。

治疗

在 SSc 中尚无通过随机、安慰剂对照的 III 期临床试验证实的有效治疗。因此，需适当监测患者的内脏

TABLE 5.2 Scleroderma Mimics

Disorder	Distinguishing Features
Other Diseases	
Morphea	One or more discrete lesions; patchy or linear in distribution
Eosinophilic fasciitis	Finger flexures without sclerodactyly; characteristic groove sign when the arms are raised; puckering or dimpling of the upper arm and thigh skin; peripheral blood eosinophilia; fascia and deep subcutaneous fibrosis
Scleredema (Buschke disease)	Prominent involvement of neck, shoulders, and upper arms; hands spared; associated with diabetes
Scleromyxedema	Association with gammopathy; skin lichenoid and thickened but not tethered; may have Raynaud's phenomenon
Graft-versus-host disease	Skin changes similar to scleroderma; vasculopathy
Nephrogenic fibrosing dermopathy	Indurated plaques or nodules on the legs or arms, sparing the face; administration of gadolinium in the setting of renal dysfunction; often preceded by edema
Reactions to Environmental Agents and Drugs	
Bleomycin	Skin and lung fibrosis similar to scleroderma
L-Tryptophan (1980s)	Eosinophilia-myalgia syndrome from L-tryptophan contaminant or metabolite (first described in the 1980s); fever, eosinophilia, neurologic manifestations
Organic solvents (e.g., trichloroethylene)	Clinically indistinguishable from idiopathic systemic sclerosis
Pentazocine	Localized lesions at injection sites
Toxic oil syndrome	Contaminated rapeseed oil (Spanish epidemic in 1981); similar to eosinophilia myalgia syndrome
Vinyl chloride	Vascular lesions, acro-osteolysis, sclerodactyly, no visceral disease
Gadolinium	Nephrogenic fibrosing dermopathy

be appropriately monitored for visceral involvement to allow early identification and therapy targeted at specific organ complications. Consultation with a rheumatologist is helpful in this respect. Generally, patients with early diffuse or evolving diffuse scleroderma are likely to be considered for treatment with immunosuppression and treatment options specifically for those SSc patients with ILD include an anti-fibrotic agent. Given the lack of US Food and Drug Administration (FDA)- or EMA-approved therapy, SSc is an active area of therapeutic research; multiple international clinical trials are either ongoing or planned. Given this, patients should be considered for referral to a dedicated scleroderma center early in disease to have the advantage of these opportunities. Autologous stem cell transplant has been tested in the United States and Europe and has demonstrated an improvement in event-free and overall survival in patients with moderate to severe and early diffuse SSc. Treatment-related mortality must be weighed when considering stem cell therapy as an option, and we do not advise it for skin management alone.

With respect to evaluation and monitoring, all patients should undergo screening evaluation for ILD and pulmonary hypertension throughout the course of their disease. Current expert recommendations suggest that patients with early, diffuse disease should be monitored at least yearly for these complications. Patients with active dcSSc, particularly if they have tendon friction rubs, should undergo weekly blood pressure monitoring because the abrupt appearance of hypertension suggests SRC. Early dcSSc patients should also have skin thickness scores assessed for progression or regression of cutaneous disease. For dcSSc and lcSSc, initial esophageal motility studies should be considered, and further objective studies should be ordered on the basis of symptoms.

Education of patients and family members regarding the disease and an accurate prognosis based on disease subtype and stage can be helpful in management. Educational programs are available through foundations across the world. This includes the Scleroderma Foundation in the United States, Scleroderma Canada, Scleroderma and Raynaud's UK, Scleroderma Australia, and the World Scleroderma Foundation.

Raynaud's Phenomenon

Nonpharmacologic measures such as cold avoidance, warming measures, avoidance of vibratory tools, and smoking cessation are encouraged in all patients. Pharmacologic measures are recommended, because ongoing vascular injury may play a role in pathogenesis.

Calcium-channel blockers have been widely used for decades, and they are generally well tolerated by patients. Long-acting nifedipine is effective in more than one half of patients; other agents such as amlodipine are also frequently prescribed. The angiotensin-receptor blocker losartan reduced the severity and frequency of Raynaud's phenomenon attacks in a placebo-controlled trial. ACE inhibitors have not proved effective in several controlled trials. Phosphodiesterase-5 (PDE-5) inhibitors have been shown to improve Raynaud's phenomenon. Some studies have shown encouraging results with use of fluoxetine (selective serotonin reuptake inhibitor). The prostacyclin iloprost is used as a therapy for severe Raynaud's phenomenon and digital ischemia. The benefit of statin therapy for Raynaud's phenomenon has produced conflicting results, although it has benefits in endothelial dysfunction, which is a component of the vascular pathogenesis in SSc.

In patients with digital ulcerations, more aggressive therapy may be warranted. PDE-5 inhibitors have been helpful. Topical nitroglycerin as a paste, gel, or patch placed at the base of the fingers or over the dorsal wrist may be a useful adjunct. In randomized, placebo-controlled trials, bosentan, an endothelin receptor antagonist, prevented the formation of new digital ulcerations in patients with SSc and Raynaud's phenomenon, although it has not been approved by the FDA for this indication. Iloprost, an intravenous prostacyclin, has also been shown to reduce digital ulcerations and is frequently used in Europe, but it is not FDA-approved in the United States.

For patients with digital ulcers involving adjacent fingers, assessment of the ulnar and radial artery should be performed with arterial Doppler or angiography because larger arteries can become severely narrowed. Surgical interventions include sympathectomy of the digital, radial, or ulnar artery and venous bypass for ulnar or radial artery occlusion. Topical botulinum A injections are potentially helpful in

表 5.2 硬皮病样疾病

疾病	特征性表现
其他疾病	
硬斑病	一处或者多处分散的病变;分散或者线样分布
嗜酸细胞性筋膜炎	手指屈曲但不伴硬指;上肢抬起时特征性的沟槽征;上臂和大腿皮肤起皱或凹陷;外周血嗜酸细胞增多;筋膜和深部皮下组织纤维化
硬肿病(Buschke 病)	主要累及颈部、肩部和上臂;不累及手部;与糖尿病相关
硬化性黏液性水肿	与丙种球蛋白病相关;皮肤苔藓样变并增厚,但无皱褶表现;可能有雷诺现象
移植物抗宿主病	皮肤表现与硬皮病类似;血管病变
肾源性纤维化性皮肤病	下肢或上肢出现硬结样斑块或结节,不累及颜面;出现于肾功能不全时使用钆造影剂的情况;通常先出现水肿
环境因素和药物反应	
博来霉素	皮肤和肺纤维化类似于硬皮病
L-色氨酸(1980s)	L-色氨酸污染物或者代谢物导致嗜酸细胞增多性肌痛综合征(在 20 世纪 80 年代首次描述);发热,嗜酸细胞增多,神经系统表现
有机溶剂(如三氯乙烯)	与特发性系统性硬化症临床上无法区分
喷他佐辛	注射部位的局灶病变
毒油综合征	污染的菜籽油(1981 年在西班牙流行);类似于嗜酸细胞增多性肌痛综合征
氯乙烯	血管病变,肢端骨质溶解,硬指,无内脏受累
钆	肾源性纤维化性皮肤病

受累来早期发现,并对特定的脏器并发症进行针对性治疗。这方面咨询风湿免疫科专家会有帮助。一般来说,早期弥漫型或者正在发展为弥漫型硬皮病的患者可能需考虑免疫抑制治疗,SSc 合并 ILD 的患者治疗中特别加入抗纤维化药物。由于尚缺乏获得美国食品药物管理局(FDA)或 EMA 许可通过的治疗,SSc 为治疗研究的活跃领域;多个国际性的临床试验正在进行或计划进行中。鉴于此,应考虑在疾病早期将患者转诊至专科的硬皮病中心,以使患者有可能获得这些机会。自体干细胞移植在美国和欧洲已进行试验,证实在中重度以及早期弥漫型 SSc 患者中可改善患者无事件生存和总体生存。在考虑干细胞治疗作为选择时,需权衡治疗相关的死亡风险,不推荐该方案单独用于皮肤病变的治疗。

关于评估和监测,所有患者在整个病程中均需筛查评估 ILD 和肺动脉高压。目前的专家意见建议对于早期弥漫型病变患者应至少需每年监测上述并发症。对于活动性 dcSSc 患者,特别是具有肌腱摩擦感患者,应每周监测血压,因为突然发生的高血压提示 SRC。早期 dcSSc 患者还需进行皮肤厚度评分,以评价皮肤病变是否进展或者好转。对于 dcSSc 和 lcSSc 患者,建议在病初行食管动力学检查,进一步的客观评估应在出现症状的基础上相应安排。

对患者及其家庭成员进行病情宣教,以及根据疾病的亚类和阶段进行准确的预后评估均有助于疾病的诊治。全世界多个协会/基金会均提供教育方案,包括美国硬皮病基金会、加拿大硬皮病协会、英国硬皮病和雷诺现象协会、澳大利亚硬皮病协会,以及世界硬皮病基金会。

雷诺现象

在所有的患者中鼓励非药物治疗措施,如避免受凉,保暖措施,避免使用震动工具,以及戒烟。考虑到进展性血管损伤在疾病发生中可能起作用,也推荐药物治疗措施。

钙通道阻滞剂在过去数十年中已被广泛使用,患者整体耐受良好。长效的硝苯地平在半数以上患者中有效;其他药物如氨氯地平也经常使用。在一项安慰剂对照的试验中,血管紧张素受体阻滞剂氯沙坦可降低雷诺现象发生的严重程度和频率。在几项对照试验中未证实 ACE 抑制剂有效。5 磷酸二酯酶(PDE-5)抑制剂已被显示可改善雷诺现象。有研究显示氟西汀(选择性 5-羟色胺再摄取抑制剂)有令人鼓舞的效果。前列环素类药物伊洛前列素可用于治疗严重雷诺现象和指缺血。虽然他汀类药物有益于改善内皮功能障碍,后者是 SSc 血管病变发病机制的一部分,但他汀类药物在雷诺现象中的治疗效果目前还存在争议。

在指溃疡的患者中需进行更积极的治疗。PDE-5 抑制剂有一定作用。将硝酸甘油以凝胶、凝膏或者斑贴置于手指根部或者腕关节背侧也为一种有效的辅助治疗。尽管还没有被 FDA 批准适应证,但在随机、安慰剂对照的研究中,内皮素受体拮抗剂波生坦可预防 SSc 和雷诺现象患者中新发指溃疡。伊洛前列素是一种静脉使用的前列环素类药物,也可以减少指溃疡,在欧洲经常被使用,但在美国并未被 FDA 批准。

对指溃疡累及相邻手指的患者,因可能存在较大动脉的严重狭窄,应使用动脉多普勒超声或血管造影对尺动脉和桡动脉进行评估。外科治疗包括手指动脉、桡动脉或尺动脉的交感神经切除术,以及在尺或桡动脉闭塞时行静脉搭桥术。对于部分不能耐受其他治疗

selected patients who are unable to tolerate other treatments. In SSc patients with recurrent digital ulcers or other thrombotic events, evaluation for a hypercoagulable state, particularly for lupus anticoagulant, should be performed. In this circumstance, aspirin or other anticoagulants are indicated.

Cutaneous Disease

No therapeutic agent has been found to achieve a clinically significant improvement in skin thickening as measured by the modified Rodnan skin score in a randomized, placebo-controlled trial for patients with dcSSc. The Rodnan skin score was developed by Dr. Gerald Rodnan at the University of Pittsburgh. It is calculated by estimating skin thickness on a scale of 0 to 3 in 17 skin areas. Negative findings in therapeutic trials have been attributed to the type of drugs chosen, the patient populations, and trial designs. In the past, considerable attention was given to methotrexate and D-penicillamine, but no trials demonstrate a clinically significant improvement in skin score. Case series with historical controls have suggested a benefit for mycophenolate mofetil, although it has not been studied in a randomized setting. Subset analysis from the Scleroderma Lung Study 2 suggested that both mycophenolate and cyclophosphamide therapy were associated with an improvement in the skin thickness of patients with dcSSc. More recently, two studies with tocilizumab failed to demonstrate a statistically significant improvement in skin score, although there was clinical improvement during the extended open label trial. Currently, mycophenolate mofetil and methotrexate are commonly used as first-line agents in dcSSc.

Scleroderma Renal Crisis

Early diagnosis and prompt initiation of ACE inhibitors are the keys to improved survival and outcomes of SRC. ACE inhibitors should be titrated to maintain a normal blood pressure, preferably less than 125/75 mm Hg, and lifelong treatment is recommended. Second-line agents to maintain blood pressure control include calcium-channel blockers (CCB). β-Blockers are relatively contraindicated because there is concern for worsening of Raynaud's phenomenon as well as for potential vascular complications.

Even if patients with SRC become dialysis dependent initially, some may experience a slow reversal of renal vascular damage if ACE inhibitor therapy is maintained. Because up to 50% of SRC patients can spontaneously come off dialysis, transplantation evaluation should be delayed until at least 2 years after SRC onset.

Interstitial Lung Disease

Early recognition of inflammatory ILD is important if treatment is to prevent progression to distortion of lung architecture and irreversible fibrosis. Controlled clinical trials support the potential benefit of mycophenolate mofetil, particularly with early detection of underlying ILD associated with SSc and initiation of treatment. Although the choice of mycophenolate mofetil has not been proven to be more effective compared to cyclophosphamide, there is overall better tolerance of the drug and a relatively safer side-effect profile. In addition, small trials have shown hopeful results in terms of using rituximab, an anti-CD20 monoclonal antibody, for fibrotic lung complications associated with underlying scleroderma. Two randomized controlled trials of tocilizumab revealed encouraging results regarding preservation of lung function. A recent trial of nintedanib in SSc-related ILD demonstrated that the annual rate of decline in FVC was lower with nintedanib than with placebo; nearly half the patients in this trial were taking background mycophenolate therapy. Lung transplantation can be considered for end-stage ILD. In all settings, management of ILD should include management of esophageal disease.

Pulmonary Hypertension

Several agents have been approved for the treatment of PAH (see Chapter 18). Subset analyses of several placebo-controlled drug trials have shown improvement in established SSc or connective tissue disease–related PAH. They have included phosphodiesterase-5 inhibitors (e.g., sildenafil, tadalafil), endothelial receptor antagonists (e.g., bosentan, ambrisentan, macitentan), soluble guanylate cyclase inhibitors (riociguat), and prostacyclin analogues (e.g., treprostinil, epoprostenol, selexipag). There is growing interest in the potential benefit of immunosuppressive therapies for SSc-PAH in addition to vasodilators.

Theoretically, treatment of patients with early, less severe disease should improve outcomes. Because patients with SSc-related PAH have a worse prognosis than those with idiopathic PAH despite modern therapies, SSc patients with PAH should be recommended to a tertiary care facility with a dedicated pulmonary hypertension clinic.

Cardiac Manifestations

Combined corticosteroids and immunosuppression can be used for myocarditis. Conventional treatment is recommended for symptomatic pericarditis (see Chapter 10), arrhythmias (see Chapter 9), and diastolic heart failure (see Chapter 5).

Gastrointestinal Manifestations

Gastroesophageal reflux, which occurs in most SSc patients, can be treated with proton pump inhibitors and conservative measures, including elevation of the head of the bed and avoidance of alcohol and caffeine. If untreated, reflux esophagitis can progress to distal esophageal stricture formation.

Patients with severe esophageal, gastric, or small bowel dysmotility may improve with the use of prokinetic drugs such as metoclopramide, erythromycin, or octreotide. Rotating antibiotics may be of assistance for bacterial overgrowth. For advanced small bowel involvement with malabsorption, supplementation of iron, calcium, and fat-soluble vitamins may be required. Occasionally, total parental nutrition is necessary. Unexplained iron deficiency anemia in SSc patients suggests the possibility of gastric antral vascular ectasias (i.e., watermelon stomach), which are treated with laser photocoagulation as first-line therapy.

Skeletal Muscle, Joint, and Tendon Manifestations

Bland myopathy usually is nonprogressive and is treated with physical therapy. If there is evidence of myositis with elevated serum levels of muscle enzymes or abnormal electromyography or muscle biopsy, corticosteroids and immunosuppressive therapy (e.g., methotrexate, azathioprine) may be helpful.

Patients with lcSSc or dcSSc can develop contractures of the hands due to tendon involvement. Physical therapy with daily stretching exercises directed at the finger joints should be instituted as soon as possible to prevent further loss of finger motion.

For a deeper discussion of these topics, please see Chapter 251, "Systemic Sclerosis (Scleroderma)," in *Goldman-Cecil Medicine*, 26th Edition.

SPECIAL CONSIDERATIONS

Patients with SSc are at increased risk for development of cancer, particularly hematologic malignancies such as lymphoma as well as lung and breast cancer. There is ongoing research focused on understanding the exact pathogenetic mechanisms. Underlying inflammation is thought to play a major role. The existence of specific autoantibodies

的选择性患者，肉毒杆菌 A 局部注射可能有帮助。在反复指溃疡或其他血栓事件的 SSc 患者中，应评估高凝状态，特别是狼疮抗凝物。在这种情况下，需考虑使用阿司匹林或其他抗凝药物。

皮肤病变

对于 dcSSc 患者，在随机、安慰剂对照研究中，以改良 Rodnan 皮肤评分为评价标准，目前没有治疗药物被证明能达到皮肤厚度上临床有意义的改善。Rodnan 皮肤评分是由匹兹堡大学的 Gerald Rodnan 医生提出的。该评分在人体的 17 个部位进行皮肤厚度评分，每个部位 0~3 分。治疗研究的阴性结果可能归因于被选择药物的类型、患者人群，以及研究设计。过去常考虑使用甲氨蝶呤和青霉胺，但是没有研究证实在皮肤评分上达到临床有意义的改善。历史对照的病例系列研究表明吗替麦考酚酯有效，虽然没有随机试验的证实。硬皮病肺研究 2 的亚组分析显示吗替麦考酚酯和环磷酰胺治疗均可改善 dcSSc 患者的皮肤厚度。更近期的两项关于托珠单抗的研究中，尽管在扩展的开放标签试验期间显示有临床改善，但未证实其在皮肤评分上达到有统计学意义的改善。目前吗替麦考酚酯和甲氨蝶呤是 dcSSc 患者的常用一线药物。

硬皮病肾危象

早期诊断并尽快开始使用 ACE 抑制剂是改善 SRC 生存和预后的关键。ACE 抑制剂应进行滴定，以维持正常血压，最好在 125/75 mmHg 以下，并推荐终身使用。二线控制血压的药物包括钙通道阻滞剂（CCB）。β 受体阻滞剂相对禁用，因为担心其加重雷诺现象及可能的血管并发症。

即使 SRC 患者一开始需要透析，部分患者在经过 ACE 抑制剂持续治疗后可能会缓慢恢复。由于高达 50% 的 SRC 患者能自发地脱离透析，因此应延迟到 SRC 开始后至少 2 年再行肾移植评估。

间质性肺病

如果治疗可阻止进展到肺结构破坏和不可逆的纤维化，则炎症性 ILD 的早期识别非常重要。对照的临床研究支持吗替麦考酚酯可能有效，特别是早期发现与 SSc 相关的 ILD 并开始治疗。尽管并未证实吗替麦考酚酯比环磷酰胺更有效，但是总体来说吗替麦考酚酯有更好的耐受性，相对更安全的副作用。此外，关于使用抗 CD20 单克隆抗体利妥昔单抗治疗硬皮病相关的纤维化肺并发症，小规模的研究已显示出有前景的结果。两项使用托珠单抗的随机对照研究发现其在保护肺功能方面有令人鼓舞的结果。最近的一项关于尼达尼布治疗 SSc 相关 ILD 的研究表明，尼达尼布组的 FVC 年下降率较安慰剂组更低；该研究中近一半患者接受了吗替麦考酚酯的基础治疗。对于终末期 ILD 患者可考虑行肺移植。在所有情况下，ILD 的治疗方案中需包括针对食管病变的治疗。

肺动脉高压

几种药物已被批准用于 PAH 的治疗（见第 18 章）。在确诊的 SSc 或者结缔组织病相关 PAH 中，多项安慰剂对照药物试验的亚组分析已显示出改善。这包括 5 磷酸二酯酶抑制剂（如西地那非、他达拉非），内皮素受体拮抗剂（如波生坦、安利生坦、马西替坦），可溶性鸟苷酸环化酶抑制剂（利奥西呱），以及前列环素类似物（如曲前列尼尔、依前列醇、司来帕格）。除了血管扩张治疗，免疫抑制治疗对 SSc-PAH 的可能获益引起了愈来愈多的关注。

理论上讲，早期病变较轻患者的治疗应该能改善预后。尽管有先进的疗法，SSc 相关 PAH 患者较原发性 PAH 有更差的预后，因此 SSc 伴 PAH 患者应转诊至具有肺动脉高压专科门诊的三级医疗中心。

心脏表现

皮质类固醇联合免疫抑制剂可用于治疗心肌炎。推荐常规处理有症状的心包炎（见第 10 章）、心律失常（见第 9 章）和舒张性心力衰竭（见第 5 章）。

胃肠道表现

大多数 SSc 患者发生胃食管反流，可使用质子泵抑制剂以及保守措施治疗，包括抬高床头，避免饮酒和咖啡因。若不予治疗，反流性食管炎会发展为食管远端狭窄。

严重食管、胃或者小肠动力障碍患者，可使用促动力药物改善症状，如甲氧氯普胺、红霉素或者奥曲肽。对于细菌过度增长的情况，轮换使用抗生素可能有帮助。对于小肠受累进展并吸收不良的情况，需补充铁、钙和脂溶性维生素。在少数情况下，需要进行全胃肠外营养。SSc 患者出现难以解释的缺铁性贫血提示可能存在胃窦血管扩张症（即西瓜胃），应使用激光光凝治疗作为一线治疗。

骨骼肌肉、关节和肌腱表现

轻度肌病一般为非进展性，可进行物理疗法。如果存在肌炎的证据，伴血清肌酶升高或肌电图异常，或肌活检异常，糖皮质激素和免疫抑制剂治疗（如甲氨蝶呤、硫唑嘌呤）可有帮助。

由于肌腱受累，lcSSc 或者 dcSSc 患者可发展为手挛缩。为阻止手指运动功能的进一步丧失，需尽快开始物理疗法，每日进行手指关节伸展运动。

有关此专题的深入讨论，请参阅 *Goldman-Cecil Medicine* 第 26 版第 251 章"系统性硬化症（硬皮病）"。

特殊注意事项

SSc 患者出现肿瘤的风险增加，特别是血液系统肿瘤，如淋巴瘤以及肺癌和乳腺癌。有正在进行的研究关注于其确切发病机制。潜在的炎症被认为起主要作用。除了

in addition to the use of certain immunosuppressive agents also have been implicated in playing role. Pending clarification of the pathophysiology leading to malignancy, it is important to perform age-appropriate screening in SSc patients.

SUGGESTED READINGS

Kowal-Bielecka O, Landewé R, Avouac J, et al: EULAR recommendations for the treatment of systemic sclerosis: a report from the EULAR scleroderma trials and research group (EUSTAR), Ann Rheum Dis 68:620–628, 2009.

Maurer B, Distler O: Emerging targeted therapies in scleroderma lung and skin fibrosis, Best Pract Res Clin Rheumatol 25:843–858, 2011.

Mayes MD: The scleroderma book: a guide for patients and families, New York, 1999, Oxford University Press.

Medsger TA: Natural history of systemic sclerosis and the assessment of disease activity, severity, functional status, and psychologic well-being, Rheum Dis Clin North Am 29:255–275, 2003.

特定免疫抑制剂的使用，特异性自身抗体的存在也在其中发挥作用。由于导致肿瘤的病理生理机制有待明确，在 SSc 患者中进行适合相应年龄的筛查非常重要。

推荐阅读

Kowal-Bielecka O, Landewé R, Avouac J, et al: EULAR recommendations for the treatment of systemic sclerosis: a report from the EULAR scleroderma trials and research group (EUSTAR), Ann Rheum Dis 68:620–628, 2009.

Maurer B, Distler O: Emerging targeted therapies in scleroderma lung and skin fibrosis, Best Pract Res Clin Rheumatol 25:843–858, 2011.

Mayes MD: The scleroderma book: a guide for patients and families, New York, 1999, Oxford University Press.

Medsger TA: Natural history of systemic sclerosis and the assessment of disease activity, severity, functional status, and psychologic well-being, Rheum Dis Clin North Am 29:255–275, 2003.

Systemic Vasculitis

Kimberly P. Liang, Kelly V. Liang

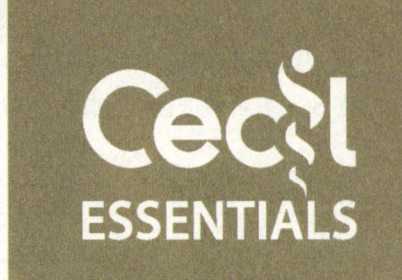

DEFINITION AND EPIDEMIOLOGY

The primary systemic vasculitides are inflammatory disorders of blood vessels that are characterized by immune-mediated injury leading to vessel necrosis, thrombosis, stenosis, or some combination of these. Vessels in any organ may be affected, but each vasculitis is characterized by different preferential vessel size or territory and tissue targeting. Although these disorders are rare, they may be organ- or life-threatening, so prompt diagnosis and treatment are necessary. The vasculitides are defined according to the 1990 American College of Rheumatology (ACR) classification criteria and the 1994 Chapel Hill Consensus Conference (revised in 2012) (CHCC) based on generally affected vessel size (small, medium, or large). Antineutrophil cytoplasmic antibody (ANCA)–associated vasculitides (AAVs) have known associations with characteristic autoantibodies. Fig. 6.1 shows the major types of vasculitides. Although the ACR and CHCC definitions were not designed as diagnostic criteria, classification criteria such as these are important in clinical research study design, treatment, and prognosis. The ACR and the European League Against Rheumatism (EULAR) are currently in the process of refining diagnostic and classification criteria for primary vasculitides.

Determining the incidence and prevalence of each of the vasculitides is challenging given the rarity of the disorders, imperfect classification criteria and definitions for epidemiologic purposes, and some clinicopathologic overlaps that occur between certain types (e.g., AAVs).

Small Vessel Vasculitis
ANCA-Associated Vasculitides

Granulomatosis with polyangiitis (GPA; previously known as Wegener's granulomatosis), microscopic polyangiitis (MPA), eosinophilic granulomatosis with polyangiitis (EGPA; previously known as Churg-Strauss syndrome), and renal-limited vasculitis (RLV) affect small and medium-sized blood vessels and may be associated with ANCA. Various studies have shown AAVs to have an incidence of approximately 10 to 20 per million. The peak age at onset is 65 to 74 years, with a female-to-male ratio of 1.5:1. EGPA is the least common of the AAVs, with an incidence of approximately 1.0 to 3.0 per million, and it also has a weaker association with ANCA than GPA and MPA.

Henoch-Schönlein Purpura

Henoch-Schönlein purpura (HSP) is a small vessel vasculitis that occurs most frequently in young children, with a peak age at onset of 4 to 6 years, but can also occur in adults. HSP accounts for almost half of all cases of childhood vasculitis. In children younger than 17 years of age, the annual incidence of HSP is approximately 20 per 100,000. Males are more commonly affected than females (approximately 2:1), and HSP occurs more frequently during the winter and spring months.

Medium Vessel Vasculitis

Polyarteritis nodosa (PAN) is a medium vessel vasculitis that is characterized by arterial aneurysmal and stenotic lesions of muscular arteries, often located at segmental and branch points. In contrast to small vessel vasculitis, renal involvement in PAN is not characterized by glomerulonephritis but rather by aneurysms and stenoses of renal arteries that may result in hypertension or renal dysfunction or both. In addition, ANCAs are usually negative in PAN. PAN may occur either as a primary vasculitis or secondary to viral infections, mainly hepatitis B or C, or human immunodeficiency virus (HIV). Determining the incidence of this vasculitis is difficult, because PAN and MPA were not differentiated until 1994.

Kawasaki disease is a medium vessel vasculitis most often seen in boys younger than 5 years of age. It is the second most common vasculitis in childhood after HSP, accounting for about 23% of all childhood vasculitis cases. In the United States, the annual incidence in children younger than 5 years old is 20 per 100,000.

Large Vessel Vasculitis

Giant cell arteritis (GCA), also known as temporal arteritis, is the most common form of vasculitis in adults. It is a large vessel vasculitis that typically affects patients of Eastern European descent, with a mean age at onset of 70 to 75 years. It affects women more commonly than men (3:1). About 40% of patients with GCA have the related condition, polymyalgia rheumatica (PMR), which is characterized by subacute onset of aching and stiffness in the muscles of the neck, shoulder girdle, and hip girdle. However, only 10% to 25% of patients with PMR have or will develop GCA.

Takayasu's arteritis (TAK), or "pulseless disease," is a rare large vessel vasculitis that was initially identified in young women from East Asia but is now described worldwide. In adults, the female-to-male ratio is about 8:1, with an average age at diagnosis in the mid-20s.

PATHOLOGY

For most of the systemic vasculitides, the etiology and pathogenesis of disease are largely unknown. It has been proposed that a number of diverse mechanisms contribute to the development of vascular inflammation and subsequent injury on the background of genetic susceptibility (Fig. 6.2). Proposed triggers of disease include infection and environmental exposures (e.g., chemicals, pollutants). For most vasculitides, these associations remain speculative.

Humoral and cellular immune responses, cytokine release, chemokine activation, and immune complex deposition are important in disease pathogenesis. Normal protective and repair processes in the vessel can also contribute to injury and ischemia. For example, after injury, cellular migration and proliferation occurring as

系统性血管炎

靳尚宜 译　田新平 徐东 审校　李梦涛 通审

定义和流行病学

原发性系统性血管炎是一组以免疫介导损伤引起的血管坏死、血栓形成、管腔狭窄或上述病变组合为特征的炎性疾病。全身任何器官的血管均可受累，但每种血管炎在主要受累血管的大小、部位和靶向组织等方面具有不同的特点。系统性血管炎虽较为罕见，但可能危及器官功能乃至生命安全，因此，需要对血管炎进行及时的诊断与治疗。

目前系统性血管炎采用的是 1990 年美国风湿病学会（ACR）制定的分类标准和 1994 年 Chapel Hill 共识会议（CHCC）上根据主要受累血管的大小（大、中、小）制定的标准（2012 年修订）来进行分类的。已知抗中性粒细胞胞质抗体（ANCA）相关血管炎（AAV）与特征性的自身抗体有关联。图 6.1 显示了主要的几类血管炎。虽然 ACR 与 CHCC 标准均非作为诊断标准而设计的，但这些分类标准对血管炎的临床研究设计、治疗和预后都非常重要。目前，ACR 和欧洲抗风湿病联盟（EULAR）正在重新制定原发性血管炎的诊断与分类标准。

由于血管炎的罕见性、其分类标准和流行病学定义的不完美性以及在一些类型血管炎（如各类 AAV）之间存在临床病理的重叠等原因，确定每一种血管炎的发病率和患病率极具挑战性。

小血管血管炎

ANCA 相关性血管炎（AAV）

肉芽肿性多血管炎（GPA，既往称为韦格纳肉芽肿）、显微镜下多血管炎（MPA）、嗜酸性肉芽肿性多血管炎（EGPA，既往称为 Churg-Strauss 综合征）和肾脏局限性血管炎（RLV）主要累及小到中等大小的血管，可能与 ANCA 相关。多项研究显示，AAV 的发病率约为每百万人 10～20 例。发病的高峰年龄为 65～74 岁，男女比例为 1.5∶1。EGPA 是 AAV 中最为少见的一种，发病率仅为每百万人 1～3 例，此外，与 GPA 和 MPA 相比，EGPA 与 ANCA 的关联性较弱。

过敏性紫癜

过敏性紫癜（HSP）是一种好发于儿童的小血管炎，发病高峰年龄为 4～6 岁，但成人亦可发病。过敏性紫癜几乎占所有儿童血管炎病例的一半。在 17 岁以下儿童中，过敏性紫癜的年发病率约为每 10 万人 20 例。男性发病多于女性（比例约为 2∶1），且过敏性紫癜更易在冬季和春季发病。

中等血管血管炎

结节性多动脉炎（PAN）是一种以肌性动脉的动脉瘤和狭窄病变为特征的中等大小血管炎。病变通常好发于血管分叉处。与小血管炎不同的是，PAN 肾脏受累主要是肾动脉狭窄或动脉瘤形成所致，而非肾小球肾炎。肾动脉狭窄或动脉瘤形成可能会引起高血压或肾功能损害，或两者同时出现。此外，PAN 患者的 ANCA 检测常为阴性。PAN 既可以为原发性的血管炎，亦可以继发于病毒感染，主要包括乙型肝炎、丙型肝炎或人类免疫缺陷病毒（HIV）。PAN 的发病率难以确定，因为直到 1994 年后，PAN 和 MPA 这两种血管炎才被区分开来。

川崎病是一种好发于 5 岁以下男孩的中等大小血管炎。它是继过敏性紫癜之后在儿童中第二常见的血管炎，约占所有儿童血管炎病例的 23%。在美国，5 岁以下儿童的川崎病年发病率为每 10 万人 20 例。

大血管血管炎

巨细胞性动脉炎（GCA）又称颞动脉炎，是成年人最常见的血管炎类型。GCA 是一种大血管炎，在东欧发病率最高，平均发病年龄为 70～75 岁，女性患者多于男性（比例为 3∶1）。大约 40% 的 GCA 患者伴有风湿性多肌痛（PMR），PMR 的典型表现为颈部、肩胛带和骨盆带肌肉的亚急性疼痛与僵硬。然而，只有 10%～25% 的 PMR 患者患有或未来会发展为 GCA。

大动脉炎（TAK）或"无脉病"是一种罕见的大血管炎，最初在东亚的年轻女性中发现，目前在全球各地均有报道。在成年患者中，女性与男性患者比例约为 8∶1，诊断时的平均年龄为 20 岁中旬。

病理学

大多数系统性血管炎的病因和发病机制不明。曾有人提出多种不同机制在遗传易感的背景下共同参与了血管炎症与后续的血管损伤（图 6.2）。已提出的可能触发系统性血管炎的因素包括感染和环境暴露（如化学物质、污染物）。对于大多数血管炎而言，这些相关性仍停留在推测阶段。

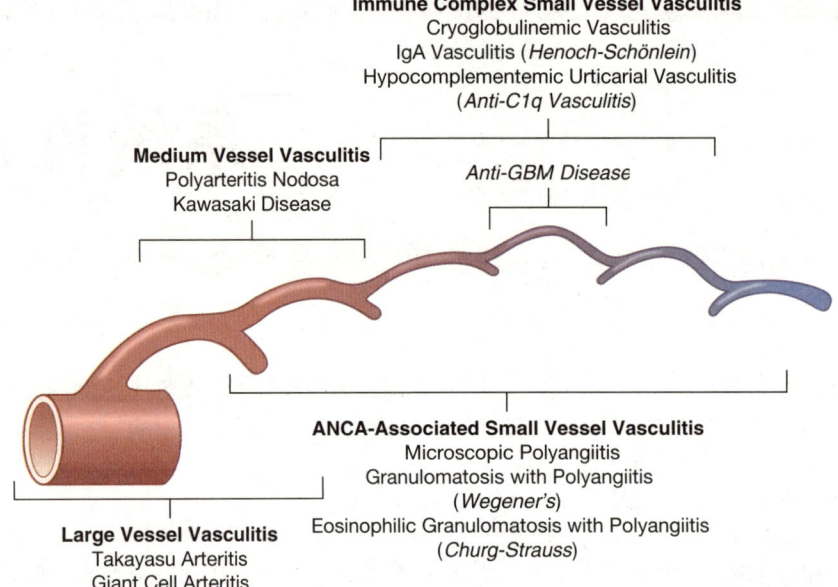

Fig. 6.1 The vascular spectrum of the vasculitides. (From Jennette JC, Falk RJ, Bacon PA, et al: 2012 revised International Chapel Hill Consensus Conference Nomenclature of Vasculitides. *Arthritis Rheum* 2013;65:1-11.)

part of vessel repair can result in intimal hyperplasia, and the procoagulant milieu that is protective against hemorrhage may lead to thrombosis and vessel occlusion. Impairment of blood flow in injured vessels results in tissue ischemia and damage. The degree of blood flow impairment varies along a broad spectrum of severity and may depend on the type of vasculitis as well as the size and location of the vessels involved.

Among the AAVs, the pathology of GPA is typically characterized by necrotizing granulomatous inflammation of small blood vessels supplying the upper and lower respiratory tract. In both GPA and MPA, renal pathology shows a pauci-immune necrotizing crescentic glomerulonephritis. In EGPA, there is a strong association with allergic and atopic disorders, including allergic rhinitis, nasal polyposis, and asthma. Approximately 70% of patients with EGPA have elevated levels of immunoglobulin E (IgE) and eosinophilia of peripheral blood and tissue. Small vessel histopathology typically reveals transmural eosinophilic infiltrates with scattered plasma cells and lymphocytes and extravascular granulomas.

The pathology of HSP is characterized by a leukocytoclastic vasculitis of small vessels with IgA deposition seen on immunofluorescence. Various infectious agents, including bacteria and viruses, have been reported as triggers for HSP.

The pathology of GCA and TAK are very similar histologically. In both, large vessels demonstrate a lymphoplasmacytic inflammatory infiltrate. Giant cells and granulomas may be seen in the media, and lumen-occlusive arteritis may occur from exuberant intimal hyperplasia. Additional pathologic features include proliferation of vascular smooth muscle cells and fragmentation of the internal elastic lamina.

CLINICAL PRESENTATION AND DIAGNOSIS

Clinical manifestations of the systemic vasculitides are diverse and differ not only among disorders but also among patients. Typical clinical manifestations associated with the size of the affected vessel are detailed in Table 6.1. Fever, weight loss, malaise, anorexia, arthralgias, and myalgias may occur with all vasculitides.

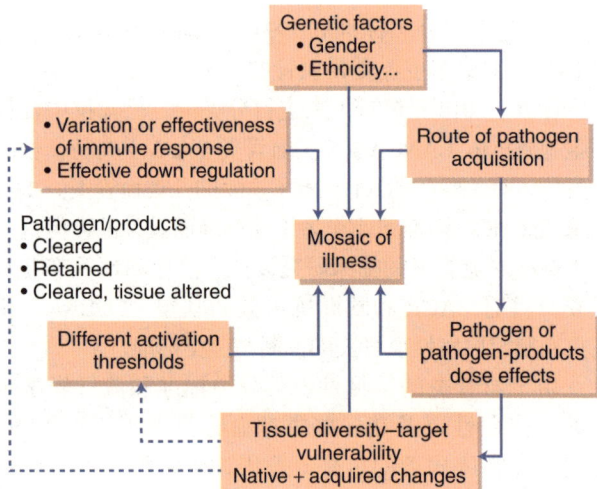

Fig. 6.2 Factors affecting disease vulnerability and expression.

Small Vessel Vasculitis
ANCA-Associated Vasculitides

GPA most commonly affects the sinuses and upper airway, the lungs, and the kidneys, although almost any organ system may be affected. Chronic refractory sinusitis, nasal crusting and ulcers, epistaxis, septal perforations, and otitis media are common presenting manifestations. Chronic nasal cartilaginous inflammation and destruction may lead to the characteristic "saddle nose" deformity. Lung involvement in GPA or MPA can include pulmonary nodules (often cavitary in GPA), infiltrates, or diffuse alveolar hemorrhage due to capillaritis. Importantly, life-threatening pulmonary hemorrhage may manifest simply as progressive acute dyspnea with hypoxia or respiratory failure, and not necessarily hemoptysis. Laryngotracheal disease may manifest as hoarseness or subglottic stenosis; orbital pseudotumors can also occur from GPA, and they may cause optic nerve compression, proptosis, and/or extraocular muscle palsies.

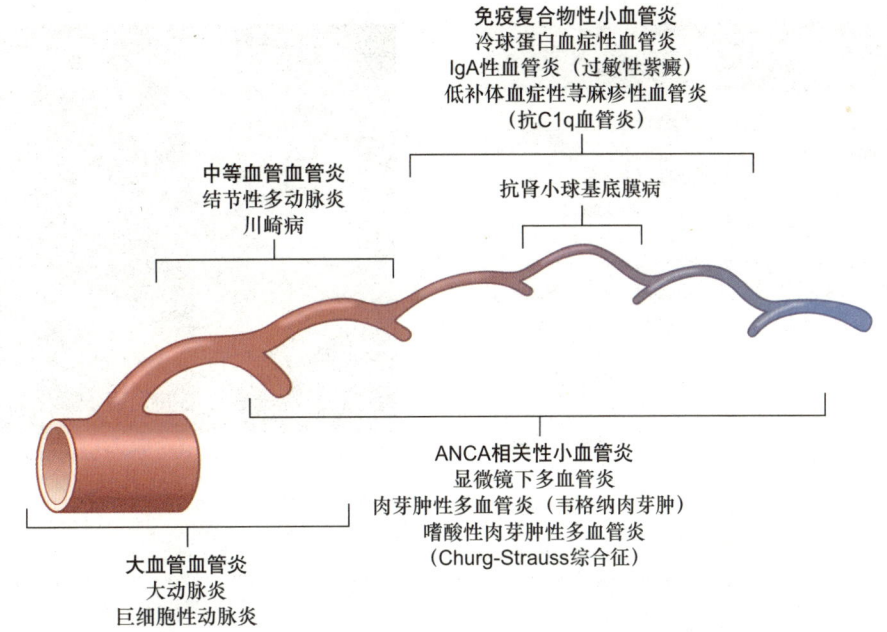

图6.1 系统性血管炎的分类（引自 Jennette JC，Falk RJ，Bacon PA，et al：2012 revised International Chapel Hill Consensus Conference Nomenclature of Vasculitides. Arthritis Rheum 2013；65：1-11.）

体液与细胞免疫反应、细胞因子的释放、趋化因子的激活以及免疫复合物的沉积在血管炎的发病机制中起着重要作用。此外，血管的正常保护和修复过程也可能导致损伤与缺血。例如，在血管损伤后，作为血管修复的一部分的细胞迁移和增殖可能导致内膜增生，而防止出血的促凝环境可能引发血栓形成与管腔闭塞。受损血管的血流异常会导致组织缺血与损伤。血流异常的严重程度依血管炎的类型和受累血管的大小与受累血管部位的不同而变化很大。

在 AAV 中，GPA 的典型病理特征是上呼吸道和下呼吸道的小血管的坏死性肉芽肿性炎症。GPA 和 MPA 两种 AAV 的肾脏病理均表现为寡免疫复合物性坏死性新月体性肾小球肾炎。EGPA 与过敏性疾病具有很强的相关性，包括过敏性鼻炎、鼻息肉和哮喘等。近70%的 EGPA 患者会出现免疫球蛋白 E（IgE）水平升高和外周血及组织中嗜酸性粒细胞增多。小血管的组织病理通常可见血管壁全层嗜酸性粒细胞浸润，伴有散在的浆细胞和淋巴细胞，以及血管外肉芽肿。

过敏性紫癜的病理特征为小血管的白细胞破碎性血管炎，免疫荧光检查可见 IgA 沉积。据报道，多种感染原，包括细菌和病毒，都可能是过敏性紫癜的诱发因素。

GCA 和 TAK 在组织病理学上非常相似。在两种疾病中，受累大血管均表现出淋巴浆细胞性炎性细胞浸润。在血管中膜可见到巨细胞和肉芽肿。内膜过度增生可能造成管腔闭塞性动脉炎。其他的病理特征包括血管平滑肌细胞增殖与内弹性板破碎。

临床表现和诊断

系统性血管炎的临床表现多种多样，不同疾病间与患者个体之间均存在差异。表6.1列出了与各种大小受累血管相对应的典型临床表现。所有血管炎患者均可出现发热、体重下降、全身不适、食欲减退、关节痛、肌痛等表现。

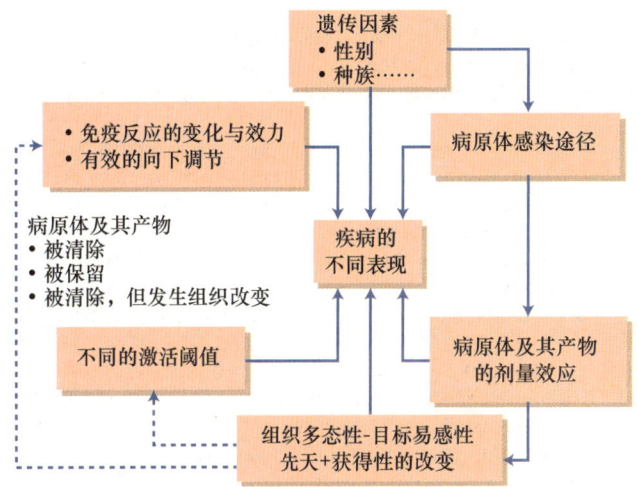

图6.2 影响疾病易感性与表现的因素

小血管血管炎

ANCA 相关性血管炎

虽然 GPA 可以累及全身所有器官，但最常累及器官包括鼻窦、上呼吸道、肺与肾脏。常见的首发症状包括慢性难治性鼻窦炎、鼻痂和溃疡、鼻衄、鼻中隔穿孔和中耳炎。慢性鼻软骨炎与软骨破坏可能导致特征性的"鞍鼻"畸形。GPA 或 MPA 的肺部受累可表现为肺部结节（GPA 常为空洞）、浸润或毛细血管炎引起的弥漫性肺泡出血。重要的是，危及生命的肺出血并不一定出现咯血，可仅表现为进行性加重的急性呼吸困难伴低氧或呼吸衰竭。GPA 也可出现喉气管病变，表现为声音嘶哑或声门下狭窄。GPA 还可以造成眼眶炎性假瘤，引起视神经压迫、眼球突出和（或）眼外肌麻痹等表现。

TABLE 6.1	Typical Clinical Features Based on Vessel Size[a]	
Large	Medium	Small
Limb claudication	Cutaneous nodules	Purpura
Asymmetrical blood pressures	Ulcers	Vesiculobullous lesions
Absence of pulses	Livedo reticularis	Alveolar hemorrhage
Bruits	Digital gangrene	Glomerulonephritis
Aortic dilatation	Mononeuritis multiplex	Mononeuritis multiplex
Aortic primary branch stenoses and/or aneurysms	Microaneurysms of mesenteric and/or renal branch arteries	Cutaneous extravascular necrotizing granulomas
		Splinter hemorrhages
		Scleritis, episcleritis, uveitis

[a]Constitutional symptoms in all types are fever, weight loss, malaise, anorexia, arthralgias, and myalgias.

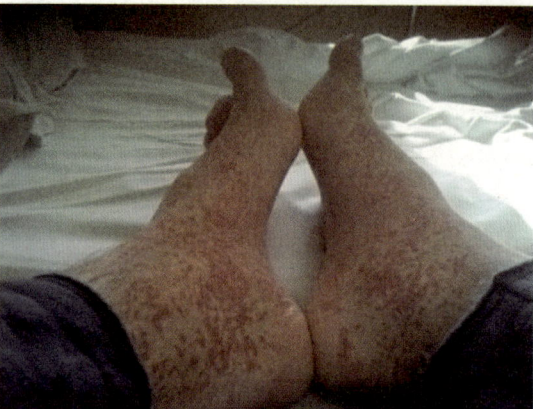

Fig. 6.3 Palpable purpura on the lower extremities of a patient with small vessel vasculitis affecting the skin. These lesions are "palpable" because they are slightly raised (i.e., palpable even with the eyes closed), and they are typically nonblanching when palpated. (Modified from Molyneux ID, Moon T, Webb AK, Morice AH: Treatment of cystic fibrosis associated cutaneous vasculitis with chloroquine, *J Cystic Fibrosis* 9:439-441, 2010. Copyright 2010 European Cystic Fibrosis Society.)

The renal manifestations in GPA, MPA, or RLV are those of nephritic syndrome, including acute renal failure, hematuria, hypertension, and subnephrotic proteinuria. Urine microscopy may reveal dysmorphic red blood cells. Renal biopsy reveals pauci-immune necrotizing crescentic glomerulonephritis. Additional organ manifestations that may occur in either GPA or MPA include neurologic, cutaneous, musculoskeletal, cardiovascular, and constitutional signs and symptoms. Patients may have subacute symptoms (weeks to months of sinusitis, arthralgias, and fatigue) or may exhibit acute "pulmonary-renal syndrome" with rapidly progressive glomerulonephritis and life-threatening alveolar hemorrhage with respiratory failure.

In EGPA, the clinical features comprise severe asthma, eosinophilia (>1500 cells/mL), and vasculitis involving two or more organs. Additional organ involvement in EGPA may include the nervous system, kidneys, skin, heart, and gastrointestinal tract. Sinus involvement in EGPA is typically not destructive as in GPA, and pulmonary infiltrates may be fleeting.

The diagnosis of any of the AAVs is most frequently established by tissue biopsy (e.g., kidney, lung, skin, sinus, nerve). ANCA testing plays an important diagnostic role in suspected small vessel vasculitis and is helpful in differentiating between GPA and MPA. Almost 90% of patients with renal disease have positive ANCA on testing. Most GPA patients have the cytoplasmic (cANCA) antiproteinase 3 (anti-PR3) type, whereas most MPA patients have the perinuclear (pANCA) antimyeloperoxidase (anti-MPO) type. The differential diagnosis for positive ANCA testing includes drug-induced effects, infections, and other autoimmune conditions. EGPA can be distinguished from other AAVs on the basis of a prior history of adult-onset asthma or allergic rhinitis and blood or tissue eosinophilia.

The differential diagnosis for any small vessel vasculitis includes infection, disorders of coagulation, drug toxicity, atherosclerotic and embolic disease, malignancy, and secondary vasculitides associated with other autoimmune diseases.

Henoch-Schönlein Purpura

Patients with HSP have lower extremity purpura, arthritis (typically of the large joints), abdominal pain, and renal disease at presentation (Fig. 6.3). In children, arthritis and abdominal pain affect about 75% of patients; the gastrointestinal manifestations may precede the purpura by up to 2 weeks and include hematochezia. The most common renal manifestation is microscopic hematuria with or without proteinuria.

The diagnosis of HSP is most often based on clinical and laboratory evidence, although skin or renal biopsy revealing IgA deposition may be helpful in solidifying the diagnosis. By classification criteria from the EULAR, patients with HSP must have purpura or petechiae with lower limb predominance and at least one of the following: arthritis or arthralgias; abdominal pain; histopathology demonstrating IgA deposition; and renal involvement. The differential for HSP includes other causes of abdominal pain, other causes of purpura in childhood, and hypersensitivity vasculitis. Hypersensitivity vasculitis is also a small vessel vasculitis that may occur in both children and adults and may be idiopathic or triggered by infections or drug exposures. It typically manifests as an isolated cutaneous leukocytoclastic (neutrophils and neutrophil debris in small vessels) vasculitis that is self-limited with treatment of the underlying cause (e.g., treatment of infection, discontinuation of drug culprit).

Medium Vessel Vasculitis
Polyarteritis Nodosa

The most common organ systems affected in PAN are the gastrointestinal, renal, and nervous systems. Mesenteric aneurysms or stenoses resulting in gut ischemia lead to symptoms of abdominal pain or "intestinal angina" (pain after eating). Renal artery aneurysms or stenoses result in hypertension or renal dysfunction, rather than glomerulonephritis as in MPA. Neurologic involvement may manifest as mononeuritis multiplex (painful asymmetrical sensory and motor peripheral neuropathy involving at least two separate nerve areas). Orchitis may be seen, manifesting as acute testicular pain. Anemia, elevated erythrocyte sedimentation rate or C-reactive protein or both, and hypertension (if renal artery involvement is present) are common. As in all vasculitides, constitutional symptoms may also be present.

The diagnosis of PAN is made based on angiographic or biopsy findings in the appropriate clinical setting. ANCAs typically are absent in PAN. A work-up for infection, including tests for hepatitis B and C and HIV, is warranted, given their known associations with PAN. The differential diagnosis includes MPA and mixed cryoglobulinemic vasculitis (defined by the presence of cryoglobulins in the blood). The latter vasculitis shares many clinical features with PAN, including peripheral neuropathy, arthralgias, myalgias, purpura, and association with hepatitis C.

表 6.1 不同大小受累血管的典型临床表现[a]

大血管	中等血管	小血管
肢体跛行	皮肤结节	紫癜
血压不对称	溃疡	水疱大疱性皮损
无脉	网状青斑	肺泡出血
血管杂音	肢端坏疽	肾小球肾炎
主动脉扩张	多发性单神经炎	多发性单神经炎
主动脉主要分支狭窄或动脉瘤	肠系膜和（或）肾分支动脉微动脉瘤	皮肤血管外坏死性肉芽肿
		裂片形出血
		巩膜炎、巩膜外层炎、虹膜炎

[a] 所有血管炎的全身症状均为发热、体重下降、全身不适、食欲减退、关节痛和肌痛。

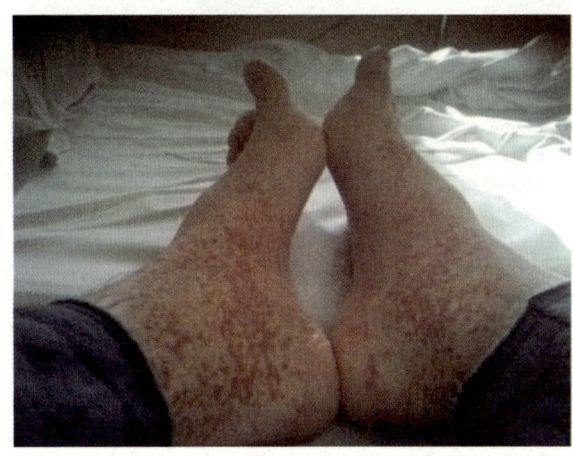

图 6.3 小血管血管炎累及皮肤引起下肢可触性紫癜。这些病变之所以"可触及"，是因为它们略微隆起（即使闭上眼睛也能触及），通常在触诊时不会褪色（改编自 Molyneux ID, Moon T, Webb AK, Morice AH: Treatment of cystic fibrosis associated cutaneous vasculitis with chloroquine, J Cystic Fibrosis 9: 439-441, 2010. Copyright 2010 European Cystic Fibrosis Society.）

GPA、MPA 或 RLV 的肾脏受累常表现为肾炎综合征，包括急性肾功能衰竭、血尿、高血压和亚肾病范围的蛋白尿。尿液镜检可以发现异形红细胞。肾活检病理表现为寡免疫复合物性坏死性新月体性肾小球肾炎。GPA 或 MPA 的其他受累脏器的临床表现包括神经、皮肤、肌肉骨骼、心血管和全身症状。患者可能有亚急性症状（如持续数周至数月的鼻窦炎、关节痛与疲劳），或者表现为急性"肺肾综合征"，伴有急进性肾小球肾炎和危及生命的肺泡出血与呼吸衰竭。

EGPA 的临床特点包括严重的哮喘、嗜酸性粒细胞增多症（>1500/ml）和累及两个及以上器官的血管炎。EGPA 的其他受累器官包括神经系统、肾脏、皮肤、心脏和胃肠道。EGPA 的鼻窦受累通常不像 GPA 那样具有破坏性，肺部浸润也可能是短暂性的。

AAV 最常通过组织活检（如肾、肺、皮肤、鼻窦、神经）来确诊。ANCA 检测在疑似小血管炎的诊断中发挥着重要作用，也有助于区分 GPA 与 MPA。约 90% 的肾脏受累患者 ANCA 检测阳性。大多数 GPA 患者为胞质型 ANCA（cANCA）抗蛋白酶 3（anti-PR3）抗体阳性，而大多数 MPA 患者为核周型 ANCA（pANCA）抗髓过氧化物酶（anti-MPO）抗体阳性。ANCA 检测阳性的鉴别诊断包括药物反应、感染和其他自身免疫性疾病。EGPA 可以通过成年发病的哮喘或过敏性鼻炎等既往病史、血液或组织中的嗜酸性粒细胞增多来与其他 AAV 进行鉴别。

小血管血管炎的鉴别诊断包括感染、凝血异常性疾病、药物毒性、动脉粥样硬化和栓塞性疾病、恶性肿瘤，以及与其他自身免疫性疾病相关的继发性血管炎。

过敏性紫癜

HSP 的患者发病时可表现为下肢紫癜、关节炎（典型者为大关节）、腹痛和肾脏损害（图 6.3）。在儿童患者中，约 75% 的患者会出现关节炎和腹痛；胃肠道症状可能在紫癜出现前 2 周或更早出现，可表现为血便。最常见的肾脏表现是镜下血尿，伴或不伴蛋白尿。

HSP 的诊断主要依靠临床和实验室证据，虽然皮肤或肾活检发现 IgA 沉积可能有助于确诊。根据 EULAR 的分类标准，HSP 患者必须有以下肢为主的紫癜或出血点，同时伴至少一项下列表现：关节炎或关节痛、腹痛、组织病理学 IgA 沉积、肾脏受累。HSP 的鉴别诊断包括其他原因引起的腹痛、其他原因引起的紫癜和过敏性血管炎。过敏性血管炎也是一种可发生在儿童或成人中的小血管炎，可能是特发性的，也可能由感染或药物诱发。典型的表现为孤立的皮肤白细胞破碎性（小血管中的中性粒细胞和中性粒细胞碎片）血管炎，在对潜在病因进行治疗（如抗感染、停用可疑药物等）后，这种血管炎通常是自限性的。

中等血管血管炎

结节性多动脉炎

在结节性多动脉炎（PAN）中，最常受累的器官系统包括胃肠道、肾脏和神经系统。肠系膜动脉瘤或狭窄可导致肠缺血，引起腹痛或"肠绞痛"（进食后出现的疼痛）。肾动脉瘤或狭窄可导致高血压或肾功能不全，而非像 MPA 一样引起肾小球肾炎。神经系统受累可表现为多发性单神经炎（至少累及两个不同神经区域的不对称的痛性感觉异常和运动周围神经病）。可能会出现睾丸炎，表现为急性睾丸疼痛。贫血、红细胞沉降率（血沉）或 C 反应蛋白升高（或两者均升高）、高血压（如病变累及肾动脉）在 PAN 中也很常见。与所有血管炎一样，PAN 也可以引起全身症状。

在出现相关临床表现时，基于血管造影或活检结果可做出 PAN 的诊断。PAN 患者的 ANCA 检测往往为阴性。由于已知 PAN 与一些感染性疾病相关，因此需对患者进行感染相关检查，包括乙型、丙型肝炎及 HIV 检测。PAN 的鉴别诊断主要包括 MPA 与混合型冷球蛋白血症性血管炎（因血液中存在冷球蛋白而命名）。后者与 PAN 具有许多相似的临床特征，包括周围神经病、关节痛、肌痛、紫癜以及与丙型肝炎相关等。

Kawasaki Disease

The clinical presentation of Kawasaki disease includes fever lasting longer than 5 days, conjunctival injection, oropharyngeal changes (strawberry tongue, mucous membrane desquamation), peripheral extremity changes (cutaneous desquamation), polymorphous rash, and cervical lymphadenopathy. Arthralgias, abdominal pain, hepatitis, aseptic meningitis, and uveitis have also been reported. Coronary artery aneurysms, one of the most serious complications of this vasculitis, appear within the first 4 weeks after onset of disease and are often detectable with echocardiography. Although areas of ectasia and small aneurysms may regress, larger aneurysms often persist and can result in coronary ischemia at any time after development, even into adulthood. Kawasaki disease is a triphasic disease, consisting of an acute febrile period lasting up to 14 days, a subacute phase of 2 to 4 weeks, and a convalescent phase that can last months to years. In the acute phase, the fever is persistent and high (>38.5° C) and is minimally responsive to antipyretics.

The differential diagnosis is wide and includes viral infections, toxin-mediated illnesses (e.g., toxic shock syndrome, scarlet fever), systemic juvenile idiopathic arthritis, hypersensitivity reactions, and drug reactions (e.g., Stevens-Johnson syndrome).

Large Vessel Vasculitis
Giant Cell Arteritis or Temporal Arteritis

At presentation, patients with GCA most commonly have new continuous headache, jaw claudication, visual disturbances (e.g., amaurosis fugax, diplopia), fatigue, and arthralgias. They are usually older than 50 years of age, have tender or thickened temporal arteries, and have an elevated erythrocyte sedimentation rate (>50 mm/hr by the Westergren method). Disease onset may be insidious or acute. Blindness due to anterior ischemic optic neuropathy occurs in 10% to 15% of patients with GCA and can occur at disease onset. Given the association between GCA and PMR, patients with PMR should be educated regarding signs and symptoms of GCA, and patients with GCA should be monitored for symptoms of PMR.

The diagnosis of GCA is often made by a biopsy of the superficial temporal artery. It is important to obtain a sufficient length of tissue (2 to 3 cm) because the vasculitis can have "skip lesions."

Takayasu's Arteritis

The typical clinical manifestations of TAK include a systolic blood pressure difference of greater than 10 mm Hg between the arms, decreased brachial or radial artery pulses, bruits auscultated over the subclavian arteries or aorta, claudication of extremities, neck or jaw pain, headache, dizziness, hypertension, constitutional symptoms, arthralgias, and myalgias.

The diagnosis of TAK is often based on vascular imaging studies that demonstrate long, tapering stenotic lesions or aneurysmal lesions in the aorta and primary branches. The differential diagnosis includes syphilis, spondyloarthropathies, rheumatoid arthritis, inflammatory bowel disease, and connective tissue disorders. Vascular imaging studies including computed tomography angiography and magnetic resonance angiography are typically performed for both diagnosis and disease surveillance.

TREATMENT AND PROGNOSIS
Small Vessel Vasculitis
ANCA-Associated Vasculitides

Glucocorticoids, often with other agents, are uniformly used to induce and maintain remission in AAV. They are typically initiated at a prednisone equivalent dose of 1 mg/kg/day with or without pulse methylprednisolone (1 g IV daily × 3 days), followed by a gradual taper over approximately 6 to 12 months. In addition, the standard of care in both GPA and MPA has traditionally been cyclophosphamide, either oral or intravenous, for 3 to 6 months. This yields remission rates varying from 30% to 93% in GPA and from 75% to 89% in MPA.

Rituximab, an anti-CD20 chimeric monoclonal antibody that depletes B cells, was shown to be noninferior to cyclophosphamide in remission induction for AAV in several randomized controlled trials (RITUXVAS and RAVE trials).

Plasmapheresis, or plasma exchange therapy (PLEX), is often used in combination with remission induction therapy in patients with life-threatening disease such as alveolar hemorrhage, or rapidly progressive glomerulonephritis (pulmonary-renal syndrome). The MEPEX study was a randomized controlled trial comparing plasmapheresis with high-dose methylprednisolone for severe renal vasculitis. PLEX was shown to be superior to methylprednisolone in reducing the number of patients remaining dependent on dialysis. The PEXIVAS trial is an ongoing multicenter randomized trial evaluating adjunctive PLEX and two oral glucocorticoid regimens in severe AAV.

For limited (early) GPA, such as disease confined to the upper respiratory tract, methotrexate may be used for remission induction, rather than cyclophosphamide; this conclusion was supported by evidence in the NORAM trial. Trimethoprim-sulfamethoxazole was shown in two randomized controlled trials to be helpful in preventing relapses after remission induction in GPA.

For EGPA, mepolizumab, an anti–interleukin-5 monoclonal antibody, has recently been shown in a multicenter double-blind placebo-controlled trial to be superior to placebo in producing a higher proportion of patients in remission and longer duration of remission in those who were relapsing or refractory to standard therapy. Only 47% of those in the mepolizumab group relapsed, compared to 81% of those in the placebo group, over 52 weeks. Hence, mepolizumab is now being used as a steroid-sparing therapy in EGPA patients who are relapsing or refractory to standard therapy.

Remission maintenance therapies in AAV include methotrexate, azathioprine, mycophenolate mofetil, and rituximab (RTX). Because there are known risks of bladder cancer, hemorrhagic cystitis, and bone marrow suppression with cumulative use of cyclophosphamide, it no longer has a role in remission maintenance in AAV. The role of RTX in remission maintenance has recently shown strong evidence of efficacy based on the MAINRITSAN Trial. In this study, patients with newly diagnosed or relapsing GPA, MPA, or renal-limited ANCA-associated vasculitis (RLV) in complete remission were recruited after a cyclophosphamide-glucocorticoid regimen. Patients were randomly assigned to receive either 500 mg of RTX on days 0 and 14 and at months 6, 12, and 18 after study entry, or daily azathioprine until month 22. At month 28, major relapse had occurred in 29% in the azathioprine group and 5% in the RTX group. RTX is now also being used to maintain remission in AAV.

Although AAVs were once considered diseases with considerable mortality (80% at 2 years if left untreated), the prognosis has improved significantly over the last 30 years because of improved treatments. Patient survival is now reported to be as high as 45% to 91% at 5 years. Among AAV patients with renal involvement at presentation, 20% develop end-stage renal disease within 5 years.

川崎病

川崎病的临床表现包括持续 5 天以上的发热、结膜充血、口咽部改变（草莓舌、黏膜脱皮）、四肢末端变化（皮肤脱皮）、多形性皮疹和颈部淋巴结肿大；也可出现关节痛、腹痛、肝炎、无菌性脑膜炎和葡萄膜炎等。冠状动脉瘤是川崎病最严重的并发症之一，往往在起病后 4 周内出现，常通过超声心动图检查发现。虽然冠状动脉局部扩张和小动脉瘤可能消退，但较大的动脉瘤常持续存在，可能在出现动脉瘤后的任何时间造成冠状动脉缺血，甚至在成年后造成冠状动脉缺血。川崎病是一种三相性疾病，包括持续长达 14 天的急性发热期、2～4 周的亚急性期和可能持续数月到数年的恢复期。在急性期，通常表现为持续高热（> 38.5℃），对退热药反应较差。

川崎病鉴别诊断较广，包括病毒感染、毒素介导疾病（如中毒性休克综合征、猩红热）、全身性幼年特发性关节炎、过敏反应和药物反应（如 Stevens-Johnson 综合征）等。

大血管血管炎
巨细胞动脉炎/颞动脉炎

GCA 患者在发病时最常见的症状包括新发的持续性头痛、下颌间歇性跛行、视力障碍（如一过性黑矇、复视）、疲劳和关节痛。患者年龄通常在 50 岁以上，伴有颞动脉压痛或颞动脉增厚，以及血沉增快（魏氏法测定大于 50 mm/h）。起病可以是隐匿的，也可是急性发病。10%～15% 的患者可出现眼前节缺血性视神经病导致的失明，可在 GCA 起病时即出现失明。鉴于 GCA 与 PMR 之间的相关性，我们应教育 PMR 患者了解 GCA 的症状和体征，在 GCA 患者的随访中也应监测是否出现了 PMR 的症状。

GCA 的诊断通常依靠颞浅动脉活检。由于颞动脉的病变可能呈跳跃性分布，因此在活检时取得足够长的组织标本（2～3 cm）非常重要。

大动脉炎

TAK 的典型临床表现包括双上肢收缩压差超过 10 mmHg、肱动脉或桡动脉脉搏减弱、锁骨下动脉或主动脉区听诊可闻及血管杂音、肢体间歇性跛行、颈部或下颌疼痛、头痛、头晕、高血压、全身症状、关节痛和肌痛。

TAK 的诊断主要基于血管影像学检查在主动脉及其主要分支上发现长的、逐渐加重的狭窄病变或动脉瘤形成。鉴别诊断包括梅毒、脊柱关节病、类风湿关节炎、炎症性肠病和结缔组织病。血管影像学检查，包括计算机断层成像血管造影（CTA）和磁共振血管造影（MRA）检查，常用于 TAK 的诊断与病情监测。

治疗与预后
小血管血管炎
ANCA 相关性血管炎

糖皮质激素是 AAV 诱导缓解与维持缓解治疗的一线用药，通常与其他药物联合使用。泼尼松的初始用量为 1 mg/（kg·d）（或等效剂量的其他激素），根据病情决定是否给予甲泼尼龙冲击治疗（每日 1 g 静脉输注，共 3 天），之后在 6～12 个月的时间内逐渐减量。GPA 与 MPA 的传统标准治疗方案为静脉或口服使用环磷酰胺治疗 3～6 个月。该方案治疗 GPA 的缓解率为 30%～93%，治疗 MPA 的缓解率为 75%～89%。

利妥昔单抗是一种可清除 B 细胞的抗 CD20 嵌合单克隆抗体，多项随机对照研究（RITUXVAS 与 RAVE）显示，该药在 AAV 诱导缓解治疗方面的作用不劣于环磷酰胺。

对于存在肺泡出血或快速进展性肾小球肾炎（肺肾综合征）等严重表现，病情危及生命的 AAV 患者，通常可考虑诱导治疗联合血浆置换（PLEX）。MEPEX 是一项在严重肾脏血管炎患者中进行的随机对照研究，旨在比较血浆置换与大剂量甲泼尼龙冲击治疗的疗效。结果显示，血浆置换在减少依赖透析患者的人数上优于甲泼尼龙。PEXIVAS 研究是一项正在进行的多中心随机对照研究，目的是探究联合血浆置换与两种口服糖皮质激素方案在重症 AAV 患者中的疗效。

对于局限型（早期）GPA 患者（如疾病局限在上呼吸道者）可使用甲氨蝶呤进行诱导缓解，而非环磷酰胺，NORAM 研究结果支持这一结论。两项随机对照研究显示，在 GPA 诱导缓解后，复方新诺明有助于防止疾病复发。

关于 EGPA 的治疗，在近期的一项多中心双盲安慰剂对照研究中显示，在复发或经标准治疗无效的难治性 EGPA 患者中，与安慰剂组相比，美泊利单抗（一种抗白介素 5 单克隆抗体）治疗组达到缓解的患者比例更高，且持续缓解时间更长。在长达 52 周的观察中，美泊利单抗治疗组仅有 47% 的患者复发，而安慰剂组中复发率高达 81%。因此，美泊利单抗已作为一种激素助减剂用于治疗复发或经标准治疗无效的难治性 EGPA。

AAV 的维持缓解治疗用药包括甲氨蝶呤、硫唑嘌呤、吗替麦考酚酯与利妥昔单抗。由于已知环磷酰胺累积使用发生膀胱癌、出血性膀胱炎、骨髓抑制等风险增加，因此，环磷酰胺已不再用于 AAV 的维持缓解。近期发表的 MAINRISTAN 研究中已获得的强有力证据支持利妥昔单抗在 AAV 维持治疗中的作用。这项研究中纳入的是经环磷酰胺联合激素治疗达完全缓解的新诊断或治疗后复发的 GPA、MPA 或 RLV 患者，这些患者被随机分配到两个治疗组中，分别接受利妥昔单抗（在第 0 天、第 14 天，以及进入研究后的第 6、12 和 18 个月，每次使用 500 mg，共 5 次）或每日口服硫唑嘌呤治疗至纳入研究后的第 22 个月。在第 28 个月时，硫唑嘌呤治疗组的重症复发率为 29%，而利妥昔单抗组仅为 5%。因此，目前利妥昔单抗已被用于 AAV 的维持缓解治疗。

虽然既往认为 AAV 是一种死亡率很高的疾病（未经治疗者 2 年死亡率为 80%），近 30 年来，随治疗进步，AAV 的预后已明显改善。现在的报告显示，目前 AAV 患者的 5 年生存率已达 45%～91%。20% 的在疾病初始即有肾脏受累的 AAV 患者，将在 5 年内发展为终末期肾病。

Henoch-Schönlein Purpura

In mild cases, the therapy for HSP is simply supportive care (i.e., hydration and analgesics). However, glucocorticoids are commonly used to hasten the resolution of symptoms; early use of glucocorticoids has been associated with improved outcomes, especially when there is severe gastrointestinal involvement. In life-threatening cases and in severe acute renal failure, additional immunosuppressive agents or plasmapheresis may be considered. The prognosis of HSP is generally good, with fewer than 1% of patients developing end-stage renal disease.

Medium Vessel Vasculitis
Polyarteritis Nodosa

Treatment of PAN includes glucocorticoids or nonsteroidal anti-inflammatory drugs (NSAIDs) or both. If disease is severe and persistent or relapsing, additional immunosuppressive agents are used, such as cyclophosphamide (especially for gastrointestinal or cardiac involvement), methotrexate, colchicine, or intravenous immunoglobulin (IVIG). In cases of PAN associated with hepatitis B or C, antiviral therapy is required not only for attaining control of the viral infection but also for treatment of the associated vasculitis itself. Corticosteroids and cyclophosphamide have improved patient outcomes, and the 1-year survival rate is now 85%. Prognosis is typically worse with more systemic complications such as renal or neurologic involvement.

Kawasaki Disease

Treatment of Kawasaki disease includes high-dose aspirin (30 to 100 mg/kg/day) for the first 48 hours, then 3 to 5 mg/kg/day. IVIG is standard therapy and has significantly decreased the incidence of coronary artery aneurysm complications in this disease. The initial IVIG dose is 2 g/kg within the first 10 days after presentation, with at least one repeat dose typically given if the first IVIG dose fails to improve the child's condition. The prognosis of Kawasaki disease, if promptly treated, is good; however, approximately 15% to 25% of patients develop coronary artery aneurysms that increase morbidity and mortality.

Large Vessel Vasculitis
Giant Cell Arteritis or Temporal Arteritis

Glucocorticoids are the cornerstone of therapy in GCA. To prevent vision loss, treatment should be instituted immediately (within 24 hours) if clinical suspicion for GCA is high or if visual disturbances are present. The initial dose of glucocorticoids is typically 1 mg/kg/day with a gradual taper. Most patients require a glucocorticoid treatment duration of 1 to 2 years, but it may be longer, especially in those with symptoms of PMR. In PMR without GCA, lower doses of glucocorticoids (10 to 20 mg/day of prednisone equivalent) are effective and provide prompt clinical response.

If patients experience relapse with glucocorticoid tapering, other immunosuppressive agents may be used. Methotrexate was shown in a meta-analysis of three randomized controlled trials to be a beneficial adjunctive agent in reducing risks of first and second relapses in GCA, with a significant decrease in the cumulative dose of glucocorticoids. Low-dose aspirin is an important adjunctive therapy in protecting against cranial ischemic events (level II evidence from two large retrospective studies). Recently, tocilizumab given subcutaneously weekly or every other week with a 26-week prednisone taper was found in a large 1-year randomized trial of GCA patients to result in more sustained glucocorticoid-free remission compared to either 26-week or 52-week prednisone tapering courses plus placebo. Hence, tocilizumab is now being used as an effective steroid-sparing agent to maintain remission in GCA.

Takayasu's Arteritis

Glucocorticoids are also the cornerstone of therapy for TAK; they are typically initiated at a dose of 0.5 to 1 mg/kg/day. Although most patients respond to the initial dose, relapses occur in more than 50% of patients during glucocorticoid tapering. Hence, steroid-sparing agents are often used to aid in maintaining disease remission. The most commonly used steroid-sparing agents are methotrexate and azathioprine. In TAK, unlike in GCA and PMR, the tumor necrosis factor (TNF) inhibitors have shown promise in treating refractory disease. As in GCA, low-dose aspirin is believed to play a beneficial adjunctive role in preventing ischemic complications.

Revascularization interventions are often indicated in patients with TAK whose presenting symptoms include cerebrovascular disease, coronary artery disease, moderate to severe aortic regurgitation, renovascular hypertension, progressive limb claudication, or progressive aneurysm enlargement. Elective intervention should be performed when the disease is quiescent.

In both GCA and TAK, aortitis—a common manifestation of large vessel involvement—can lead to an increased risk of aortic aneurysm and subsequent dissection and rupture. In both GCA and TAK, disease flares occur in most patients, rendering them chronic, progressive, and relapsing conditions.

ADDITIONAL CONSIDERATIONS IN TREATMENT

Immunosuppressive therapy is associated with an increased risk of infection. Patients receiving combination therapy with moderate- to high-dose glucocorticoid (>20 mg/day of prednisone equivalents) and another immunosuppressive agent should also receive prophylaxis for *Pneumocystis jirovecii* pneumonia (previously known as PCP). Furthermore, infections can often mimic or result in flares of systemic vasculitis. Glucocorticoid therapy should never be discontinued abruptly, even in the setting of infection, because of the risk of adrenal crisis or disease relapse or both. In most cases, other immunosuppressive agents should be discontinued if infection is suspected or diagnosed.

Glucocorticoid therapy is a common cause of bone loss (osteopenia, osteoporosis). Because significant bone loss can occur even within the first 6 months of therapy, calcium and vitamin D supplementation should be initiated, and a baseline bone density study should be obtained. Consideration should be given to additional bone protection therapies (e.g., bisphosphonates). Methotrexate and cyclophosphamide are teratogenic, and cyclophosphamide may result in premature ovarian failure. These factors must be considered when choosing therapies for women of child-bearing age. Immunosuppressive agents also can be associated with bone marrow suppression and with additional long-term risks such as malignancy.

Acknowledgments

The author wishes to acknowledge the assistance of Kathleen Maksimowicz-McKinnon, DO.

For a deeper discussion on this topic, please see Chapter 254, "The Systemic Vasculitides," in *Goldman-Cecil Medicine,* 26th Edition.

过敏性紫癜

对于轻症过敏性紫癜患者，通常仅需进行支持治疗（即补液和镇痛）。但通常会使用糖皮质激素来迅速控制症状；早期使用糖皮质激素有助于改善预后，特别是对于严重胃肠道受累患者。在病情危及生命或出现急性肾衰竭时，可考虑联合免疫抑制剂或血浆置换。过敏性紫癜的预后通常较好，不到1%的患者会发展为终末期肾病。

中等大小血管血管炎

结节性多动脉炎

PAN 的治疗药物主要包括糖皮质激素或 NSAID，或两者联合。如 PAN 病情严重、持续或出现复发，则需在此基础上加用免疫抑制剂，如环磷酰胺（特别是胃肠道或心脏受累时）、甲氨蝶呤、秋水仙碱或静脉注射免疫球蛋白（IVIG）。在乙型或丙型肝炎相关 PAN 患者中，需加用抗病毒治疗，这不仅是为了控制病毒感染，同时抗病毒治疗本身也可治疗感染相关的血管炎。糖皮质激素和环磷酰胺治疗改善了 PAN 患者的预后，目前 PAN 患者的1年生存率为85%。有更多系统性并发症（如肾或神经系统受累）的患者，往往预后较差。

川崎病

川崎病的治疗包括在病初48 h 应用大剂量阿司匹林 [30～100 mg/（kg·d）]，此后减为3～5 mg/（kg·d）。IVIG 是川崎病的标准治疗，可显著降低并发冠状动脉瘤概率。在起病后10天内应用 IVIG，起始剂量2 g/kg，如首剂 IVIG 未能改善患儿病情，需重复至少一剂 IVIG 治疗。如能得到及时治疗，预后通常良好。但是，约15%～25%患者会发展为冠状动脉瘤，导致病残率和死亡率增加。

大血管血管炎

巨细胞动脉炎／颞动脉炎

糖皮质激素是 GCA 治疗的基石。为预防视力丧失，对于临床高度怀疑 GCA 或已出现视力障碍患者，应立即（24 h 内）开始使用糖皮质激素，初始剂量通常为1 mg/（kg·d），然后逐渐减量。大多数患者需接受1～2年的糖皮质激素治疗，或使用更长时间，尤其在伴有 PMR 症状的患者。在未合并 GCA 的 PMR 患者中，较低剂量糖皮质激素（相当于泼尼松10～20mg/d）通常有效，且起效很快。

如患者在糖皮质激素减量过程中病情复发，可加用其他免疫抑制剂。一项纳入三项随机对照试验的荟萃分析显示，联用甲氨蝶呤有助于减少 GCA 的首次和第二次复发风险，同时也可显著降低糖皮质激素的累积剂量。低剂量阿司匹林是预防 GCA 发生脑缺血事件的重要辅助治疗（来自两项大型回顾性研究的 II 级证据）。近来在 GCA 患者中进行的一项为期1年的大规模随机临床试验显示，与泼尼松减量联合安慰剂治疗相比，无论是第26周或第52周，泼尼松减量联合托珠单抗治疗（每周或每两周皮下注射）组有更多的患者能达到无激素持续缓解。因此，目前托珠单抗已被作为一种有效的激素助减剂，应用于 GCA 的维持治疗中。

大动脉炎

糖皮质激素也是 TAK 治疗的基石，常用起始剂量为0.5～1 mg/（kg·d）。虽然大部分患者对起始激素治疗有效，但超过50%的患者会在激素减量过程中出现复发。因此，临床中常使用激素助减剂来协助维持病情缓解。最常用的激素助减剂是甲氨蝶呤和硫唑嘌呤。不同于 GCA 和 PMR，肿瘤坏死因子抑制剂在难治性 TAK 的治疗中显示出了良好的应用前景。低剂量阿司匹林在预防缺血并发症方面显示出了与在 GCA 中相似的良好辅助作用。

对已出现脑血管疾病、冠状动脉疾病、中重度主动脉瓣关闭不全、肾血管性高血压、进行性加重的肢体跛行或不断扩大的动脉瘤等表现的 TAK 患者，通常需进行血运重建治疗。应在疾病稳定期进行择期手术。

主动脉炎是 TAK 和 GCA 这两种大血管血管炎的常见表现，会增加主动脉瘤形成及继而出现主动脉夹层和破裂的风险。大多数 TAK 和 GCA 患者会出现疾病复发，使其发展为慢性、进行性加重并反复发作的疾病。

治疗方面的其他注意事项

免疫抑制治疗会增加感染风险。接受中-大剂量糖皮质激素（泼尼松＞20 mg/d 或等效剂量的其他激素）和免疫抑制剂联合治疗的患者应同时接受肺孢子菌肺炎（以前称为 PCP）预防性治疗。此外，感染常常会模仿系统性血管炎或导致系统性血管炎复发。即使在感染的情况下，也不应突然停用糖皮质激素，因为这可能导致肾上腺危象或疾病复发或两者兼而有之。在大多数情况下，如怀疑或确诊了感染，应停用其他免疫抑制剂。

糖皮质激素治疗是引起骨质流失（骨量减少、骨质疏松）的常见原因。由于在开始治疗的前6个月内即可发生严重的骨质流失，因此，应为接受糖皮质激素治疗的患者补充钙和维生素 D，并进行基线骨密度检查。应考虑使用其他的骨保护治疗（如双膦酸盐）。甲氨蝶呤和环磷酰胺具有致畸性，环磷酰胺还可能导致卵巢早衰。因此，在为育龄期女性选择治疗方案时，务必考虑到这些因素。免疫抑制剂还可能造成骨髓抑制以及其他的长期风险如恶性肿瘤等。

致谢

感谢 Kathleen Maksimowicz-McKinnon, DO 提供的帮助。

有关此专题的深入讨论，请参阅 *Goldman-Cecil Medicine* 第26版第254章"系统性血管炎"。

SUGGESTED READINGS

Bloch DA, Michel BA, Hunder GG, et al: The American College of Rheumatology 1990 criteria for the classification of vasculitis: patients and methods, Arthritis Rheum 33:1068–1073, 1990.

Guillevin L, Pagnoux C, Karras A, et al: Rituximab versus azathioprine for maintenance in ANCA-associated vasculitis, N Engl J Med 371:1771–1780, 2014.

Hoffman GS, Cid MC, Rendt-Zagar KE, et al: Infliximab for maintenance of glucocorticosteroid-induced remission of giant cell arteritis: a randomized trial, Ann Intern Med 146:621–630, 2007.

Hunder GG, Bloch DA, Michel BA, et al: The American College of Rheumatology 1990 criteria for the classification of giant cell arteritis, Arthritis Rheum 33:1122–1128, 1990.

Jennette JC, Falk RJ, Bacon PA, et al: 2012 revised International Chapel Hill Consensus Conference Nomenclature of vasculitides, Arthritis Rheum 65:1–11, 2013.

Jones RB, Tervaert JW, Hauser T, et al: Rituximab versus cyclophosphamide in ANCA-associated renal vasculitis, N Engl J Med 363:211–220, 2010.

Specks U, Merkel PA, Seo P, et al: Efficacy of remission-induction regimens for ANCA-associated vasculitis, N Engl J Med 369:417–427, 2013.

Stone JH, Merkel PA, Spiera R, et al: Rituximab versus cyclophosphamide for ANCA-associated vasculitis, N Engl J Med 363:221–232, 2010.

Stone JH, Tuckwell K, Dimonaco S, et al: Trial of tocilizumab in giant cell arteritis, N Engl J Med 337:317–328, 2017.

Wechsler ME, Akuthota P, Jayne D, et al: Mepolizumab or placebo for eosinophilic granulomatosis with polyangiitis, N Engl J Med 376:1921–1932, 2017.

Weiss PF: Pediatric vasculitis, Pediatr Clin North Am 59:407–423, 2012.

推荐阅读

Bloch DA, Michel BA, Hunder GG, et al: The American College of Rheumatology 1990 criteria for the classification of vasculitis: patients and methods, Arthritis Rheum 33:1068–1073, 1990.

Guillevin L, Pagnoux C, Karras A, et al: Rituximab versus azathioprine for maintenance in ANCA-associated vasculitis, N Engl J Med 371:1771–1780, 2014.

Hoffman GS, Cid MC, Rendt-Zagar KE, et al: Infliximab for maintenance of glucocorticosteroid-induced remission of giant cell arteritis: a randomized trial, Ann Intern Med 146:621–630, 2007.

Hunder GG, Bloch DA, Michel BA, et al: The American College of Rheumatology 1990 criteria for the classification of giant cell arteritis, Arthritis Rheum 33:1122–1128, 1990.

Jennette JC, Falk RJ, Bacon PA, et al: 2012 revised International Chapel Hill Consensus Conference Nomenclature of vasculitides, Arthritis Rheum 65:1–11, 2013.

Jones RB, Tervaert JW, Hauser T, et al: Rituximab versus cyclophosphamide in ANCA-associated renal vasculitis, N Engl J Med 363:211–220, 2010.

Specks U, Merkel PA, Seo P, et al: Efficacy of remission-induction regimens for ANCA-associated vasculitis, N Engl J Med 369:417–427, 2013.

Stone JH, Merkel PA, Spiera R, et al: Rituximab versus cyclophosphamide for ANCA-associated vasculitis, N Engl J Med 363:221–232, 2010.

Stone JH, Tuckwell K, Dimonaco S, et al: Trial of tocilizumab in giant cell arteritis, N Engl J Med 337:317–328, 2017.

Wechsler ME, Akuthota P, Jayne D, et al: Mepolizumab or placebo for eosinophilic granulomatosis with polyangiitis, N Engl J Med 376:1921–1932, 2017.

Weiss PF: Pediatric vasculitis, Pediatr Clin North Am 59:407–423, 2012.

Crystal Arthropathies

Pooja Bhadbhade, Ghaith Noaiseh

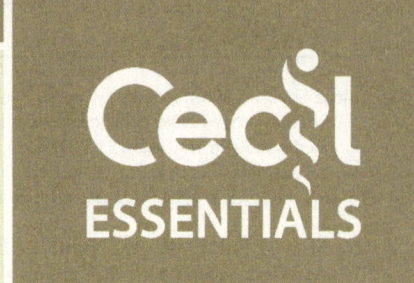

GOUT

Gout is a disorder resulting from deposition of monosodium urate (MSU) monohydrate crystals in and around the tissues of joints causing attacks of acute inflammatory arthritis. Gout is associated with hyperuricemia, which is defined as a serum urate level greater than 6.8 mg/dL. The risk of gout is strongly associated with the degree of hyperuricemia. However, it is not a sufficient causative factor for the development of gout.

Typically, the disease presents as an acute and episodic monoarthritis affecting the lower extremities but can become recurrent, chronic, and deforming, affecting multiple joints. Tophi are a pathognomonic feature of gout resulting from accumulation of urate crystals in soft tissues or joints.

Epidemiology

In the United States, the prevalence of gout is 3.9%, affecting 8.3 million adults. The incidence rate ranges from 0.45 to 1 cases per 1000 person-years. There is a trend towards increasing incidence and prevalence, thought to be related to the aging population, increased use of certain medications such as diuretics, and the increasing frequency of risk factors for hyperuricemia including obesity, hypertension, renal disease, cardiovascular disease, and metabolic syndrome.

Men are three to six times more likely to have gout than women, but the sex disparity decreases with age due to loss of the uricosuric effect of estrogen after menopause. This also explains why gout is less common in premenopausal women.

Pathogenesis
Pathophysiology of Hyperuricemia

Uric acid is the end product of purine metabolism in humans. Unlike many other species, humans lack the enzyme uricase, which catalyzes the conversion of uric acid into allantoin, a very soluble metabolite. Most individuals maintain uric acid levels between 4 and 6.8 mg/dL and a total body uric acid pool of approximately 1000 mg. However, uric acid levels may increase, leading to supersaturation of urate in blood. MSU crystals form in some patients with serum uric acid levels greater than 6.8 mg/dL. Only about 20% of hyperuricemic patients develop gout during their lifetime. Factors controlling crystal formation are poorly understood, but urate solubility may be affected by temperature, pH, salt concentration, and cartilage matrix components. Urate crystallization is a critical step in the progression from asymptomatic hyperuricemia to clinical gout. Unlike soluble urate molecules, MSU crystals are a potent promoter of acute inflammation.

The total body uric acid pool depends on the balance between dietary intake, synthesis, and excretion. About two thirds of the daily excretion of uric acid occurs in the kidneys; the rest is eliminated by the gut. Renal underexcretion is the cause for approximately 90% of hyperuricemia cases (Table 7.1). In the remaining 10%, hyperuricemia is caused by uric acid overproduction (>1000 mg in a 24-hour urine collection while on a standard Western diet) or by a combination of overproduction with renal underexcretion.

Fig. 7.1 summarizes the de novo biosynthesis and salvage pathways of purine metabolism. Abnormalities in the activities of key enzymes can lead to increased serum uric acid levels and development of gout. The de novo synthesis of purine is driven by the enzyme 5′-phosphoribosyl 1-pyrophosphate (PRPP) synthetase. In PRPP synthetase overactivity, overproduction of PRPP increases purine production. In salvage pathways, tissue-derived intermediate purine products (hypoxanthine, guanine, and adenine) are reutilized rather than undergoing further degradation to xanthine and uric acid. Deficiencies of hypoxanthine-guanine phosphoribosyltransferase (HGPRT) activity result in impaired purine salvage and increased substrate for uric acid generation (Lysch-Nyhan syndrome and Kelley-Seegmiller syndrome). Overall, inborn errors of metabolism account for a small fraction of uric acid overproduction.

Most cases of uric acid overproduction result from increased reutilization of purine bases through salvage pathways (see Fig. 7.1). The purine precursors come from exogenous (dietary) sources or endogenous metabolism (synthesis and cell turnover) Purine-rich foods such as red meat, organ meats (e.g., sweetbreads, liver), seafood, high-fructose corn syrup–sweetened beverages, and alcohol comprise a significant portion of the daily purine load and can worsen hyperuricemia. On the other hand, consumption of low-fat dairy products is associated with reduced serum urate levels and may decrease the risk of gout.

A very small proportion of serum urate is bound to plasma proteins; therefore, urate is almost completely filtered in the glomeruli. Subsequent reabsorption and secretion are controlled by various organic acid transporters located on the luminal side of the proximal convoluted tubule epithelium. Only 10% of the initially filtered uric acid is eventually excreted in the urine.

In addition to the bidirectional transport of uric acid, organic acid transporters are also responsible for eliminating other organic acids and certain medications. The function of these transporters is affected by certain medications, including thiazides, low-dose aspirin, and cyclosporine, leading to decreased uric acid excretion and hyperuricemia. Conversely, medications such as probenecid and losartan, when excreted in the tubular lumen, exert their uricosuric effect by displacing uric acid from the transporter and increasing uric acid excretion. Certain genetic mutations affecting these transporters may lead to uric acid underexcretion. Renal insufficiency can cause hyperuricemia though decreased uric acid filtration.

Pathophysiology of Acute Gouty Attack

In some patients with prolonged hyperuricemia, tissue deposits of MSU crystals, called microtophi, form in the synovium and on the

晶体性关节病

李谦华 译 戴冽 王俐 厉小梅 审校 栗占国 通审

痛风

痛风是一种单钠尿酸盐（MSU）的一水晶体在关节及周围组织中沉积引起急性炎症性关节炎发作的疾病。痛风与高尿酸血症有关，高尿酸血症是指血清尿酸盐水平＞408 μmol/L（6.8 mg/dl）。痛风的风险与高尿酸血症的程度密切相关，但高尿酸血症并不是痛风发病的唯一致病因素。

痛风的典型表现是累及下肢关节的急性发作性的单关节炎，但可进展为复发性、慢性、致残性关节炎并可累及多关节。尿酸盐晶体在软组织或关节中积聚形成的痛风石是痛风的特征性病变。

流行病学

在美国，痛风的患病率为3.9%，影响了830万成年人。其发病率介于（0.45～1）/1000人年。发病率和患病率均呈上升趋势，这被认为与人口老龄化、利尿剂等药物应用的增加以及肥胖、高血压、肾脏病、心血管疾病和代谢综合征等高尿酸血症风险因素的增加相关。

男性患痛风的风险是女性的3～6倍，但这种性别差异会随年龄的增长而逐渐缩小，因为绝经后雌激素的促尿酸排泄作用减弱，这也解释了为何痛风在绝经前的女性中较少见。

发病机制

高尿酸血症的病理生理学

尿酸是人类嘌呤代谢的最终产物。与许多其他物种不同，人类体内缺乏尿酸酶，而尿酸酶能催化尿酸转化为一种可溶性很强的代谢产物——尿囊素。大多数人的尿酸水平维持在240～408 μmol/L（4～6.8 mg/dl）之间，体内尿酸池总量约为6000 μmol。然而，尿酸水平可能会升高，导致血液中尿酸盐过饱和。某些血清尿酸水平超过408 μmol/L（6.8 mg/dl）的患者会形成MSU晶体。只有约20%的高尿酸血症患者最终发展为痛风。控制晶体形成的因素现今尚未明确，但尿酸盐的溶解度可能会受温度、pH值、盐浓度和软骨基质成分的影响。尿酸盐形成晶体是无症状性高尿酸血症发展为临床痛风的关键步骤。与可溶性尿酸盐分子不同，MSU晶体是急性炎症的强有力促进剂。

体内尿酸池的总量取决于饮食摄入、合成和排泄之间的平衡。每天约有2/3的尿酸通过肾排出，其余则由肠道排出。大约90%的高尿酸血症病例由于肾排泄不足所致（表7.1）。在其余的10%病例中，高尿酸血症是由于尿酸生成过多（在标准西方饮食下，24 h尿尿酸＞6000 μmol）引起，或尿酸生成过多和肾排泄不足共同引起。

图7.1概述了嘌呤代谢的从头合成和补救合成途径。关键酶的活性异常可导致血清尿酸水平升高和痛风的发生。嘌呤的从头合成由5′-磷酸核糖1-焦磷酸（PRPP）合成酶驱动。在PRPP合成酶过度活跃的情况下，PRPP的过度生成会增加嘌呤的产生。在补救途径中，组织来源的嘌呤代谢中间产物（次黄嘌呤、鸟嘌呤和腺嘌呤）被重新利用，而不是进一步降解为黄嘌呤和尿酸。次黄嘌呤-鸟嘌呤磷酸核糖基转移酶活性不足会导致这一嘌呤补救功能受损，尿酸生成的底物增加（Lysch-Nyhan综合征和Kelley-Seegmiller综合征）。总体而言，先天性代谢缺陷只占尿酸生成过多的一小部分。

大多数尿酸生成过多的病例都是由于嘌呤碱补救合成途径的再利用增加所致（见图7.1）。嘌呤前体来自外源性（饮食）或内源性代谢（合成和细胞代谢）。富含嘌呤的食物，如红肉、内脏（如胰腺、肝）、海鲜、高果糖玉米糖浆糖化饮料和酒精，是日常嘌呤负荷的重要组成部分，这些食物可使高尿酸血症恶化。另一方面，食用低脂乳制品与血清尿酸盐水平负相关，可能可以降低痛风的风险。

仅有极小部分的血清尿酸盐可与血浆蛋白结合，因此尿酸盐几乎完全被肾小球滤过。随后通过位于肾小管近曲小管上皮管腔侧的各种有机酸转运体进行重吸收和分泌。最初滤过的尿酸最终仅10%会随尿液排出体外。

除了双向转运尿酸，有机酸转运体还负责排出其他有机酸和某些药物。这些转运体的功能会受到某些药物的影响，包括噻嗪类利尿剂、小剂量阿司匹林和环孢素，导致尿酸排泄减少和高尿酸血症。相反，丙磺舒和氯沙坦等药物在肾小管管腔内排泄时，会将尿酸从转运体中置换出来，增加尿酸排泄，从而发挥促尿酸排泄的作用。影响这些转运体的某些基因突变可能导致尿酸排泄不足。肾功能不全可通过尿酸滤过减少引起高尿酸血症。

急性痛风发作的病理生理学

在某些长期高尿酸血症患者中，组织中的MSU晶体沉积物，即微小痛风石，会在滑膜和软骨表面形

TABLE 7.1 Causes of Hyperuricemia

Urate Overproduction	Urate Underexcretion
Metabolic Disorders	Renal insufficiency
HGPRT deficiency (homozygous or heterozygous)	Volume depletion
PRPP synthetase hyperactivity	Metabolic acidosis (lactic acidosis and ketoacidosis)
G6PD deficiency	Obesity
Glycogen storage diseases	Ethanol
Others	Medications: low-dose salicylate, diuretics (thiazides, loop diuretics), cyclosporine, tacrolimus, L-dopa, ethambutol
Myeloproliferative and lymphoproliferative disorders	Familial juvenile hyperuricemic nephropathy
Erythropoietic disorders (hemolytic anemia, megaloblastic anemia, sickle cell disease, thalassemia, other hemoglobinopathies)	Medullary cystic kidney disease
Solid tumors	Lead nephropathy
Diffuse psoriasis	
Ethanol (particularly beer)	
Medications: cytotoxic agents, nicotinic acid	
Shellfish, organ meat, red meat	
Fructose	
Obesity	

G6PD, Glucose-6-phosphate dehydrogenase; *HGPRT*, hypoxanthine-guanine phosphoribosyltransferase; *PRPP*, 5-phosphoribosyl 1-pyrophosphate.

surface of cartilage. During an acute attack, microtophi break apart, shedding a large number of MSU crystals into the joint space and activating synovial macrophages and fibroblasts that phagocytize the crystals. This, in turn, leads to the activation of a cytosolic multiprotein complex, the NALP3 (NACHT, LRR, and PYD domains–containing protein 3) inflammasome (Fig. 7.2). There is evidence that in acute gout, MSU crystals undergo phagocytosis, which activates the NLRP3 inflammasome, leading to the release of interleukin-1β, which in turn induces further production of interleukin-1β and other inflammatory mediators and activation of synovial lining cells and phagocytes.

MSU crystals undergo clearance by inflammatory cells that then undergo apoptosis. This, along with other mechanisms, eventually leads to resolution of the acute inflammatory process, typically after 10 to 14 days. Even after complete resolution of symptoms, a low-grade level of inflammation (intercritical inflammation) can persist in the otherwise asymptomatic joint. This inflammation may become clinically apparent in long-standing gout, contributing to development of tophi, chronic synovitis, cartilage loss, and bony erosions.

Clinical Features

Gout has three stages: asymptomatic hyperuricemia, acute intermittent gout, and chronic gout.

Acute Gouty Attacks

The classic picture of acute gout is rapid development of an inflammatory arthritis involving one or occasionally two joints. Severe pain, erythema, swelling, and exquisite tenderness typically occur. This clinical picture can be easily confused with that of septic arthritis or bacterial

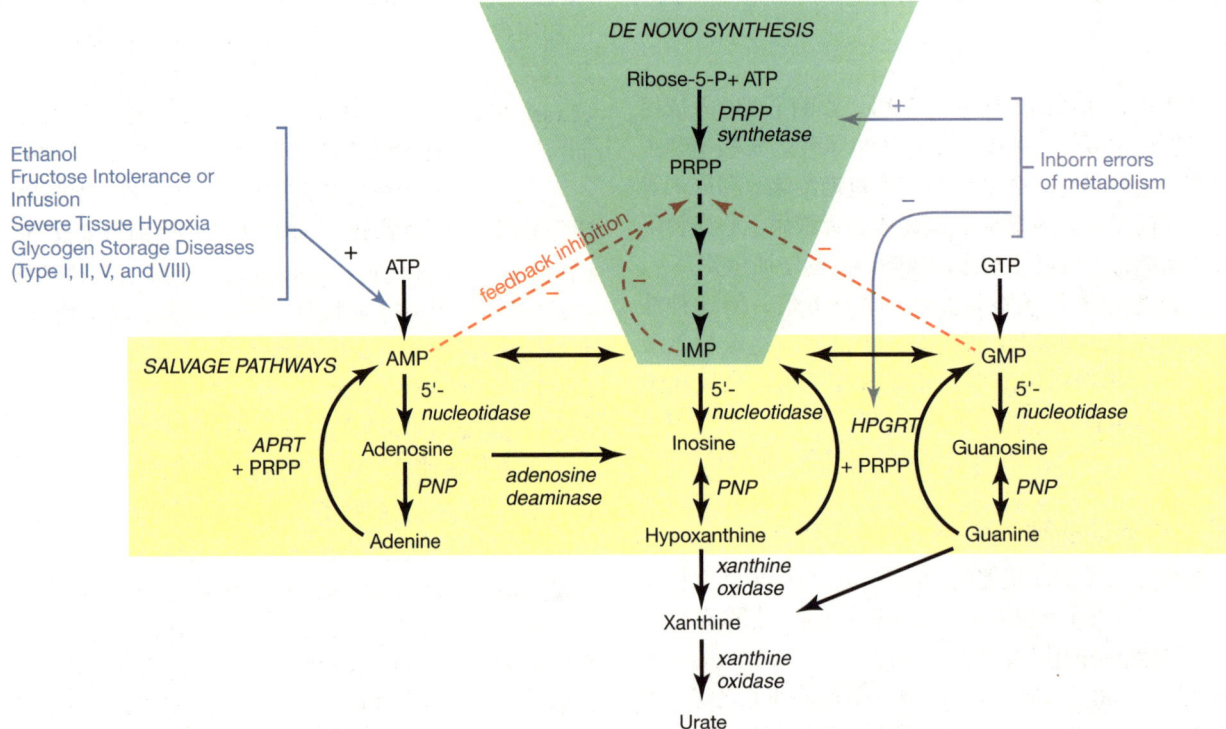

Fig. 7.1 The steps in the urate production pathways implicated in the pathogenesis of hyperuricemia and gout. *ADP*, Adenosine diphosphate; *APRT*, adenine phosphoribosyl transferase; *ATP*, adenosine triphosphate; *GMP*, guanosine monophosphate; *GTB*, guanosine triphosphate; *HPGRT*, hypoxanthine-guanine phosphoribosyl transferase; *IMP*, inosine monophosphate; *PNP*, purine nucleotide phosphorylase; *PRPP*, 5'-ribosyl 1-pyrophosphate. (From Choi HK: Epidemiology, pathology, and pathogenesis, chap 12. In Stone JH, Crofford LJ, White PH, editors: Primer on the rheumatic diseases, ed 13, New York, 2008, Springer.)

表7.1 高尿酸血症的病因

尿酸生成过多	尿酸排泄减少
代谢障碍 HGPRT缺乏（纯合或杂合） PRPP合成酶活性增强 G-6-PD缺乏 糖原贮积病	肾功能不全 容量不足 代谢性酸中毒（乳酸性酸中毒和酮症酸中毒） 肥胖 乙醇
其他 骨髓增殖和淋巴增殖性疾病 红细胞生成相关疾病（溶血性贫血、巨细胞性贫血、镰状细胞病、地中海贫血、其他血红蛋白病） 实体肿瘤 弥漫性银屑病 酒精（尤其是啤酒） 药物：细胞毒药物、烟酸 海鲜、动物内脏、红肉 果糖 肥胖	药物：低剂量水杨酸盐、利尿剂（噻嗪类、袢利尿剂）、环孢素、他克莫司、左旋多巴、乙胺丁醇 家族性青少年高尿酸血症肾病 髓质囊性肾病 铅性肾病

注：HGPRT：次黄嘌呤-鸟嘌呤磷酸核糖基转移酶；PRPP：5′-磷酸核糖1-焦磷酸；G-6-PD：葡萄糖-6-磷酸脱氢酶。

成。急性发作时，微痛风石裂解，释放大量MSU晶体到关节腔中，激活滑膜巨噬细胞和成纤维细胞吞噬晶体，结果导致细胞质多蛋白复合物NLRP3（译者注：原文NALP3等同于NLRP3）（NACHT、LRR和PYD结构域——包含蛋白3）炎症小体的激活（图7.2）。有证据表明，在急性痛风时，MSU晶体会被吞噬，从而激活NLRP3炎症小体，导致白细胞介素（interleukin, IL）-1β的释放，而IL-1β又会诱导产生更多的IL-1β和其他炎症介质，激活滑膜衬里层细胞和吞噬细胞。

MSU晶体被炎症细胞清除，然后这些炎症细胞会凋亡。这与其他机制共同最终导致通常在10～14天后急性炎症过程消退。即便症状完全缓解后，低水平的炎症状态（间歇期炎症）仍会在那些无症状的关节中持续存在。这种炎症在长期痛风患者中可能会变得明显，导致痛风石的形成、慢性滑膜炎、软骨损失和骨侵蚀。

临床特征

痛风包括三个阶段：无症状性高尿酸血症、急性间歇期痛风及慢性痛风。

急性痛风发作

急性痛风的典型表现是迅速发展的炎症性关节炎，通常累及一个关节，偶尔会累及两个关节。受累关节通常会出现剧烈疼痛、皮肤红斑、肿胀和极度压痛。这种临床表现很容易与化脓性关节炎或细菌性蜂窝织

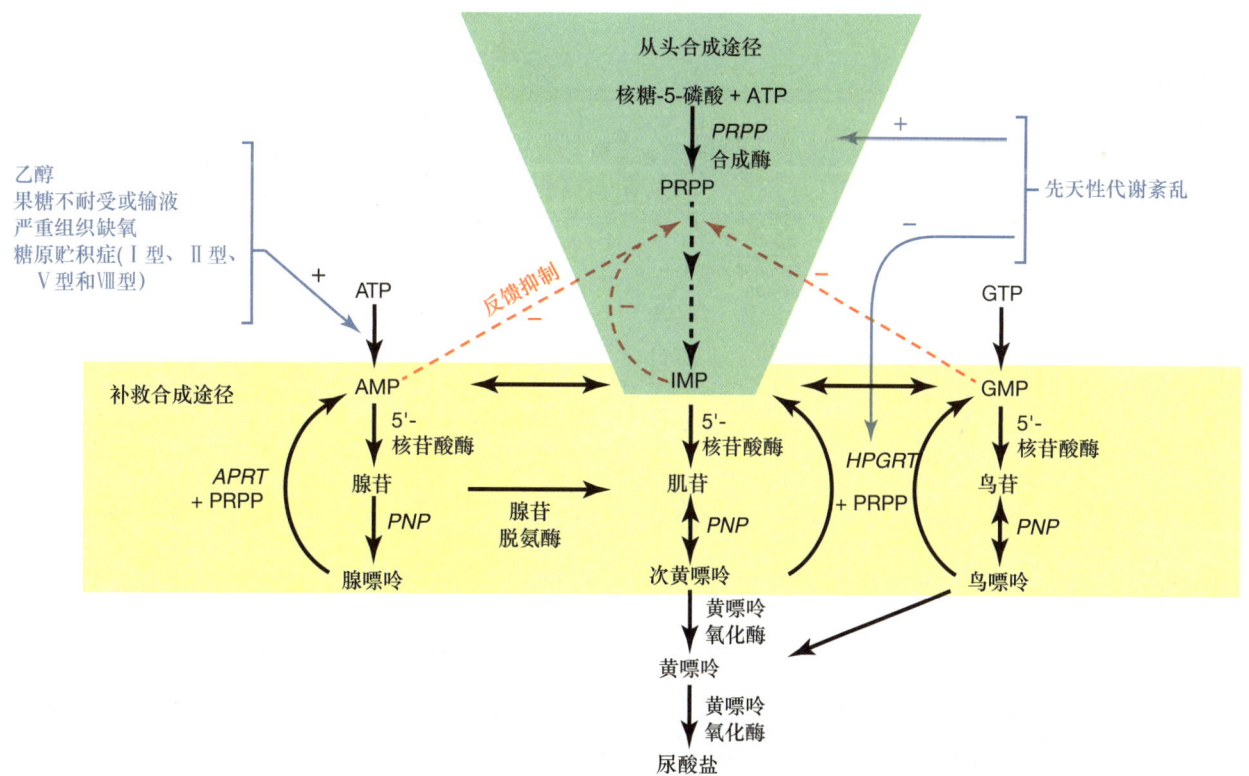

图7.1 在尿酸生成途径中涉及高尿酸血症和痛风发病机制的步骤。ADP，腺苷二磷酸；APRT，腺嘌呤磷酸核糖转移酶；ATP，腺苷三磷酸；GMP，鸟苷酸；GTP，鸟苷三磷酸（译者注：原文GTB有误）；HPGRT，次黄嘌呤-鸟嘌呤磷酸核糖基转移酶；IMP，肌苷酸；PNP，嘌呤核苷酸磷酸化酶；PRPP，5′-磷酸核糖1-焦磷酸（引自Choi HK：Epidemiology, pathology, and pathogenesis, chap 12. In Stone JH, Crofford LJ, White PH, editors：Primer on the rheumatic diseases, ed 13, New York, 2008, Springer.）

cellulitis, because many patients can mount an intense systemic inflammatory response with fever, chills, and elevated inflammatory markers. The most commonly involved joints are the first metatarsophalangeal joint (podagra), followed by the joints of the ankle, midfoot, and knee. The pain intensifies over 8 to 24 hours. Acute attacks usually resolve, even without therapy, within 5 to 14 days. The clinical resolution is complete, and the patient is asymptomatic between attacks. Subsequently, involvement of the upper extremities can occur, affecting the small joints of the hands, wrists, and elbows.

Attack-provoking factors include use of diuretics, alcohol, surgery, trauma, and consumption of foods containing high purine levels. Each of these can cause fluctuation in serum urate levels. Initiation of urate-lowering therapy can trigger attacks in the early phase by the same mechanism.

Chronic Gout

This phase, called chronic gout (also referred to as *chronic tophaceous gout* or *chronic advanced gout*), typically develops 10 or more years after the onset of acute attacks. Transition to the chronic phase occurs if hyperuricemia is inadequately treated. During this transition, the intercritical periods are no longer free of pain. The involved joints become persistently uncomfortable and swollen, although the intensity of these symptoms is significantly less pronounced compared to acute attacks. On top of this persistent background pain, acute gouty attacks continue to occur, especially in the absence of therapy. Polyarticular involvement becomes much more frequent during this time, including joints of the upper limbs.

The pathognomonic feature of chronic gout is the *tophus*, a palpable collection of MSU crystals in soft tissue or joints. It is detected in about 75% of patients who have had gout for more than 20 years. The severity and duration of hyperuricemia determine the likelihood of tophus development. While tophi most often occur over the first metatarsophalangeal joint, fingers, wrist, olecranon bursa, and helix of the ear, they can occur anywhere in the body. Infiltration of tophi into bone is thought to be the driving mechanism for bone erosion and joint damage in gout.

Diagnosis

The typical presentation of acute gouty arthritis in a characteristic joint distribution is strongly suggestive of the diagnosis, particularly if history of similar attacks that completely resolved is reported. However, detection of MSU crystals in the synovial fluid, bursa or tophus remains the diagnostic "gold standard." Arthrocentesis is not only important to confirm clinical suspicion but also to rule out septic arthritis or other crystalline arthropathies. During acute attacks, intracellular, strongly negative birefringent, needle-shaped MSU crystals are typically identified by polarized compensated microscopy. MSU crystals can also be demonstrated in tophus aspiration (Fig. 7.3A).

Septic arthritis can coexist with urate crystals in the synovial fluid; Gram stain and culture should be performed and are necessary to exclude septic arthritis. Aspirated synovial fluid appears cloudy, and analysis shows inflammatory fluid (>2000 white blood cells per microliter), usually in the 10,000 to 100,000 white blood cells per microliter range. Serum uric acid is not a diagnostically reliable test during acute flares since serum urate level may be normal or even low. Laboratory testing may reveal leukocytosis and elevated inflammatory markers, both of which are nonspecific. Between attacks, MSU crystals can often be demonstrated in previously inflamed joints, providing support to the diagnosis.

Radiologic Features

During an acute attack, a plain radiograph may only show soft tissue swelling. In chronic advanced gout, well-defined, "punched out" juxta-articular erosions characterized by a sclerotic rim and overhanging

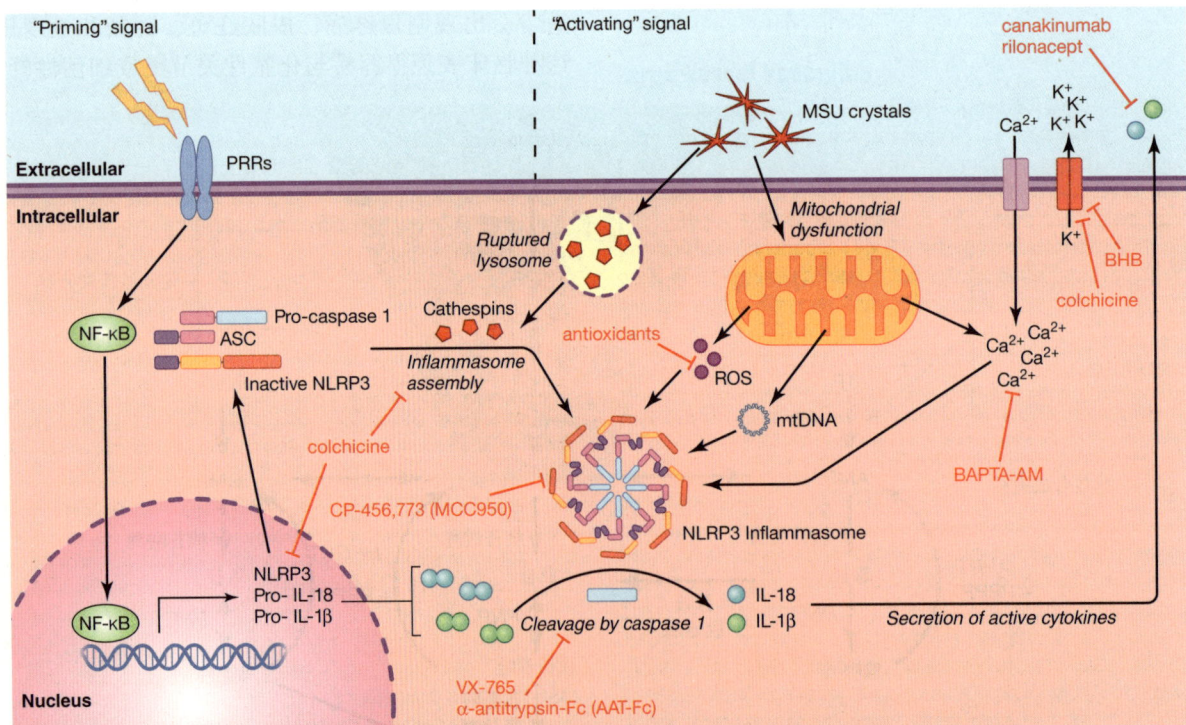

Fig. 7.2 NLRP3 inflammasome activation and potential targets in gout. *ASC*, Apoptosis-associated speck-like protein containing a CARD; *mtDNA*, mitochondrial DNA; *NF-kB*, nuclear factor kappa light-chain-enhancer of activated B cells; *PRRs*, pattern recognition receptors; *ROS*, reactive oxygen species. (From Szekanecz Z, Szamosi S, Kovács GE, et al: The NLRP3 inflammasome–interleukin 1 pathway as a therapeutic target in gout, Arch Biochem Biophys 670:82-93, 2019.)

炎相混淆，因为许多患者可出现发热、寒战和炎症指标升高等强烈的全身炎症反应。最常受累的关节是第一跖趾关节（足痛风），其次是踝关节、足背和膝关节。疼痛在 8～24 h 内加剧。即使不进行治疗，急性发作也通常会在 5～14 天内缓解。急性痛风发作可以达到临床的完全缓解，患者在两次发作的间歇期没有任何症状。随后，上肢也可能受累，影响手部的小关节、腕关节和肘关节。

诱发痛风发作的因素包括利尿剂、饮酒、手术、外伤和摄入高嘌呤食物。这些都有可能引起血清尿酸盐水平的波动。启动降尿酸治疗可能在早期阶段通过相同的机制诱发痛风发作。

慢性痛风

慢性痛风这一阶段也被称为慢性痛风石性痛风或慢性进展性痛风，通常在急性发作起病后的 10 年或更长时间出现。如果高尿酸血症没有得到充分治疗，将转变为慢性期。在这个转变过程中，发作间歇期不再没有疼痛。受累关节会持续不适和肿胀，尽管这些症状的强度明显低于急性发作。在持续的背景疼痛基础上，会继续出现急性痛风发作，尤其是在不治疗的情况下。此时，多关节受累越来越常见（包括上肢关节）。

慢性痛风的标志性特征是痛风石，即在软组织或关节中可触及的 MSU 晶体聚集。患病超过 20 年的痛风患者中约 75% 可发现痛风石。高尿酸血症的严重程度和持续时间决定了痛风石发生的风险。痛风石最常发生在第一跖趾关节、手指、手腕、鹰嘴滑囊和耳郭，但也可能发生在身体的任何部位。痛风石浸润至骨质被认为是驱动痛风患者的骨侵蚀和关节破坏的机制。

诊断

在特征性累及的关节出现急性痛风性关节炎的典型表现高度提示痛风，尤其是患者报告有类似的可以完全缓解的关节炎发作病史。然而，在滑液、滑囊或痛风石中检测出 MSU 晶体仍然是诊断的"金标准"。关节穿刺不仅对确诊很重要，而且对排除化脓性关节炎或其他晶体性关节病也很重要。在急性发作期，通过偏振光显微镜可观察到细胞内强负性双折光针状 MSU 晶体。MSU 晶体也可在痛风石的抽吸物中被检测到（图 7.3A）。

化脓性关节炎可伴有滑液中尿酸盐晶体，应进行革兰氏染色和培养以排除化脓性关节炎。本病患者所抽出的滑液外观混浊，滑液分析符合炎性液体（白细胞计数 $> 2000/\mu l$），白细胞计数通常在 10 000～100 000/μl 的范围内。急性发作时的血清尿酸不是诊断的可靠指标，因为此时血清尿酸水平可能正常甚至偏低。实验室检查可能显示血细胞分析中的白细胞增多和炎症指标升高，但两者都是非特异性的。在发作间歇期，在既往发作过的关节常可检测到 MSU 晶体，这可提供痛风诊断的支持。

影像学特征

在急性发作期间，X 线平片可能仅显示软组织肿胀。在慢性进展性痛风中，临近关节的骨质可能会出现边界清晰的"穿凿样"侵蚀，其特征为被侵蚀的骨质周围出现硬化缘和边缘增生。在本病的晚期阶段之

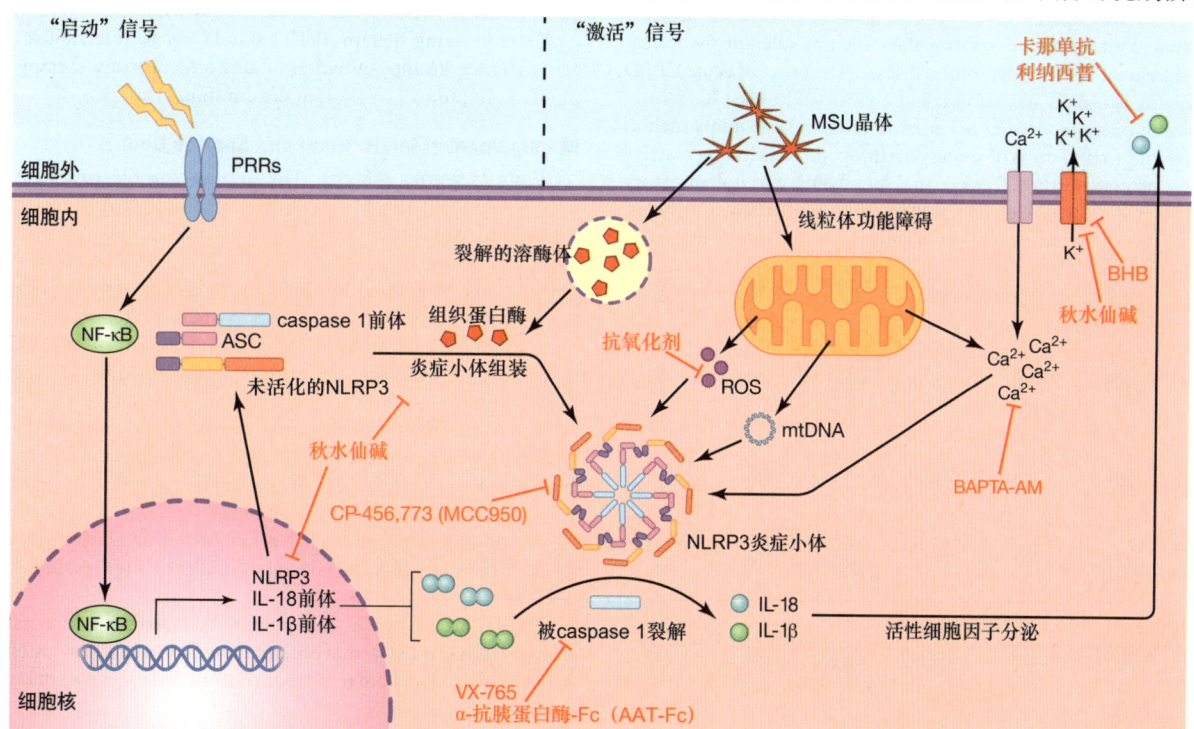

图 7.2　痛风中 NLRP3 炎症小体的激活和潜在靶点。ASC，含有胱天蛋白酶（caspase）激活募集结构域的凋亡相关斑点样蛋白；mtDNA，线粒体 DNA；NF-κB，活化 B 细胞核因子 κ 轻链增强子；PRRs，模式识别受体；ROS，活性氧（引自 Szekanecz Z, Szamosi S, Kovács GE, et al: The NLRP3 inflammasome-interleukin 1 pathway as a therapeutic target in gout, Arch Biochem Biophys 670：82-93，2019.）

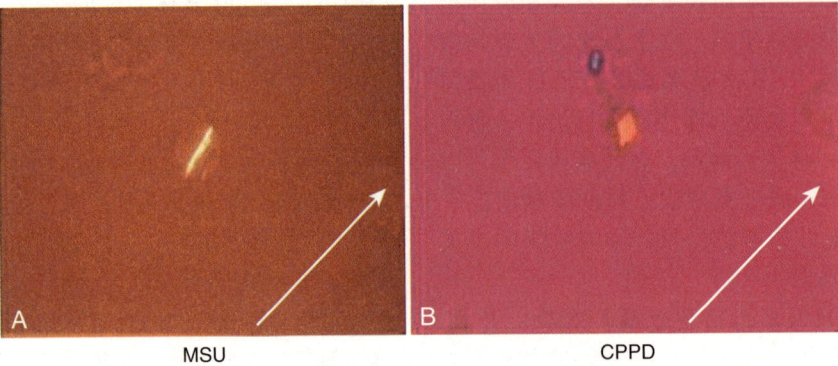

Fig. 7.3 Polarized microscopy image of (A) strongly negative birefringent monosodium urate crystals and (B) weakly positive calcium pyrophosphate dihydrate crystals. *Arrows* indicate axis of polarization. (A, Modified from the ACR Slide Collection on the Rheumatic Diseases. Available at http://images.rheumatology.org/. Accessed January 2015; B, Modified from Saadeh C, Diamond HS: Calcium pyrophosphate deposition disease. Available at: http://emedicine.medscape.com/article/330936-overview#showall.)

edges may be seen. The joint space is preserved until late in the course of the disease. Soft tissue masses may be detected in patients with tophi.

Dual-energy CT is a useful noninvasive imaging modality that can identify and color-code urate deposits in patients with gout. Ultrasound is a promising noninvasive tool in the diagnosis and management of gout.

Gout in Transplantation Patients

Hyperuricemia occurs much more frequently in transplantation patients using cyclosporine than in the normal population. Compared to patients with classic gout, transplant patients exhibit a significantly shorter period of asymptomatic hyperuricemia (0.5 to 4 years vs. 20 to 30 years), a shorter stage of acute intermittent gout (1 to 4 years vs. 10 to 15 years), and rapid development of tophi as early as 1 year after transplantation. Gouty attacks can be atypical and less severe, in part because of the concomitant use of prednisone.

Differential Diagnosis

Acute gouty arthropathy should be distinguished from septic arthritis and other crystal-induced arthropathies such as calcium pyrophosphate dihydrate (CPPD) deposition disease. The onset of acute CPPD arthropathy is usually less abrupt, and attacks tend to last longer, up to 1 month or more. Attacks occur more often in large joints such as the knee and wrist. Forms of spondyloarthropathies including reactive arthritis, psoriatic arthritis, ankylosing spondylitis, and inflammatory bowel–related arthritis can also present with monoarticular arthritis. In these disorders, synovial fluid is inflammatory, with a leukocyte count usually in the range of 10,000 to 50,000/μL, but crystals are absent and fluid culture is negative.

The diffuse and symmetric involvement of small joints in the hands and feet seen in chronic tophaceous gout can sometimes be confused with the symmetrical polyarthritis of rheumatoid arthritis and rheumatoid nodules. Aspiration of chronically inflamed joints or a tophus can help in distinguishing the two entities.

Treatment

Management strategies should focus on treating acute attacks, long-term management of hyperuricemia, patient education, and lifestyle modification.

Management of Acute Gouty Attack

Nonsteroidal anti-inflammatory drugs (NSAIDs) (such as naproxen and indomethacin) are typically used, and all seem to be equally effective. A full dose should be immediately initiated. Therapy should be continued for 7 to 10 days to ensure complete resolution of symptoms. NSAIDs are inappropriate in patients with peptic ulcer disease, inflammatory bowel disease, or renal insufficiency, and they must be used with caution in patients at risk for cardiovascular events.

Oral colchicine can be effective if used within the first 24 to 48 hours of an acute attack. A commonly prescribed dose is 1.2 mg, followed by 0.6 mg 1 hour later in the first day, followed by dose tapering until the attack is resolved. Colchicine can cause nausea and diarrhea and therapy should be stopped if symptoms are severe. Use of intravenous colchicine is discouraged due to high risk of bone marrow suppression.

Intra-articular corticosteroid administration is a very effective therapy for patients with monoarticular or oligoarticular disease in whom other systemic therapies are contraindicated. Enteral or parenteral glucocorticosteroids are effective in patients with renal insufficiency, intolerance to NSAIDs or colchicine, or treatment resistance. This approach is usually reserved for polyarticular flares when intra-articular injection is not practical (i.e., too many involved joints). Prednisone, 30 to 50 mg daily, is commonly used.

Urate-lowering therapy (ULT) should *not* be interrupted during acute attacks. Prompt initiation of anti-inflammatory therapy at the onset of symptoms may shorten the duration of attacks.

Management of Intercritical and Chronic Gout

Urate-lowering therapy. The aim of chronic treatment is to prevent recurrent attacks and to minimize joint damage by depleting tophaceous deposits in joints and soft tissue. This is achieved by lowering uric acid level below 6 mg/dL. A target level of less than 5 mg/dL should be considered in patients with chronic tophaceous gout as this may result in a faster, more effective reduction in tophus size and flare frequency. Indications for ULT include two or more attacks in a single year, presence of tophi, chronic kidney disease CKD stage 2 or more, chronic gouty arthritis, or recurrent nephrolithiasis.

Three categories of urate-lowering therapies are available: uricostatic agents that decrease uric acid production, uricosuric agents that increase renal excretion of uric acid, and uricolytic agents that break up uric acid into other metabolites.

The optimal duration of ULT is not known, and lifelong therapy is usually recommended. ULT is typically started after resolution of an acute attack.

Uricostatic therapy. Allopurinol and febuxostat are xanthine oxidase inhibitors (XOI) that prevent urate formation. They are effective in managing gout in both overproducers and undersecretors of uric acid.

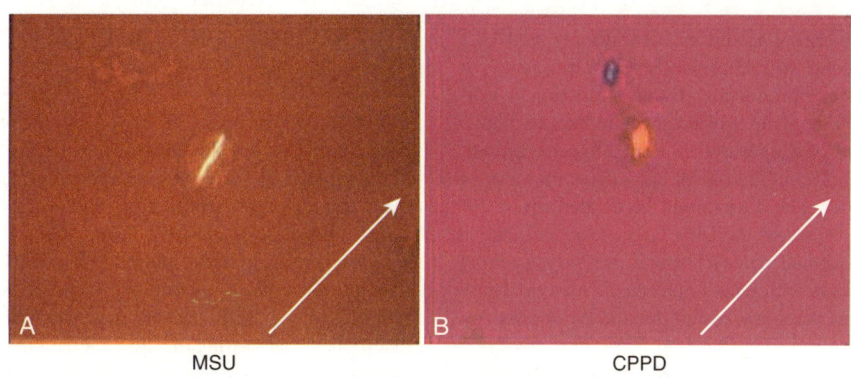

图 7.3 （A）强负性双折光单钠尿酸盐（MSU）晶体和（B）弱正性折光二羟焦磷酸钙（CPPD）晶体的偏振光显微镜图像。箭头表示偏振轴（A，改编自 the ACR Slide Collection on the Rheumatic Diseases. Available at http://images.rheumatology.org/. Accessed January 2015；B，改编自 Saadeh C，Diamond HS：Calcium pyrophosphate deposition disease. Available at：http://emedicine.medscape.com/article/330936-overview#showall.）

前，关节间隙通常可保留。在有痛风结节的患者中，可能会检测到软组织肿块。

双能 CT 是一种有用的非侵入性成像模式，可以在痛风患者中识别尿酸盐沉积并对其进行彩色编码。超声是一种在痛风诊断和管理中很有前景的无创工具。

移植相关的痛风

应用环孢素的移植患者高尿酸血症的发生率明显高于普通人群。与经典的痛风患者相比，移植患者无症状高尿酸血症的阶段明显较短（0.5～4 年 vs. 20～30 年），急性间歇期痛风的阶段也更短（1～4 年 vs. 10～15 年），并且可迅速发展出现痛风石，最早可在移植后 1 年就出现。痛风发作可能不典型且症状较轻，部分原因是移植患者同时使用了泼尼松。

鉴别诊断

急性痛风性关节病应与化脓性关节炎和其他晶体性关节病相鉴别，如二羟焦磷酸钙（CPPD）沉积病。急性 CPPD 沉积病的起病通常较为缓慢，并且发作持续时间更久，可长达 1 个月或更长。发作更多见于大关节如膝关节和腕关节等。各种脊柱关节病，包括反应性关节炎、银屑病关节炎、强直性脊柱炎和炎症性肠病相关的关节炎均可表现为单关节受累。在这些疾病中，关节液呈炎症性，白细胞计数通常在 10 000～50 000/μl 之间，但没有晶体存在且滑液培养呈阴性。

慢性痛风石性痛风的手足小关节呈弥漫性对称受累，有时会与类风湿关节炎的对称性多关节炎和类风湿结节相混淆。慢性炎症关节或痛风石的穿刺抽吸物的晶体分析可帮助鉴别这两类疾病。

治疗

管理策略的重点是治疗急性发作，高尿酸血症的长期管理，患者教育和生活方式调整。

急性痛风发作的治疗

通常推荐使用非甾体抗炎药（NSAID）（如萘普生和吲哚美辛），所有品种的疗效相近。在发作初期应立即开始足量用药，治疗应持续 7～10 天，以确保症状完全缓解。NSAID 不适用于伴有消化性溃疡、炎症性肠病或肾功能不全的患者，有心血管事件风险的患者慎用。

在急性发作的头 24～48 h 内口服秋水仙碱有效。常用的用法为第一天首剂 1.2 mg，1 h 后再服 0.6 mg，第二天起剂量逐渐减少，直至症状缓解。秋水仙碱可引起恶心和腹泻，如果症状严重，应停止服用。不推荐静脉应用秋水仙碱，原因是其骨髓抑制的风险高。

对于单关节或寡关节受累的患者，若其他全身治疗不耐受，关节内注射糖皮质激素是一种有效的治疗手段。肠内或肠外应用糖皮质激素可有效治疗合并肾功能不全、对 NSAID 或秋水仙碱不耐受或无效的患者。该治疗手段通常用于多关节发作而关节内注射不适用时（如受累关节过多），常用的剂量为泼尼松 30～50 mg/d。

急性发作期间不应中断降尿酸治疗（ULT）。在症状出现时立即开始抗炎治疗可能会缩短发作的持续时间。

间歇期和慢性痛风的治疗

降尿酸治疗（ULT） 慢性期治疗的目的是防止反复发作，消除关节和软组织中沉积的痛风石以最大限度地减少关节破坏。这可以通过尿酸水平降低至 360 μmol/L（6 mg/dl）以下来实现。慢性痛风石性痛风患者应考虑将目标定为小于 300 μmol/L（5 mg/dl），这样可以更快、更有效地减少痛风石和降低发作频率。ULT 的指征包括在 1 年内发作 2 次或以上、存在痛风石、慢性肾脏病 2 期或以上、慢性痛风性关节炎或复发性肾结石。

目前可及的 ULT 有 3 类：抑制尿酸合成药物可减少尿酸生成，促进尿酸排泄药物可增加肾尿酸排泄，尿酸溶解药物可将尿酸分解成其他代谢物。

目前，ULT 的最佳疗程尚不明确，通常推荐长期维持治疗。ULT 通常在急性发作缓解后开始。

抑制尿酸合成治疗 别嘌呤醇和非布司他作为黄嘌呤氧化酶抑制剂（XOI）可防止尿酸盐的形成，对尿酸生成过多和排泄减少的痛风患者均有效。

Allopurinol remains the first-line and most commonly used ULT agent, particularly in patients with chronic renal insufficiency, uric acid stones, or uric acid overproduction. If renal function is normal, a starting dose of 100 mg daily is recommended because higher doses may increase the risk of allopurinol-associated hypersensitivity, a potentially lethal complication. The risk of early flares may also be increased with higher doses. The dose should be titrated up by 100 mg increments every 2 to 5 weeks until the target uric acid level is reached. The maximal dose is 800 mg/day. Doses above 300 mg per day can be safely used in patients with renal impairment. Adverse events include rash (2%), hepatitis, vasculitis, eosinophilia, and bone marrow suppression.

Allopurinol-associated hypersensitivity is a serious side effect. Risk factors include concomitant use of thiazides and penicillin allergy. Fever, severe exfoliative dermatitis, eosinophilia, and hepatic and renal failure can occur. Febuxostat may be used in patients who do not achieve target uric acid levels despite adequate allopurinol dose titration or in patients with side effects to allopurinol.

Uricosuric therapy. Probenecid may be used as first-line ULT in uric acid undersecretors (<600 mg in a 24-hour urine collection) and in the setting of contraindication or intolerance to XOIs. Probenecid can be combined with an XOI to achieve target UA level, assuming adequate renal function. Probenecid is ineffective in patients with renal insufficiency (glomerular filtration rate <50 mL/minute) and is contraindicated in patients with nephrolithiasis. Patients should maintain high urine volume by drinking at least 1.5 L of fluid daily. Lesinurad is not used as monotherapy but can be combined with an XOI.

Uricolytic therapy. Pegloticase (pegylated recombinant uricase), administered intravenously every 2 weeks, is used in cases refractory to conventional ULT. Rasburicase, another recombinant uricase, is used to prevent tumor lysis syndrome but has no role in the management of gout.

Future directions. As previously mentioned, IL-1 is a proinflammatory cytokine that has been shown to play an important role in pathogenesis of acute gouty attacks. As a result, IL-1 antagonists have been a target for recent drug therapies (see Fig. 7.2). These include anakinra, rilonacept, and canakinumab. Anakinra has been shown to be effective at treating acute flares, whereas rilonacept may be more effective in preventing gout flares due to its longer half-life. Canakinumab may be effective for both acute flares and flare prophylaxis when used with ULT. More formal clinical trials are needed comparing these therapies with conventional gout treatment.

Non–urate-lowering prophylactic therapy. Anti-inflammatory prophylaxis using low-dose colchicine or NSAIDs is usually recommended in conjunction with ULT to decrease the risk of flares that often accompany initiation of ULT. Prophylactic treatment is usually continued for 6 months after the serum uric acid goal is achieved.

Lifestyle modifications and education. A patient newly diagnosed with gout should be evaluated for potentially modifiable risk factors and associated illnesses such as obesity, hypertension, and hyperlipidemia. Decreased consumption of high-purine food (e.g., shellfish, liver, sweetbreads) and fructose-containing beverages, as well as reduced alcohol intake, should be recommended. Diuretics should be avoided, if possible.

Treatment of hyperuricemia in patients without gout. Allopurinol and rasburicase have been used for treatment and prevention of tumor lysis syndrome–associated hyperuricemia following chemotherapy. Otherwise, there is no evidence to support their use in asymptomatic hyperuricemia.

CALCIUM PYROPHOSPHATE DIHYDRATE DEPOSITION DISEASE

CPPD deposition disease is a clinically heterogeneous disorder that is characterized by the presence of intra-articular CPPD crystals. These crystals are deposited primarily in the cartilage, in the normally unmineralized pericellular matrix of hyaline and fibrocartilage. Calcification of the cartilage is promoted by alterations in the metabolism of inorganic pyrophosphate (PPi) and extracellular matrix leading to extracellular accumulation of PPi, which is necessary to the formation of CPPD crystals. Crystals are phagocytized by resident synovial macrophages, activating the intracellular NALP3 inflammasome complex and leading to recruitment and influx of neutrophils into the joint space.

CPPD deposition disease typically affects the elderly population. Up to 50% of individuals older than 85 years of age have radiographic evidence of CPPD crystal accumulation in cartilage (chondrocalcinosis), but most are asymptomatic. The most commonly involved joints are the knee menisci and the triangular fibrocartilage of the wrist. It is uncommon for CPPD deposition disease to affect patients younger than 50 years of age, unless the disease is familial or related to a metabolic abnormality (e.g., hyperparathyroidism, hemochromatosis).

CPPD deposition disease can present with acute CPPD crystal arthritis (pseudogout), chronic arthropathy with structural changes of osteoarthritis, or may be asymptomatic, presenting as an incidental finding of chondrocalcinosis on imaging. The most common clinical manifestation, occurring in more than 50% of patients, is a peculiar type of osteoarthritis called pseudo-osteoarthritis; it is a noninflammatory arthritis involving joints not typically affected by osteoarthritis, such as the wrist, shoulder, and metacarpophalangeal joints. A chronic symmetric polyarticular arthritis pattern resembling rheumatoid arthritis and a severe destructive arthropathy that mimics neuropathic arthritis on radiographs may be seen.

Acute pseudogout attacks may be precipitated by trauma, surgery (particularly parathyroidectomy for hyperparathyroidism), or severe medical illness. Administration of intra-articular viscosupplementation may also trigger a CPPD flare. Attacks are usually monoarticular or oligoarticular, similar to an acute gouty attack; if left untreated, they may last from a few days to a few months. The vigorous inflammatory response to CPPD crystals manifests as warmth, erythema, and swelling in and around the affected joint resembling acute gouty arthritis. Fever, elevated erythrocyte sedimentation rate, and leukocytosis can occur.

The diagnosis is confirmed by assessing synovial fluid for the presence of intracellular rod- or rhomboid-shaped crystals, which exhibit weakly positive birefringence when examined by compensated polarized light microscopy (see Fig. 7.3B). CPP crystals can be difficult to detect in some patients and are frequently missed in clinical specimens.

The presence of chondrocalcinosis (radio-dense deposits on radiographs) is highly suggestive of the diagnosis in the appropriate clinical context. Joint aspiration should always be performed to rule out septic arthritis. Importantly, joint infection can cause crystal shedding, leading to a concomitant crystal-related inflammation. Synovial fluid is inflammatory (>2000 white blood cells per microliter).

Therapy for CPPD deposition disease is indicated for symptomatic patients. There is no effective treatment to remove CPPD deposits from synovium or cartilage. Intra-articular glucocorticoid administration to the affected joints is effective. NSAIDs are also effective, but their potential toxicity in elderly patients may limit their use. Severe polyarticular attacks may require short courses of systemic corticosteroids.

别嘌呤醇仍是一线和最常用的 ULT 药物，尤其适用于合并慢性肾功能不全、尿酸性结石或尿酸生成过多的患者。如果肾功能正常，建议起始剂量为 100 mg/d，因为剂量过大可能会增加别嘌呤醇相关超敏反应的风险，这是一种潜在致命的并发症。剂量越大，治疗早期发生急性痛风发作的风险也可能越高。别嘌呤醇剂量每 2～5 周递增 100 mg，直至达到目标尿酸水平。最大剂量为 800 mg/d。合并肾功能损害的患者可安全使用超过 300 mg/d 的剂量。不良反应包括皮疹（2%）、肝炎、血管炎、嗜酸性粒细胞增多症和骨髓抑制。

别嘌呤醇相关超敏反应是一种严重的副作用。风险因素包括同时使用噻嗪类药物和青霉素过敏。发热、严重剥脱性皮炎、嗜酸性粒细胞增多症以及肝肾功能衰竭均可能发生。别嘌呤醇滴定至最大剂量尿酸水平仍无法达标或出现不良反应的患者可使用非布司他。

促进尿酸排泄治疗 丙磺舒可作为一线 ULT 药物用于尿酸排泄不足（24 h 尿尿酸 < 3600 μmol）和对 XOI 禁忌或不耐受的患者。如果患者肾功能正常，丙磺舒可与一种 XOI 联用，以达到目标尿酸水平，但对肾功能不全（肾小球滤过率 < 50 ml/min）患者丙磺舒无效。丙磺舒禁用于有肾结石的患者。此外，患者应通过每天至少喝 1.5 L 液体来维持高尿量。雷西纳德（lesinurad）不能单药治疗，但可与一种 XOI 联合使用。

尿酸溶解治疗 对于常规 ULT 治疗反应不佳的痛风患者，可每 2 周静脉注射一次普瑞凯希（pegloticase，聚乙二醇重组尿酸酶）。拉布立海（rasburicase）是另一种重组尿酸酶，用于预防肿瘤溶解综合征，但不用于痛风的治疗。

未来展望 如前所述，IL-1 是一种促炎细胞因子，已证实其在急性痛风发作的发病机制中起重要作用。因此，IL-1 拮抗剂已成为近期药物疗法的靶点（见图 7.2）。这些药物包括阿那白滞素（anakinra）、利纳西普（rilonacept）和卡那单抗（canakinumab）。阿那白滞素已被证明能有效治疗急性发作，而利纳西普由于半衰期较长，在预防痛风发作方面可能更有效。卡那单抗与 ULT 联合可能对控制急性复发和预防复发皆有效。未来，还需要进行更多正式的临床试验来比较这些疗法与传统痛风治疗的效果。

非降尿酸预防性治疗 通常建议在进行 ULT 时联合使用小剂量秋水仙碱或 NSAID 进行抗炎预防治疗，以降低 ULT 起始阶段常伴随出现的痛风复发风险。在血清尿酸水平达标后，预防性治疗通常需持续 6 个月。

生活方式调整及教育 对于新诊断的痛风患者，应评估潜在的可改变的危险因素和相关疾病，如肥胖、高血压和高脂血症。应建议减少摄入高嘌呤食物（如贝类、肝脏、胰腺）和含果糖饮料，并减少酒精摄入。如果可能，应尽可能避免使用利尿剂。

无痛风患者的高尿酸血症的治疗 别嘌呤醇和拉布立海已被用于治疗和预防化疗后的肿瘤溶解综合征相关高尿酸血症。除此之外，尚无证据支持它们用于治疗无症状性高尿酸血症。

二羟焦磷酸钙沉积病

CPPD 沉积病是一种临床异质性疾病，其特征是关节内存在 CPPD 晶体沉积。这些晶体主要沉积在软骨以及透明软骨和纤维软骨未矿化的细胞外基质中。无机焦磷酸（PPi）和细胞外基质代谢的改变会导致细胞外 PPi 的聚集，促进软骨的钙化，这是 CPPD 晶体形成所必需的步骤。晶体被常驻滑膜巨噬细胞吞噬，激活细胞内的 NLRP3 炎症小体复合物，并募集中性粒细胞进入关节间隙。

CPPD 沉积病通常好发于老年人群。在 85 岁以上的老年人中，接近 50% 的人有 CPPD 晶体在软骨沉积（软骨钙质沉着症）的放射学证据，但大多数无症状。最常受累的关节是膝关节半月板和腕关节三角纤维软骨。CPPD 沉积病影响 50 岁以下患者的情况并不常见，除非该病是家族性或与代谢异常（如甲状旁腺功能亢进症、血色病）有关。

CPPD 沉积病可表现为急性 CPPD 晶体性关节炎（假性痛风）、伴有骨关节炎结构变化的慢性关节病，但也可能没有症状，仅在进行影像学检查时偶然发现软骨钙化。最常见的临床表现（发生在超过一半的患者）是一种特殊类型的骨关节炎，称为假性骨关节炎。这是一种非炎症性关节炎，累及的关节不是骨关节炎典型受累关节，如腕关节、肩关节和掌指关节。此外，也可表现为类似类风湿关节炎的慢性对称性多关节炎和一种在放射学上模拟神经病性关节炎的严重的损毁性关节病。

外伤、手术（尤其是甲状旁腺功能亢进症的甲状旁腺切除术）或严重的内科疾病都可能诱发急性假性痛风发作。关节内的黏弹性补充疗法也可能促发 CPPD 沉积病的复发。发作往往是单关节或寡关节，类似于急性痛风发作。若不及时治疗，症状可持续数天至数月。CPPD 晶体的剧烈炎症反应与急性痛风性关节炎相似，表现为受累关节及其周围皮温升高、皮肤红斑和肿胀，也可出现发热、红细胞沉降率增快和白细胞增多。

在偏振光显微镜下发现滑液中存在弱正性双折光的细胞内棒状或菱形晶体可明确诊断（见图 7.3B）。然而，这些晶体在一些患者中可能难以被检测到，并且常常在临床标本中被遗漏。

在临床表现相符合的情况下，有软骨钙质沉着症（放射学上的放射性高密度沉积）高度提示诊断。应常规进行关节腔穿刺排除化脓性关节炎。重要的是，关节感染可导致晶体脱落，从而引起伴随的晶体相关的炎症。滑液分析呈炎症性（白细胞计数 > 2000/μl）。

CPPD 沉积病的治疗针对有症状的患者进行。目前尚无有效治疗去除滑膜或软骨中沉积的 CPPD。受累关节关节腔内注射糖皮质激素有效。NSAID 也很有效，但在老年患者中的潜在毒性可能限制了其使用。严重的多关节发作可能需要短期应用全身性糖皮质激素治

In patients with frequent attacks, prophylactic daily low-dose colchicine may decrease the attack frequency.

APATITE-ASSOCIATED ARTHROPATHY

Abnormal accumulation of apatite (basic calcium phosphate, or BCP) may occur in hypercalcemic states and other illnesses. Unlike MSU or CPPD crystals, individual BCP crystals are not identifiable by polarized microscopy and can only be seen using electron microscopy. The most common presentation is calcific periarteritis, which typically occurs in the shoulder.

Milwaukee shoulder is an extremely destructive BCP-associated arthropathy that tends to affect elderly women. It is characterized by a large noninflammatory effusion (i.e., <2000 white blood cells per microliter) causing destruction of the rotator cuff and marked instability of the glenohumeral joint.

Other manifestations include acute reversible inflammatory arthropathies that resemble gout, referred to as *pseudo-pseudogout*, and ossifications along the anterolateral aspect of spinal vertebrae, termed *diffuse idiopathic skeletal hyperostosis* (DISH). Acute attacks of arthritis or bursitis may be self-limited. Intra-articular or periarticular injection of corticosteroids or the use of NSAIDs may shorten the duration and intensity of symptoms.

CALCIUM OXALATE DEPOSITION DISEASE

In calcium oxalate deposition disease, or oxalosis, calcium oxalate crystals are deposited in tissue. In primary oxalosis, a hereditary metabolic disorder, this leads to nephrocalcinosis, renal failure, and early mortality. Secondary oxalosis complicates long-term hemo- and peritoneal dialysis; crystals are deposited in bone, cartilage, synovium, and periarticular tissue. Crystal shedding into the joint space may result in inflammatory arthritis of peripheral joints. Chondrocalcinosis or soft tissue calcifications can be seen on plain radiographs. The presence of strongly birefringent bipyramidal crystals in synovial fluid is characteristic. Treatment with NSAIDS, intra-articular corticosteroids, or colchicine usually results in moderate improvement.

SUGGESTED READINGS

Choi HK: Epidemiology, pathology, and pathogenesis, chap 12. In Stone JH, Crofford LJ, White PH, editors: Primer on the rheumatic diseases, ed 13, New York, 2008, Springer.

Dalbeth N, Merriman TR, Stamp LK: Gout, Lancet 388:2039–2052, 2016.

Khanna D, Fitzgerald JD, Khanna PP, et al: 2012 American College of Rheumatology guidelines for management of gout. Part 1: systematic nonpharmacologic and pharmacologic therapeutic approaches to hyperuricemia, Arthritis Care Res 64:1431–1446, 2012.

Khanna D, Khanna PP, Fitzgerald JD, et al: 2012 American College of Rheumatology guidelines for management of gout. Part 2: therapy and anti-inflammatory prophylaxis of acute gouty arthritis, Arthritis Care Res 64:1447–1461, 2012.

疗。对于频繁发作患者，每天预防性服用小剂量秋水仙碱可能会降低发作频率。

磷灰石相关性关节病

磷灰石（碱性磷酸钙，BCP）的异常堆积可能发生在高钙血症和其他疾病的患者。与 MSU 或 CPPD 晶体不同，偏振光显微镜无法识别单个的 BCP 晶体，只能通过电子显微镜才能观察到。最常见的表现是钙化性动脉周围炎，通常发生在肩部。

密尔沃基肩病是一种极具破坏性的 BCP 相关性关节病，多发于老年女性。其特征是大量非炎症性渗出（如白细胞计数 < 2000/μl），并且导致肩袖破坏和盂肱关节的明显不稳定。

其他表现还包括类似于痛风的急性可逆性炎症性关节病，称为假-假性痛风（pseudo-pseudogout），以及沿着脊柱椎体前外侧骨化的弥漫性特发性骨肥厚症（DISH）。关节炎或滑囊炎的急性发作可能是自限性的。关节内或关节周围注射糖皮质激素或使用 NSAID 可能缩短症状持续时间和减轻症状。

草酸钙沉积病

在草酸钙沉积病或草酸盐病中，草酸钙晶体沉积在组织中。原发性草酸盐病是一种遗传性代谢疾病，会导致肾钙盐沉着症、肾衰竭和早期死亡。继发性草酸盐病是长期血液透析和腹膜透析的并发症；晶体会沉积在骨骼、软骨、滑膜和关节周围组织中。晶体脱落到关节腔可能导致外周关节的炎症性关节炎。在放射学平片上可以看到软骨钙质沉着症或软组织钙化。滑液中出现强双折光双锥体形状的晶体是其特征性表现。NSAID、关节内糖皮质激素或秋水仙碱治疗通常会在一定程度上改善病情。

推荐阅读

Choi HK: Epidemiology, pathology, and pathogenesis, chap 12. In Stone JH, Crofford LJ, White PH, editors: Primer on the rheumatic diseases, ed 13, New York, 2008, Springer.

Dalbeth N, Merriman TR, Stamp LK: Gout, Lancet 388:2039–2052, 2016.

Khanna D, Fitzgerald JD, Khanna PP, et al: 2012 American College of Rheumatology guidelines for management of gout. Part 1: systematic nonpharmacologic and pharmacologic therapeutic approaches to hyperuricemia, Arthritis Care Res 64:1431–1446, 2012.

Khanna D, Khanna PP, Fitzgerald JD, et al: 2012 American College of Rheumatology guidelines for management of gout. Part 2: therapy and anti-inflammatory prophylaxis of acute gouty arthritis, Arthritis Care Res 64:1447–1461, 2012.

8

Osteoarthritis

Joanne S. Cunha, Zuhal Arzomand, Philip Tsoukas

DEFINITION AND EPIDEMIOLOGY

Osteoarthritis, also known as degenerative joint disease, is the most common type of arthritis and musculoskeletal disease. It is a disease of synovial joints that encompasses the pathophysiologic changes that result from alterations in joint structure due to failed repair of joint damage and the individual's experience of illness, which is most often characterized by pain.

Osteoarthritis affects more than 300 million people worldwide. The prevalence of osteoarthritis continues to rise with the aging population, obesity epidemic, and increased numbers of joint injuries. Currently, more than 30 million adult Americans have some form of osteoarthritis.

The hands, knees, and hips are commonly affected joints in osteoarthritis. Hand and knee osteoarthritis is more common among women, especially after 50 years of age. Radiographic prevalence of osteoarthritis varies by the joint involved and often predates symptomatic osteoarthritis, with higher prevalence for knee and hand osteoarthritis than hip osteoarthritis.

Osteoarthritis is associated with major morbidity, reduced quality of life, and disability. There is increasing evidence of an association between osteoarthritis and cardiovascular disease. Osteoarthritis is one of the leading causes of long-term disability in the United States. Lower extremity osteoarthritis is the most common cause of difficulty with walking or climbing stairs, preventing an estimated 100,000 elderly Americans from independently walking from their bed to the bathroom.

Osteoarthritis has a large economic impact because of direct medical costs (e.g., physician visits, laboratory tests, medications, surgery) and indirect costs (e.g., lost wages, home care). With the aging of the US population, the burden of osteoarthritis is expected to increase in the coming years.

PATHOLOGIC FACTORS

The causes of osteoarthritis are complex and heterogeneous. Osteoarthritis may be classified as primary, or idiopathic, without a specific cause. Secondary osteoarthritis has an identifiable cause and is pathologically identical to primary osteoarthritis. Causes of secondary osteoarthritis include biomechanical factors, congenital or developmental deformities of the joint that alter its shape, traumatic events, metabolic disorders, and inflammatory conditions. Genetic predisposition, age, gender, and obesity are prominent risk factors as well.

The pathophysiology of osteoarthritis is not well understood. The cardinal feature in the pathogenesis of osteoarthritis is an imbalance between the destruction and repair of the joint tissues, with failure of the repair process and progressive loss of articular cartilage with associated remodeling of subchondral bone. In normal cartilage, there is continuous extracellular matrix turnover with a balance between synthesis and degradation. In osteoarthritis, there is disproportion between these two processes, with an excess of matrix degradation that exceeds ongoing matrix synthesis. Excess degradation results from overproduction of catabolic factors such as proinflammatory cytokines and reactive oxygen species (Fig. 8.1).

Osteoarthritis is best defined as joint failure, a disease process that involves the total joint, including the subchondral bone, ligaments, joint capsule, synovial membrane, periarticular muscles, and articular cartilage. After bone trauma or repetitive injury, joint failure may result from joint instability caused by muscle weakness and ligamentous laxity, nerve injury and neuronal sensitization or hyperexcitability, or both.

Biomechanical contributors include repetitive or isolated joint trauma related to certain occupations or physical activities that involve repeated joint stress and predispose to early osteoarthritis. Altered joint shape may contribute to osteoarthritis through biomechanical factors, as may be seen with chronic patellar maltracking and the development of knee osteoarthritis and cam deformity or acetabular dysplasia in the development of hip osteoarthritis.

Obesity may contribute to osteoarthritis biomechanically or systemically through subacute or overt metabolic syndromes, both of which are associated with low-grade systemic inflammation. Age-related changes in habitus result in decreased muscle mass with a relative increase in visceral adiposity. This contributes to abnormal joint mechanics and low-grade systemic inflammation. Other age-related factors include changes in the extracellular matrix composition and structure leading to susceptibility for degeneration, mitochondrial dysfunction with increase in oxidative stress and promotion of catabolic activity, and chondrocyte dysfunction.

Inflammatory joint diseases, such as rheumatoid arthritis, may result in cartilage degradation and biomechanical effects that lead to secondary osteoarthritis. Crystal deposition diseases, osteonecrosis, Paget's disease, and metabolic disorders such as hemochromatosis, ochronosis, Wilson's disease, and Gaucher's disease are also associated with secondary osteoarthritis. High bone mineral density is associated with hip and knee involvement. Estrogen deficiency may be a risk factor for hip or knee disease, showcasing a hormonal influence. Candidate gene studies and genome-wide scans have identified several potential genetic markers. Patients often have a family history of osteoarthritis or joint replacement.

The destruction of the joint, including articular cartilage damage, osteophyte formation, and subchondral bone remodeling, is best viewed as joint failure and the final product of a variety of etiologic factors.

The earliest finding is fibrillation of the most superficial layer of the articular cartilage. Over time, disruption of the articular surface becomes deeper, with fibrillations extending to subchondral bone,

骨关节炎

王俐 译 厉小梅 贾园 审校 栗占国 通审

定义和流行病学

骨关节炎也称为退行性关节病，是最常见的关节炎和肌骨疾病。它是一种滑膜关节疾病，关节损伤修复失败，导致关节结构改变引起病理生理变化，疼痛是其最常见的临床症状。

骨关节炎影响全球超过3亿人。随着人口老龄化、肥胖症流行以及关节损伤增多，骨关节炎的发病率持续上升。目前，超过3000万美国成年人患有某种形式的骨关节炎。

骨关节炎通常累及手、膝和髋。手和膝骨关节炎在女性更常见，50岁以后尤为明显。骨关节炎影像学特征通常早于其症状，不同关节的患病率存在差异，膝和手骨关节炎的患病率高于髋骨关节炎。

骨关节炎患病率高，与生活质量降低以及残疾相关。越来越多的证据表明骨关节炎和心血管疾病之间存在联系。骨关节炎是导致美国人长期残疾的主要原因之一。下肢骨关节炎是导致步行或走楼梯困难的最常见原因，约有10万美国老年人无法从床边独立走到浴室。

骨关节炎相关的直接医疗费用（如医生就诊、实验室检查、药物、手术）和间接费用（如工资损失、家庭护理）对经济产生巨大影响。随着美国人口老龄化，预计未来几年骨关节炎的负担将继续增加。

病理因素

骨关节炎的病因复杂，存在异质性。骨关节炎可分为原发性或称为特发性，即没有特定发病原因；以及继发性骨关节炎，继发性骨关节炎有明确的原因，病理上与原发性骨关节炎相同。继发性骨关节炎的原因包括生物力学因素、先天性或发育性关节畸形、创伤事件、代谢紊乱和炎症。遗传易感性、年龄、性别和肥胖症也是突出的危险因素。

骨关节炎的病理生理学机制尚不清楚。骨关节炎发病机制的主要特征是关节组织的破坏和修复之间的不平衡，修复过程失败，关节软骨的进行性丢失和软骨下骨重塑。在正常软骨中，细胞外基质持续更新，合成和降解之间保持平衡。在骨关节炎中，这两个过程不均衡，基质降解过度，超过了基质合成。分解代谢因子如前炎症细胞因子和活性氧导致基质过度降解（图8.1）。

骨关节炎最好的定义是一种涉及整个关节的关节衰退过程，累及软骨下骨、韧带、关节囊、滑膜、关节周围肌肉和关节软骨。骨损伤或重复损伤后，肌无力和韧带松弛引起关节不稳定；神经损伤和神经元敏感或过度兴奋可能导致关节衰退。关节不稳与神经损伤可能独立或同时存在。

生物力学的损伤包括与职业或体育活动相关的重复性或单次关节创伤，重复关节应力易导致早期骨关节炎。关节形状改变可能通过生物力学导致骨关节炎，如慢性髌骨炎导致膝骨关节炎，凸轮畸形或髋臼发育不良促进髋骨关节炎。

肥胖症可能通过生物力学促进骨关节炎，也可能通过明显的或缓慢的代谢综合征导致骨关节炎，这两种综合征都存在低水平全身炎症。年龄相关的体质变化导致肌肉减少，内脏脂肪相对增加。这一变化引起关节力学异常和低水平全身炎症。其他与年龄相关的因素有细胞外基质组成和结构改变更容易出现关节衰退、线粒体功能障碍、氧化应激增加、分解代谢活性增强，以及软骨细胞功能障碍。

炎症性关节疾病如类风湿关节炎，因软骨退化和生物力学效应，能够出现继发性骨关节炎。晶体沉积病、骨坏死、佩吉特（Paget）病和代谢紊乱如血色素沉着病、黄褐病、威尔逊（Wilson）病和戈谢（Gaucher）病也能够出现继发性骨关节炎。高骨密度与髋、膝关节受累有关。雌激素缺乏可能是髋关节或膝关节疾病危险因素，激素对骨关节炎存在影响。基因研究和全基因组扫描已经确定了几个潜在的遗传标记。骨关节炎患者通常有骨关节炎或关节置换家族史。

骨关节炎的关节破坏包括：关节软骨损伤、骨赘形成和软骨下骨重塑。该过程是关节衰退和多种病因的最终结局。

骨关节炎最早的表现是关节软骨最上层纤维化。随时间推移，关节表面破坏加深，纤维化延伸到软骨

fragmentation of cartilage with release into the joint, fragmentation of cartilage with release into the joint, matrix degradation, and eventually, complete loss of cartilage, leaving only exposed bone.

Early in the process, the cartilage matrix demonstrates increased water and decreased proteoglycan content, unlike the dehydration of cartilage that occurs with aging. The tidemark zone, separating the calcified cartilage from the radial zone, is invaded by capillaries. Chondrocytes initially are metabolically active and release a variety of cytokines and metalloproteinases, contributing to matrix degradation. In the later stages, this results in the penetration of fissures to the subchondral bone and the release of fibrillated cartilage into the joint space.

An imbalance between tissue inhibitors of metalloproteinases and the production of metalloproteinases may be operative in osteoarthritis. Subchondral bone remodels and increases in density. Cystlike bone cavities containing myxoid, fibrous, or cartilaginous tissue may form. Osteophytes or bony proliferations at the margin of joints at the site of the bone-cartilage interface may form at capsule insertions. Osteophytes contribute to joint motion restriction and are thought to be the result of new bone formation in response to the degeneration

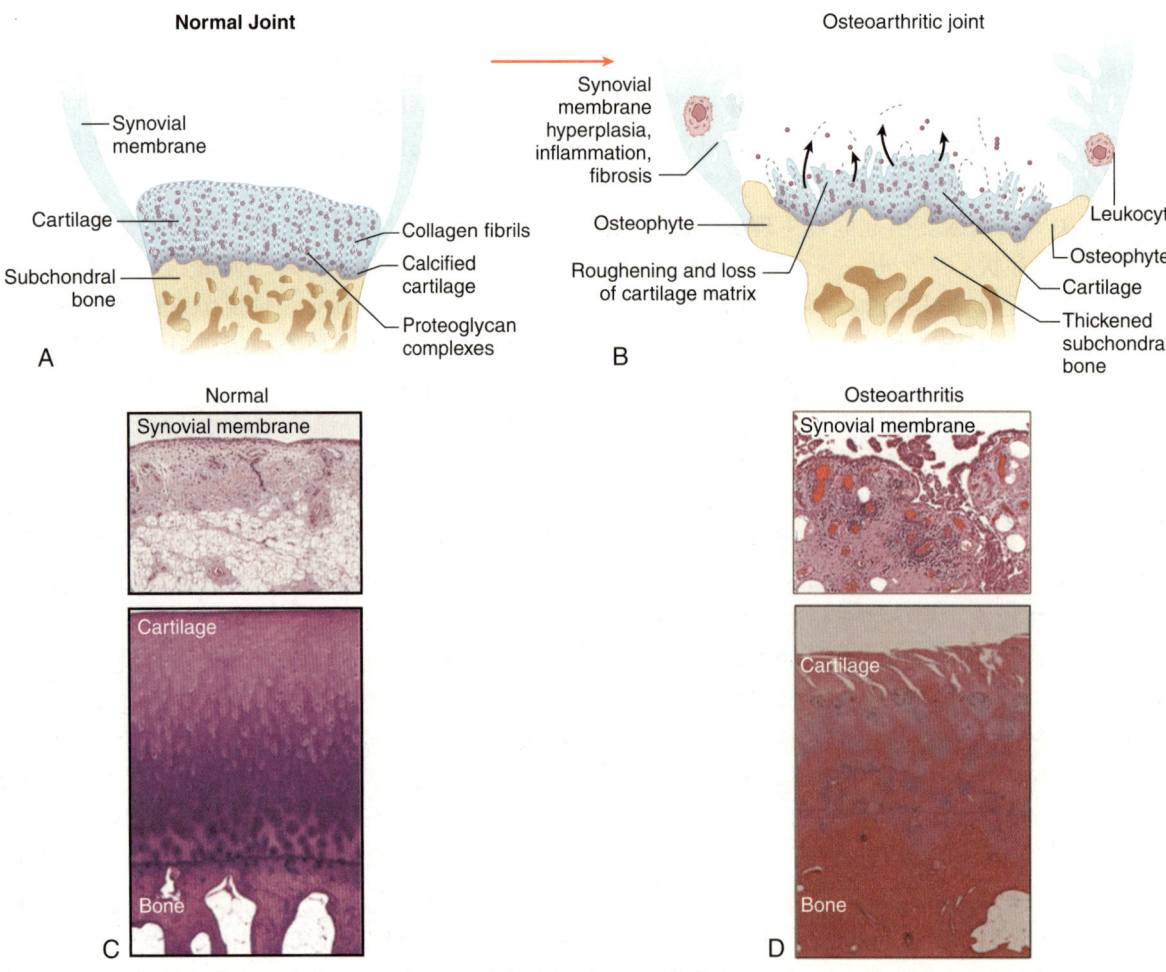

Fig. 8.1 Pathologic features of osteoarthritic joint tissues. (A) Features of a normal adult synovial joint. Healthy adult articular cartilage is characterized by a smooth surface and extracellular matrix (ECM) composed of a collagen type II fibrillar network and large proteoglycan complexes. The ECM is produced and maintained by the cellular components of cartilage, chondrocytes. The subchondral bone consists of a thin cortical layer and underlying trabecular bone. The synovial membrane lines the joint capsule and attaches at the cartilage-bone interface. In the normal state, it consists of a lining layer one or two cells thick, with underlying vascularized loose connective tissue. (B) Typical changes to tissues seen in osteoarthritis (OA). Enzymatic activities (ADAMTS4,5 and MMP-13 in particular) cleave proteoglycan and collagen components of the ECM, leading to loss of these molecules from the matrix. As the process advances, the articular cartilage thins and fibrillates, and eventually fissures down to the underlying bone are seen. Simultaneously, a remodeling response in the bone is observed. Thickening of the cortical subchondral bone layer occurs, and new bone growth at the margins appears as osteophytes. The synovial membrane changes observed in OA patients include lining layer hyperplasia, inflammation in the form of leukocyte infiltration, and fibrosis, which can be seen to varying degrees. Photomicrographs of human joint tissues showing these features are depicted in C (normal tissues) and D (OA tissues). (C and D, Courtesy Edward F. DiCarlo, MD, Hospital for Special Surgery, New York, NY.)

下骨，软骨碎裂，碎片被释放到关节中，基质降解，最终软骨完全丧失，只留下暴露的骨组织。

此过程早期表现为软骨基质水分增加，以及蛋白多糖含量减少，这一特征与伴随衰老出现的软骨脱水不同。钙化软骨与软骨深层放射带之间是软骨潮线区，其被毛细血管侵袭。起初，软骨细胞代谢活性增强，释放多种细胞因子和金属蛋白酶，促进基质降解。后期，软骨损伤的裂缝穿透到软骨下骨，纤维化的软骨碎片被释放到关节间隙中。

金属蛋白酶的产生与抑制间的不平衡可能在骨关节炎中发挥作用。软骨下骨重塑，骨密度增加。囊状骨腔形成，其中含有黏液样、纤维样或软骨样组织。在关节边缘骨-软骨交界面的关节囊附着点，有骨赘或骨增生形成。骨赘导致关节活动受限，被认为是软骨

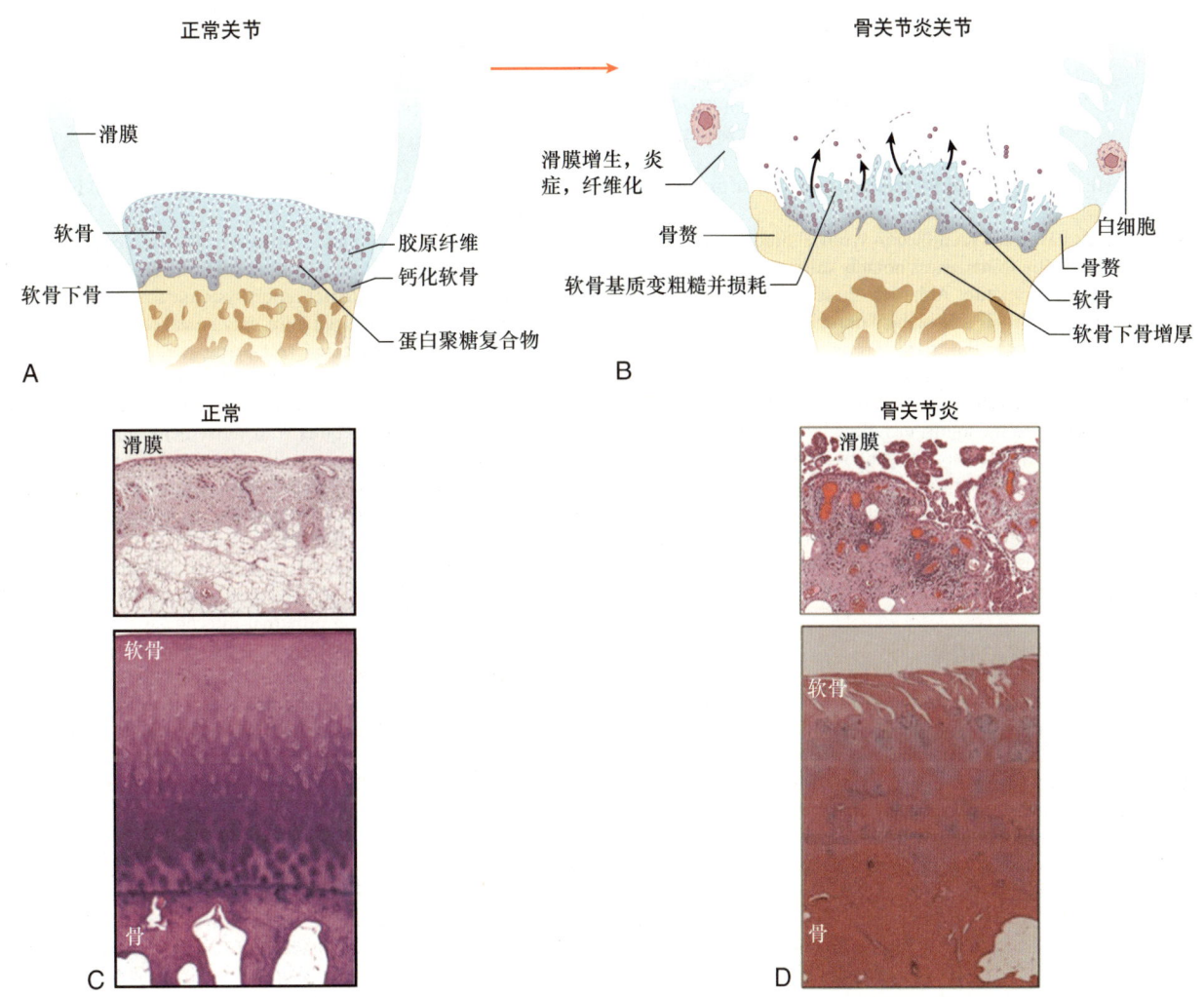

图 8.1　骨关节炎关节组织病理特征。（**A**）正常成人关节和滑膜特征。正常成人关节软骨的特征是表面光滑，Ⅱ型胶原纤维网和蛋白聚糖复合物组成细胞外基质（ECM）。ECM 由软骨中的软骨细胞产生并维持。软骨下骨由一薄层皮质层和下层的小梁骨组成。滑膜衬在关节囊内部，并贴于软骨-骨界面上。正常状态下，它由一或两个细胞厚度的内衬层组成，下有血管化的疏松结缔组织。（**B**）骨关节炎（OA）典型组织改变。一些酶（特别是 ADAMTS 4、5 和 MMP-13）裂解了 ECM 中的蛋白聚糖和胶原蛋白，导致这些分子从基质中丢失。随之进展，关节软骨变薄并纤维化，最终可见裂缝向下延伸达骨面。与此同时，可见骨的重塑反应。软骨下骨的皮质层增厚，边缘的新骨生长为骨赘。OA 患者滑膜改变包括内衬层增生、白细胞浸润出现炎症，以及不同程度纤维化。上述人类关节组织的显微照片见图 **C**（正常组织）和图 **D**（OA 组织）（C 和 D，授权自 Edward F. DiCarlo，MD，Hospital for Special Surgery，New York，NY.）

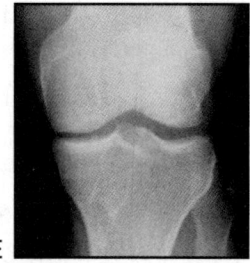 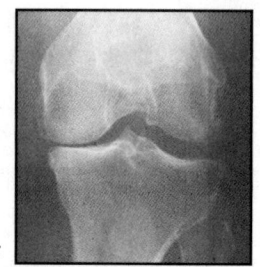

Fig. 8.1, cont'd (E and F) Radiographic features of osteoarthritic joint. Patient baseline (E) vs. 3 years later (F) showing typical features of OA progression including the development of medial joint space narrowing and osteophyte (spur outgrowth) at joint margins. The classical Kellgren and Lawrence grading system scores radiographs by five categories (scores 0–4) as follows: 0 = no osteoarthritis; 1 = small osteophyte of doubtful significance; 2 = definite osteophyte(s), possible joint space narrowing; 3 = multiple osteophytes, definite joint space narrowing, some subchondral sclerosis and possible deformity of bony ends; 4 = large osteophytes, marked narrowing of joint space, severe sclerosis of subchondral bone, and definite deformity of bone ends. (From Byers VV, Vincent TL: Osteoarthritis. In Goldman-Cecil Medicine, 26th edition, eds. Goldman L, Schafer AI, Goldman-Cecil Medicine, 1698-1703.e2, Fig. 246-3.)

of articular cartilage, but the precise mechanism for their production remains unknown.

Several crystals have been identified in synovial fluid and other tissues from osteoarthritic joints, most notably calcium pyrophosphate dehydrate and hydroxyapatite. Although these crystals have potent inflammatory potential, their role in the pathogenesis of osteoarthritis remains unclear. Frequently, the crystals are asymptomatic and do not correlate with extent or severity of disease.

The diversity of risk factors predisposing to osteoarthritis suggests that many insults to the joints, including biomechanical trauma, chronic articular inflammation, and genetic and metabolic errors, can contribute to or trigger the cascade of events that results in the characteristic pathologic features described earlier. At some point, the cartilage degradation process becomes irreversible. With progressive changes in articular cartilage, joint mechanics become altered, perpetuating the degradative process.

CLINICAL PRESENTATION

Pain is the characteristic feature of osteoarthritis and the most common presenting symptom. Pain is usually worse with activity or weight bearing and better with rest. In later stages, pain may also occur at rest. Early in the disease course, pain tends to be transient, intermittent, and unpredictable. The pain may be characterized as severe, and its unpredictable nature is an extremely bothersome feature that limits activity and affects quality of life. With disease progression, pain tends to become constant but is reported to be less severe and have an aching quality. Other prominent symptoms, such as stiffness, gelling, fatigue, and sleep disturbance, often lead to functional limitation and disability.

Pain tends to be localized to the specific joint involved, but it may be referred to a more distant site. The cause of pain is unclear but is likely to be heterogeneous. Pain may result from interactions among structural pathology; the motor, sensory, and autonomic innervation of the joint; and pain signal processing at the spinal and cortical levels. Specific individual and environmental factors also may be important. A subset of patients may have neuropathic pain.

Patient-specific factors may modify pain reception and pain reporting. Patients' affective status, such as depression, anxiety, and anger, may influence the level of pain reported. Their cognitive status, including pain beliefs, expectations, and memories of past pain, and their communication skills may determine how pain is perceived and reported. Studies have shown that demographic factors such as age, sex, socioeconomic status, race or ethnicity, and cultural background may affect pain reporting.

Patients may have stiffness, particularly after prolonged inactivity, but it is not a major feature of osteoarthritis and usually lasts for less than 30 minutes. Patients do not report systemic features such as fever.

Examination of an involved joint may reveal tenderness and bony enlargement. Joint effusion and soft tissue swelling may occur with knee involvement, but they tend to be intermittent. Persistent inflammation with joint warmth, erythema, effusion, and soft tissue swelling is usually not seen. Crepitus with movement, limitation of joint motion, and joint deformity, malalignment, and joint laxity or instability may be detected on evaluation. Joint deformity as manifested by lateral subluxation is fixed and not reducible. Muscle weakness and gait abnormalities may be seen.

Several subtypes of osteoarthritis have been identified. The nodal form involves the distal interphalangeal joints (DIPs), also known as Heberden nodes, and the proximal interphalangeal joints (PIPs), also known as Bouchard nodes. It is most common in middle-aged women, typically those with a strong family history among first-degree relatives. Erosive, inflammatory osteoarthritis is associated with prominent destructive changes, especially in the finger joints, and it is often quite symptomatic. Generalized osteoarthritis is characterized by involvement of the DIP, PIP, and first carpal-metacarpal joints, as well as the knees, feet, and hips.

DIAGNOSIS AND DIFFERENTIAL DIAGNOSIS

The diagnosis of osteoarthritis is based on the signs and symptoms previously outlined. Although there are characteristic radiographic features, they are not necessary to make the clinical diagnosis. Imaging may be used to confirm the diagnosis and exclude other diseases, but radiographs are insensitive and may not show findings early in the disease course. Despite radiographic findings of osteoarthritis, pain may have other sources, such as bursitis, tendonitis, or referred pain. For example, hip disease may manifest as knee pain.

Osteoarthritis must be distinguished from inflammatory joint diseases such as rheumatoid arthritis and the spondyloarthropathies. This is accomplished by identifying the characteristic pattern of joint involvement and the nature of the individual joint deformity. Joints commonly involved in osteoarthritis include the DIPs, PIPs, first carpal-metacarpal, cervical and lumbar spine facet joints, hips, knees, and first metatarsophalangeal joints. Involvement of the metacarpal phalangeal joints (MCPs), wrist, elbows, shoulders, and ankles is

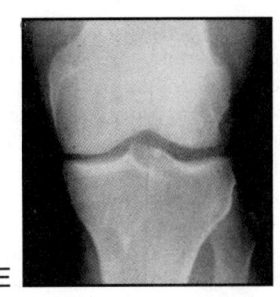 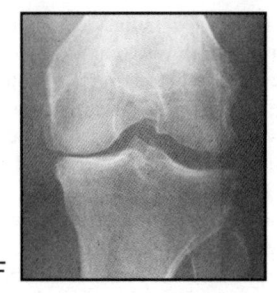

图 8.1 续（E 和 F）骨关节炎的关节影像学特征。患者基线（E）与 3 年后（F）显示 OA 进展的典型特征，包括内侧关节间隙狭窄和关节边缘骨赘（骨刺生长）的进展。经典的凯尔格伦和劳伦斯（Kellgren and Lawrence）分级系统将 X 线片分为 5 级（0～4 分）：0 ＝ 无骨关节炎；1 ＝ 可疑的小骨赘；2 ＝ 明确的骨赘，可能的关节间隙狭窄；3 ＝ 多发骨赘，关节间隙狭窄，部分软骨下骨硬化，骨末端可能畸形；4 ＝ 大的骨赘，关节间隙明显狭窄，软骨下骨严重硬化，骨末端明显畸形（引自 Byers VV, Vincent TL: Osteoarthritis. In Goldman-Cecil Medicine, 26th edition, eds. Goldman L, Schafer AI, Goldman-Cecil Medicine, 1698-1703.e2, Fig. 246-3.）

降解后新骨形成的结果，然而骨赘形成的精确机制尚不清楚。

在骨关节炎关节的滑液和其他组织中鉴定出几种晶体，最显著的是焦磷酸钙脱水物和羟基磷灰石。虽然这些晶体有强大的炎症潜能，但它们在骨关节炎发病机制中的作用尚不清楚。晶体通常不引起症状，与疾病严重程度无关。

多种危险因素诱发骨关节炎，生物力学创伤、慢性关节炎症以及遗传和代谢问题都可能引起或触发一连串事件导致上述典型病理特征。软骨降解达到某一程度则不可逆。关节软骨持续变化，关节力学发生了改变，则进入了永久化退化过程。

临床表现

疼痛是骨关节炎的典型特征，也是最常见的症状。疼痛通常在活动或负重时加重，休息时减轻。在后期，休息时也可能疼痛。疾病早期，疼痛往往是短暂的、间歇的、不可预测的。不期而遇的严重疼痛限制了患者的活动，严重影响生活质量。随疾病进展，疼痛往往持续存在，但减轻成为隐痛。其他突出的症状如僵硬、胶着感、疲劳、睡眠障碍，通常会导致功能受限和残疾。

疼痛往往局限在受累的特定关节，也能牵涉到更远的部位。疼痛的原因尚不清楚，但很可能存在多种不同原因。疼痛可能是由关节病理结构相互作用导致；可能是关节的运动、感觉和自主神经支配异常导致；也可能是脊髓和皮质水平的疼痛信号处理异常导致。具体的个人和环境因素也可能很重要。部分患者可能患有神经痛。

特定因素可能会改变患者对疼痛的感受和描述。患者的情感状态，抑郁、焦虑和愤怒可能会影响其疼痛程度。他们的认知状态，包括疼痛信念、期望、过去疼痛的记忆，以及沟通技巧，可能决定了他们如何感知和描述疼痛。研究表明，人口统计学因素，如年龄、性别、社会经济地位、种族或民族以及文化背景等可能影响患者对疼痛的描述。长期不活动后患者可能出现关节僵硬，僵硬不是骨关节炎的主要特征，通常持续时间小于 30 min。患者没有发热等全身症状。

受累关节查体可出现压痛和骨膨大。膝关节受累时可能出现关节积液和软组织肿胀，多为间歇性。通常见不到关节温度增高、红斑、积液和软组织肿胀的持续炎症表现。查体时可有关节活动伴捻发音，活动受限，关节畸形，对位不良，关节松弛或不稳定。外侧半脱位表现为关节固定畸形，不可复位。可见肌肉无力和步态异常。

骨关节炎有几种亚型。远端指间关节（DIP）结节亦称为赫伯登（Heberden）结节，近端指间关节（PIP）结节亦称为布夏尔（Bouchard）结节。它们在中年女性中最多见，尤其是直系亲属中有强家族史的女性。侵蚀性、炎症性骨关节炎可出现显著的关节破坏性变化，手指关节尤为突出，通常有显著症状。广泛性骨关节炎的特征是累及 DIP、PIP、第一腕掌关节，以及膝、足和髋关节。

诊断和鉴别诊断

骨关节炎诊断基于前文概述的体征和症状。临床诊断可以不需要特征性放射学表现。影像学可以确诊并排除其他疾病，但放射线平片不敏感，可能无法显示早期病程。即使放射学发现骨关节炎，疼痛也可能源于其他原因，如滑囊炎、肌腱炎或牵涉痛。例如，髋关节病变可表现为膝关节疼痛。

骨关节炎必须与炎症性关节病（如类风湿关节炎和脊柱关节病）区分。骨关节炎可通过关节受累的特征、单关节畸形性质被识别。骨关节炎常累及 DIP、PIP、第一腕掌关节、颈椎和腰椎小关节、髋关节、膝关节和第一跖趾关节。除了外伤、先天性疾病或合并内分泌或代谢疾病以外，掌指关节（MCP）、手腕、肘部、

uncommon, except in the case of trauma, congenital disease, or coexisting endocrine or metabolic disease.

The characteristic radiographic features of osteoarthritis include joint space narrowing as a surrogate for cartilage loss; osteophytes and subchondral sclerosis as an indicator of new bone formation, which is characteristic of osteoarthritis; and subchondral cysts as a manifestation of myxoid or fibrous degeneration of subchondral bone. Bone attrition and subchondral bone remodeling may result in changes in bone shape. Magnetic resonance imaging (MRI) can demonstrate additional morphologic abnormalities, such as bone marrow lesions in subchondral bone, meniscal degeneration, and synovitis. Musculoskeletal ultrasonography is an alternative imaging modality used to identify osteoarthritic pathologic changes within the joint space, soft tissue, cartilage, and bone surfaces. Ultrasound can identify osteoarthritis features such as osteophytes, morphologic degeneration in cartilage, synovitis, and synovial fluid.

The pain and swelling of erosive hand osteoarthritis may suggest rheumatoid arthritis, although systemic inflammatory signs and other typical features of rheumatoid arthritis are absent. Patients with osteoarthritis typically have a negative rheumatoid factor, normal inflammatory markers such as erythrocyte sedimentation rate and c-reactive protein, normal complete blood count, and normal antinuclear antibody tests. Synovial fluid examination is typically noninflammatory with clear viscous fluid and normal white blood cell count. The prevalence of false-positive findings of rheumatoid factor and antinuclear antibody, sometimes in significant titers, is higher with increasing age. Osteoarthritis more commonly affects the distal small joints in the hands (DIPs > PIPs > MCPs and wrists), whereas rheumatoid arthritis more commonly affects proximal small joints in the hands (MCPs and wrists > PIPs > DIPs).

TREATMENT

The natural history of osteoarthritis includes periods of relative stability interspersed with rapid deterioration. Management should be individually tailored and may include a combination of nonpharmacologic, pharmacologic, and surgical approaches. The primary goal of treatment is to improve pain and function and reduce disability.

Patients should be educated regarding the objectives of treatment and the importance of lifestyle changes, exercise, pacing of activities, and other measures to unload the damaged joints. The initial focus should be on self-help and patient-driven treatments rather than on passive therapies. Patients should be encouraged to adhere to non-pharmacologic and pharmacologic therapies. Physical therapists may be helpful in providing instruction in appropriate exercises to reduce pain and preserve functional capacity. For knee and hip osteoarthritis, assistive devices such as walking aids may be useful. In patients with first carpometacarpal joint osteoarthritis, hand orthoses are recommended. Graded regular aerobic, aquatic exercise, muscle-strengthening, and range-of-motion exercises are beneficial. Tai chi has been shown to have beneficial effects not only in the treatment of knee and hip osteoarthritis, but also in improving quality of life and depression.

Overweight patients should be encouraged to lose weight. A combination of dietary weight loss in conjunction with exercise results in improvement of both pain and function compared to either intervention alone, though long-term weight management may be challenging for patients. A knee brace can reduce pain, improve stability, and diminish the risk of falling for patients with knee osteoarthritis and mild or moderate varus or valgus instability. Advice concerning appropriate footwear is also important. Spinal orthoses may provide benefit to patients with significant cervical or lumbar involvement. Local applications of heat, ultrasound, or transcutaneous electrical nerve stimulation (TENS) may provide short-term benefit in these patients. In patients with knee and hip osteoarthritis, TENS is not recommended as there have been limited studies and lack of benefit. Acupuncture may also offer symptomatic benefit for patients with osteoarthritis, but its efficacy in knee, hip, and hand osteoarthritis is still debatable as studies have shown variable results.

Pharmacologic therapy provides symptomatic relief but does not alter the course of the disease. Pharmacologic therapy should therefore be selected based on its relative efficacy and safety. The use of concomitant medications in the setting of comorbidities should be taken into account.

Acetaminophen (up to 3 g/day with caution) may be an effective initial oral analgesic for mild to moderate pain, though it may not provide sufficient benefit on its own. In patients with symptomatic osteoarthritis, nonsteroidal anti-inflammatory drugs (NSAIDs) should be used at the lowest effective dose, although their long-term use should be avoided if possible. If patients are at risk for increased gastrointestinal toxicity, a cyclooxygenase-2 (COX2)–selective agent or a nonselective NSAID with co-prescription of a proton pump inhibitor or misoprostol for gastroprotection should be considered. All NSAIDs, including nonselective and COX2-selective agents, should be used with caution in patients with cardiovascular risk factors and chronic kidney disease. Topical NSAIDs and capsaicin may be effective alternatives to oral analgesic or anti-inflammatory agents in knee and hand osteoarthritis and may be used as adjunctive agents, particularly in elderly patients. If patients fail the aforementioned, find other therapies ineffective, and are not surgical candidates, then tramadol, a weak opioid receptor agonist, may also be used in these select cases. Non-tramadol opiates are discouraged as they pose risk for an increase of adverse effects that typically outweighs their benefits. In select patients that have exhausted other therapies and medications, non-tramadol opioids may be used for the shortest possible length of time, given the limited pain control with longer duration of these medications.

Despite the popularity of these products, meta-analyses have shown that oral glucosamine and chondroitin sulfate have limited benefit in patients with knee osteoarthritis and are currently not recommended in knee, hip or hand osteoarthritis.

Other agents, such as duloxetine, when compared to placebo, were shown to reduce pain and improve function in a meta-analysis. Duloxetine can be used in pain management and studies have shown efficacy in the treatment of osteoarthritis.

Occasional injection of intra-articular corticosteroids (usually no more than once every 4 months) may provide modest short-term symptomatic benefit with minimal toxicity, especially in the knee. Studies have shown that patients given more frequent corticosteroid injections (i.e., every 3 months) lose greater cartilage volume than those given a corticosteroid injection every 4 months, but the significance of this cartilage loss is unclear. Patients with moderate to severe pain and effusion or other local signs of inflammation may be more responsive to these injections. Intra-articular hyaluronate appears to have little or no benefit based on current evidence. Recent trials evaluated platelet-rich plasma injections and mesenchymal stem cell injections in osteoarthritis, but these are not currently recommended because there is a concern in the techniques used for these injections as well as the heterogeneity and lack of standardization of available preparations.

Surgical management includes total joint replacement, which is extremely effective in relieving pain, decreasing disability, and improving function. With improvements in surgical technique and technology, the indications for total joint replacement have expanded to include younger and older age groups. Other surgical options include osteotomy and uni-compartmental knee replacement.

肩部和脚踝的受累不常见。

骨关节炎的特征性放射学表现包括：关节间隙变窄（体现软骨丢失）；骨赘和软骨下硬化（提示新骨形成），这是骨关节炎的特征性表现；软骨下囊肿（为软骨下骨黏液样或纤维变性的表现）。骨磨损和软骨下骨重塑可能导致骨骼外形改变。磁共振成像（MRI）可以显示其他形态学异常，如软骨下骨的骨髓病变、半月板变性和滑膜炎。肌肉骨骼超声是另一种可供选择的成像模式，可以识别骨关节炎关节间隙、软组织、软骨和骨表面的病理变化。超声可以识别骨关节炎的特征，如骨赘、软骨形态退化、滑膜炎和滑膜积液。

侵蚀性手骨关节炎出现的疼痛、肿胀提示类风湿关节炎，即便没有类风湿关节炎的全身炎症体征和其他典型特征。骨关节炎患者通常类风湿因子为阴性，红细胞沉降率（血沉）、C反应蛋白等炎症标志物正常，血常规、抗核抗体均正常。关节滑液检查通常为非炎症性，滑液清澈黏稠，白细胞计数正常。随年龄增长，类风湿因子和抗核抗体假阳性率越来越高，有时显著增高。骨关节炎更多见于手部远端小关节（DIP > PIP > MCP 和腕），而类风湿关节炎更多见于手部近端小关节（MCP 和腕 > PIP > DIP）。

治疗

骨关节炎的自然病程包括相对稳定期和快速恶化期。个体化管理应结合非药物治疗、药物治疗和手术治疗。治疗的主要目标是缓解疼痛，改善功能，减少残疾。

教育患者认识治疗目标，重视改变生活方式、锻炼、活动节奏，采取措施减轻受损关节负荷。治疗初始应聚焦在患者主动的自助治疗，优于被动治疗。应鼓励患者坚持非药物和药物治疗。理疗师帮助患者恰当的锻炼，减轻关节疼痛，维持关节功能。辅助行走等辅助设备可能有利于膝、髋骨关节炎。第一腕掌关节受累的骨关节炎患者推荐使用手矫形器。分级有氧运动、水上运动、肌力增强和关节活动度训练（range-of-motion exercises）均有益。已证实，太极拳不仅有利于治疗膝、髋骨关节炎，也可改善生活质量，并缓解抑郁。

鼓励超重患者减轻体重。长期体重管理对于患者是一种挑战，饮食减重与运动相结合，比两者单独应用更有利于缓解关节疼痛，改善关节功能。护膝可以减轻膝骨关节炎患者的疼痛，提高关节稳定性，减小轻/中度膝关节内翻或外翻不稳定患者跌倒的风险。建议患者穿着合适的鞋子也很重要。脊柱矫形器对颈椎或腰椎明显受累的患者有价值。局部热疗、超声波或经皮电神经刺激（TENS）对于患者短期有益。不建议膝和髋骨关节炎患者使用TENS，相关研究有限且无益。针灸可缓解骨关节炎患者症状，但其对膝、髋和手骨关节炎的疗效仍有争议，研究结果各不相同。

药物治疗可以缓解症状，但不能改变疾病进程。应根据相对疗效和安全性选择药物治疗。针对合并症考虑应用辅助药物。

对乙酰氨基酚（谨慎应用，最高可达 3 g/d）是治疗轻度至中度疼痛的有效初始口服止痛药，但其镇痛效果可能有限。对症状性骨关节炎患者，非甾体抗炎药（NSAID）应使用最低有效剂量，并尽可能避免长期使用。如果患者有胃肠道毒性风险，应考虑使用环氧合酶-2（COX2）选择性药物，或非选择性NSAID联合质子泵抑制剂或米索前列醇来护胃。存在心血管危险因素和慢性肾病的患者应慎用所有NSAID，包括非选择性和COX2选择性药物。局部NSAID和辣椒素可能是口服镇痛或抗炎药的有效替代品，也可作为辅助药物，特别适合老年患者。如果患者不能接受上述治疗，其他治疗无效，且无手术指征，曲马多是一种弱阿片受体激动剂，可用于这些特定病例。不推荐曲马多以外的阿片类药物，它们的副作用可能会增加，并超过其获益。对于其他疗法和药物治疗欠佳者，可在尽可能最短时间内应用曲马多之外的阿片类药物，这类药物随用药时间延长，镇痛能力降低。

虽然，口服葡萄糖胺和硫酸软骨素很受欢迎，但荟萃分析显示这类药物对于骨关节炎患者的益处有限，目前不推荐用于膝、髋或手骨关节炎患者。

一项荟萃分析显示，度洛西汀比安慰剂更好地减轻疼痛和改善功能。度洛西汀可用于疼痛管理，研究显示了其治疗骨关节炎的疗效。

针对膝关节，关节腔内注射皮质类固醇（通常不超过每4个月1次）可短期适度改善关节症状，且毒性最低。研究表明，与每4个月注射1次皮质类固醇的患者相比，更频繁地注射皮质类固醇（即每3个月1次），患者软骨体积损失更多，但其意义尚不清楚。中重度疼痛、关节积液或有其他局部炎症征象的患者可能对关节腔注射更敏感。现有的证据显示，关节内注射透明质酸似乎少有或没有益处。最近的试验评估了骨关节炎患者于关节腔注射富血小板血浆、间充质干细胞的效果，但由于这些关节腔注射技术及注射制剂存在异质性，并缺乏标准化，目前不推荐这些治疗方式。

包括全关节置换的手术治疗在缓解疼痛、减少残疾以及改善功能方面疗效显著。随着手术技术和工艺的进步，全关节置换术的适应证已拓展到了更年轻和更年长的群体。其他术式有截骨和膝关节单髁置换术。如已

Referral to an orthopedic surgeon should be considered in cases where other treatment options have been exhausted and quality of life is greatly reduced, including joint pain disrupting sleep, restriction of walking distance, and limiting participation in daily activities. Arthroscopy is not recommended for the management of knee osteoarthritis.

PROGNOSIS

Given the obesity epidemic and the marked contact loads that increased weight places on the knee, obesity is likely the most important modifiable risk factor for the development and progression of knee osteoarthritis. One kilogram of weight loss decreases the load on the knee by 4 kg. Varus and valgus malalignments have also been identified as important risk factors for the progression of knee osteoarthritis.

SUGGESTED READINGS

Blagojevic M, Jinks C, Jeffery A, et al: Risk factors for onset of osteoarthritis of the knee in older adults: a systematic review and meta-analysis, Osteoarthritis Cartilage 18:24–33, 2013.

Helmick CG, Felson DT, Kwoh CK, et al: Estimates of the prevalence of arthritis and other rheumatic conditions in the United States. Part I, Arthritis Rheum 58:15–25, 2008.

Hochberg MC, Altman RD, April KT, et al: American College of Rheumatology 2012 recommendations for the use of nonpharmacologic and pharmacologic therapies in osteoarthritis of the hand, hip, and knee, Arthritis Care Res 64:465–474, 2012.

Hunter DJ, Bierma-Zeinstra S: Osteoarthritis, Lancet 393(10182): 1745–1759, 2019.

Kolasinski SL, Neogi T, Hochberg MC, et al: 2019 American College of Rheumatology/Arthritis Foundation guidelines for the management of osteoarthritis of the hand, hip and knee, Art Rheum 72(2):220–233, 2019.

Litwic A, Edwards MH, Dennison EM, et al: Epidemiology and burden of osteoarthritis, Br Med Bull 105:185–199, 2013.

McAlindon TE, LaValley MP, Harvey WF, et al: Effect of intra-articular triamcinolone vs saline on knee cartilage volume and pain in patients with knee osteoarthritis: a randomized clinical trial, J Am Med Assoc 317:1967–1975, 2017.

Okano T, Mamoto K, Di Carlo M, et al: Clinical utility and potential of ultrasound in osteoarthritis, Radiol Med 124:1101–1111, 2019.

Wang ZY, Shi SY, Li SJ, et al: Efficacy and safety of duloxetine on osteoarthritis knee pain: a meta-analysis of randomized controlled trials, Pain Med 16(7):1373–1385, 2015.

Zhang W, Moskowitz RW, Kwoh CK, et al: OARSI recommendations for the management of hip and knee osteoarthritis, part I: critical appraisal of existing treatment guidelines and systematic review of current research evidence, Osteoarthritis Cartilage 15:981–1000, 2007.

Zhang W, Moskovitz RW, Nuki G, et al: OARSI recommendations for the management of hip and knee osteoarthritis, part II: OARSI evidence-based, expert consensus guidelines, Osteoarthritis Cartilage 16:137–162, 2008.

穷尽其他治疗方案，生活质量大幅降低，包括关节疼痛影响睡眠、步行距离受限和日常活动受限，应考虑转诊给骨科医生。不推荐关节镜用于膝骨关节炎治疗。

预后

肥胖症流行和体重增加显著增加了膝关节的接触性负荷，肥胖症可能是膝骨关节炎发生和进展最重要、可改变的危险因素。体重减轻 1 kg 可减少 4 kg 膝关节负荷。关节内翻和外翻错位也是膝骨关节炎进展的重要危险因素。

推荐阅读

Blagojevic M, Jinks C, Jeffery A, et al: Risk factors for onset of osteoarthritis of the knee in older adults: a systematic review and meta-analysis, Osteoarthritis Cartilage 18:24–33, 2013.

Helmick CG, Felson DT, Kwoh CK, et al: Estimates of the prevalence of arthritis and other rheumatic conditions in the United States. Part I, Arthritis Rheum 58:15–25, 2008.

Hochberg MC, Altman RD, April KT, et al: American College of Rheumatology 2012 recommendations for the use of nonpharmacologic and pharmacologic therapies in osteoarthritis of the hand, hip, and knee, Arthritis Care Res 64:465–474, 2012.

Hunter DJ, Bierma-Zeinstra S: Osteoarthritis, Lancet 393(10182): 1745–1759, 2019.

Kolasinski SL, Neogi T, Hochberg MC, et al: 2019 American College of Rheumatology/Arthritis Foundation guidelines for the management of osteoarthritis of the hand, hip and knee, Art Rheum 72(2):220–233, 2019.

Litwic A, Edwards MH, Dennison EM, et al: Epidemiology and burden of osteoarthritis, Br Med Bull 105:185–199, 2013.

McAlindon TE, LaValley MP, Harvey WF, et al: Effect of intra-articular triamcinolone vs saline on knee cartilage volume and pain in patients with knee osteoarthritis: a randomized clinical trial, J Am Med Assoc 317:1967–1975, 2017.

Okano T, Mamoto K, Di Carlo M, et al: Clinical utility and potential of ultrasound in osteoarthritis, Radiol Med 124:1101–1111, 2019.

Wang ZY, Shi SY, Li SJ, et al: Efficacy and safety of duloxetine on osteoarthritis knee pain: a meta-analysis of randomized controlled trials, Pain Med 16(7):1373–1385, 2015.

Zhang W, Moskowitz RW, Kwoh CK, et al: OARSI recommendations for the management of hip and knee osteoarthritis, part I: critical appraisal of existing treatment guidelines and systematic review of current research evidence, Osteoarthritis Cartilage 15:981–1000, 2007.

Zhang W, Moskovitz RW, Nuki G, et al: OARSI recommendations for the management of hip and knee osteoarthritis, part II: OARSI evidence-based, expert consensus guidelines, Osteoarthritis Cartilage 16:137–162, 2008.

Nonarticular Soft Tissue Disorders

Niveditha Mohan

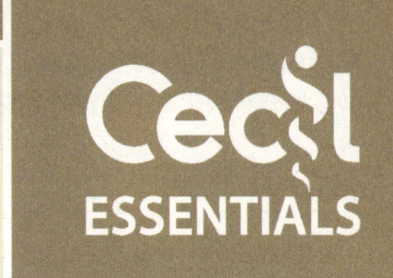

INTRODUCTION

The nonarticular soft tissue disorders account for most musculoskeletal complaints in the general population. These disorders include a large number of anatomically localized conditions (e.g., bursitis, tendinitis) and fibromyalgia syndrome, a generalized pain disorder. For most nonarticular soft tissue conditions, the etiologic factors and pathogenesis are poorly understood.

Once the location of the symptom is defined, (e.g., shoulder pain), the specific structure that is involved should be identified (e.g., supraspinatus tendon, subacromial bursa) using a careful history and physical examination. In the case of back pain, precise anatomic delineation of the structure involved (e.g., intervertebral disk, facet joint, ligament, paraspinal muscle) is more likely to require advanced imaging. When the patient complains of diffuse pain, it is imperative to evaluate for contribution of local pain that may be driving the diffuse pain, with a thorough physical examination.

EPIDEMIOLOGY

Precise data for prevalence or incidence of most nonarticular soft tissue syndromes are not available, but these conditions account for up to 30% of all outpatient visits. Fibromyalgia is considered to be the most common cause of generalized musculoskeletal pain in women between the ages of 20 and 55 years. The global mean prevalence is 2.7%.

ETIOLOGIC FACTORS AND PATHOGENESIS

The precise pathophysiology of most nonarticular soft tissue disorders remains unknown, although predisposing factors, such as trauma, overuse, repetitive activities (e.g., tennis elbow, lateral epicondylitis) or biomechanical factors (e.g., leg-length discrepancy in trochanteric bursitis), can be identified in many cases.

The term *tendinitis* implies tendon sheath inflammation, but small tendon tears, periostitis, and nerve entrapment have been proposed as potential mechanisms. Similarly, although the term *bursitis* implies bursal inflammation, demonstrable inflammation is difficult to find. In some cases (e.g., acute bursitis of the olecranon or prepatellar bursa), the mechanism is an acute inflammatory response to sodium urate crystals deposited in the soft tissue, an extra-articular manifestation of gout. The favorable response of tendinitis and bursitis to anti-inflammatory agents, including corticosteroids, supports the view that at least one component of these syndromes is the result of an inflammatory process.

Fibromyalgia is the current term for chronic widespread musculoskeletal pain for which no alternative cause can be identified. The underlying pathology is due to alterations in central nervous system (CNS) function leading to augmented nociceptive (caused by pain) processing that leads to the development of CNS-mediated somatic symptoms of fatigue, sleep, memory and mood difficulties in addition to the chronic widespread pain. There may also be alterations in the immune system leading to an enhanced inflammatory state with emerging evidence that some of the pathobiology of fibromyalgia may involve altered nociceptor sensitivity. This disorder often begins in childhood or adolescence, and individuals who eventually go on to develop FM are more likely to experience headaches, dysmenorrhea, temporomandibular joint disorder, chronic fatigue, irritable bowel syndrome and other functional gastrointestinal tract disorders, interstitial cystitis/painful bladder syndrome, endometriosis, and other regional pain syndromes (especially back and neck pain).

CLINICAL PRESENTATION

Many of the soft tissue rheumatic syndromes involve bursae, tendons, ligaments, and muscles. Bursae are closed sacs lined with mesenchymal cells that are similar to synovial cells; the sacs are strategically located to facilitate tissue gliding. Subcutaneous bursae (e.g., olecranon, prepatellar) form after birth in response to normal external friction. Deep bursae (e.g., subacromial bursa) usually form before birth in response to movement between muscles and bones and may or may not communicate with adjacent joint cavities. Adventitious bursae (e.g., over the first metatarsal head) form in response to abnormal shearing stresses and are not uniformly found. Although most forms of bursitis involve isolated, local conditions, some may be the result of systemic conditions such as gout.

Tendinitis, bursitis, and myofascial disorders should be distinguished from articular disorders. In most cases, this can be accomplished by a careful examination of the involved structure (Table 9.1). General principles of the musculoskeletal examination are as follows:

1. Observation: If deformity or soft tissue swelling is detected, is it fusiform (i.e., surrounding the entire joint in a symmetrical fashion) or is it localized? Local rather than fusiform deformity distinguishes nonarticular disorders from articular disorders.
2. Palpation: Is tenderness localized or in a fusiform distribution? Is there an effusion? Local (not fusiform or joint line) tenderness distinguishes nonarticular disorders from articular disorders. An effusion typically indicates an articular disorder.
3. Assessing range of motion: The musculoskeletal examination includes the assessment of active range of motion (i.e., patient attempts to move the symptomatic structure) and passive range of motion (i.e., examiner moves the symptomatic structure). Articular disorders usually are characterized by equal impairment in active and passive movements as a result of the mechanical limitation

非关节软组织疾病

孙兴 译　贾园 何菁 审校　粟占国 通审

引言

非关节软组织疾病是一般人群中大多数肌肉骨骼问题的主要来源，包括许多以解剖定位的疾病（如滑囊炎、肌腱炎）和纤维肌痛综合征，后者是一种全身性疼痛疾病。大多数非关节软组织疾病的病因和发病机制尚不清楚。

一旦症状被定位（如肩部疼痛），应详细询问病史和体格检查来识别受累的特定结构（如冈上肌腱、肩峰下滑囊）。如果出现背痛，需要进一步完善影像学检查来明确受累的解剖结构（如椎间盘、关节突关节、韧带、脊柱旁肌肉）。当患者主诉弥漫性疼痛时，必须通过完善的体格检查来评估可能促发弥漫性疼痛的局部疼痛位点。

流行病学

大多数非关节软组织综合征的发病率或患病率的精确数据尚不清楚，这些状况可占门诊就诊的30%。纤维肌痛被认为是20～55岁女性中最常见的全身性肌肉骨骼疼痛原因。全球平均患病率为2.7%。

病因和发病机制

尽管创伤、过度使用、重复活动（如网球肘、外上髁炎）或生物力学因素（如腿不等长引起转子滑囊炎）可能是大多数非关节软组织疾病的易感因素，但确切病理生理学机制尚不明确。

肌腱炎意味着肌腱腱鞘炎症，但小的肌腱撕裂、骨膜炎和神经卡压是其潜在的机制。同样，尽管滑囊炎一词意味着滑囊炎症，但很难找到明显的炎症。在某些情况下（如肘部或髌前滑囊的急性滑囊炎），滑囊炎的发生机制是对软组织中沉积的尿酸钠盐晶体的急性炎症反应，这是痛风的关节外表现。肌腱炎和滑囊炎对包括皮质类固醇在内的抗炎药物反应良好，证明炎症过程在这些综合征中占据一席之地。

在无法识别其他可能病因时，纤维肌痛是目前用于描述慢性全身性肌肉骨骼疼痛的术语。其潜在病理是由于中枢神经系统（CNS）功能改变导致由疼痛引起的伤害增强，进而中枢神经系统介导出躯体症状，如疲劳，睡眠、记忆和情绪障碍以及慢性全身性疼痛。免疫系统也可能发生改变，导致炎症活化，新证据表明纤维肌痛可能涉及痛觉感受器敏感性的改变。这种疾病通常始于儿童或青少年时期，最终发展为纤维肌痛的个体更有可能经历头痛、痛经、颞下颌关节疾病、慢性疲劳、肠易激综合征和其他功能性胃肠道疾病、间质性膀胱炎/疼痛性膀胱综合征、子宫内膜异位症和其他区域性疼痛综合征（特别是背部和颈部疼痛）。

临床表现

许多软组织风湿综合征涉及滑囊、肌腱、韧带和肌肉。滑囊是内衬有类似于滑膜细胞的间充质细胞的封闭囊，位于关键位置以助于组织滑动。皮下滑囊（如肘部、髌前滑囊）是在出生后对正常的外来摩擦做出反应所形成的。深部滑囊（如肩峰下滑囊）则通常是在出生前对肌肉和骨骼之间的运动做出反应形成的，可能或可能不与邻近关节腔相通。不定囊（如第一跖骨头上方滑囊）是针对异常剪切应力形成的，临床表现各异。尽管大多数滑囊炎的形式以孤立的局部表现为主，但有些可能是系统性疾病的结果，如痛风。

肌腱炎、滑囊炎和肌筋膜疾病应与关节疾病区分开来。大多数情况下，可以通过仔细检查受累结构来区分上述疾病（表9.1）。肌肉骨骼检查的一般原则如下：

1. 观察：如果有畸形或软组织肿胀，需判断是呈梭形（即以对称的方式环绕整个关节）还是局部的。局部而非梭形的畸形可以帮助将非关节性疾病从关节性疾病中区分出来。

2. 触诊：判断压痛是局部的还是梭形分布？有无积液？局部压痛（非梭形或沿关节线分布）可以将非关节性疾病从关节性疾病中区分出来。积液通常表明关节受累。

3. 关节活动范围评估：肌肉骨骼检查包括评估关节主动活动范围（即患者尝试移动有症状的结构）和被动活动范围（即检查者移动有症状的结构）。关节性疾病通常由于滑膜增生、积液或关节内结构紊乱导致关节活

TABLE 9.1 Differentiating Nonarticular Soft Tissue Disorders From Articular Disease

Manifestation	Nonarticular Soft Tissue Disorders	Articular Disease
Limitation of motion	Active > passive	Active = passive
Crepitus of articular surfaces (structural damage)	0	+/0
Tenderness		
Synovial (fusiform pattern)	0	+
Local	+	0
Swelling		
Synovial (fusiform pattern)	0	+
Local	+/0	0

+, Present; 0, absent.

TABLE 9.2 Bursitis Syndromes

Location	Symptom	Finding
Subacromial	Shoulder pain	Tender subacromial space
Olecranon	Elbow pain	Tender olecranon swelling
Iliopectineal	Groin pain	Tender inguinal region
Trochanteric	Lateral hip pain	Tender at greater trochanter
Prepatellar	Anterior knee pain	Tender swelling over patella
Infrapatellar	Anterior knee pain	Tender swelling lateral or medial to patellar tendon
Anserine	Medial knee pain	Tender medioproximal tibia (below joint line of knee)
Ischiogluteal	Buttock pain	Tender ischial spine (at gluteal fold)
Retrocalcaneal	Heel pain	Tender swelling between Achilles tendon insertion and calcaneus
Calcaneal	Heel pain	Tender central heel pad

of joint motion resulting from proliferation of the synovial membrane, an effusion, or derangement of intra-articular structures. Impairment of active movement characterizes nonarticular disorders to a much greater degree than passive movement.

Clinical symptoms include pain, warmth, and swelling over the site of the bursa that are worse with activity and better with rest. Bursitis can be distinguished from tendinitis by the pain during active and passive range of movement; in tendinitis, pain is elicited only during active range of movement. However, for many patients there is concomitant bursitis and tendinitis.

Muscle sprains or strains are typically diagnosed based on a history of preceding activity causing the symptom along with pain and limitation of movement when the muscle is contracted against resistance. The clinical signs and symptoms of chronic myofascial pain are more nonspecific and characterized by a distribution that is frequently nonanatomic and associated with hyperalgesia in the involved area.

Fibromyalgia syndrome is characterized by widespread pain and a host of other symptoms, including insomnia, cognitive dysfunction, depression, anxiety, recurrent headaches, dizziness, fatigue, morning stiffness, extremity dysesthesia, irritable bowel syndrome, and irritable bladder syndrome.

DIAGNOSIS AND TREATMENT

Septic Bursitis

Superficial forms of bursitis, particularly olecranon bursitis and prepatellar and occasionally infrapatellar bursitis, are more frequently infected or involved with crystal deposition than are deep forms of bursitis, presumably due to direct extension of organisms through subcutaneous tissues. Most commonly, *Staphylococcus aureus* is isolated from infected superficial bursae. Septic bursitis should be suspected when there is cellulitis, erythema, fever, and peripheral leukocytosis.

Definitive diagnosis and exclusion of infection of subcutaneous bursae usually require aspiration of the distended bursa. The bursal fluid should be assessed for cell count, Gram stain, and culture and examined for crystals.

Nonseptic Bursitis

Nonseptic bursitis frequently appears as an overuse condition associated with sudden or unaccustomed repetitive activity of the associated extremity. The two most common types of bursitis are subacromial and trochanteric bursitis (Table 9.2).

Subacromial bursitis is the most common overall cause of shoulder pain over the lateral upper arm or deltoid muscle that is exacerbated with abduction of the arm. It occurs as a result of compression of the inflamed rotator cuff tendon between the acromion and humeral head. Because the rotator cuff forms the floor of the subacromial bursa, bursitis in this location often results from tendinitis of the rotator cuff. Occasionally, subacromial bursitis or rotator cuff tendinitis results from osteophyte compression of the rotator cuff tendon originating from the acromioclavicular joint. The differential diagnosis includes tears of the rotator cuff, intra-articular pathologic mechanisms of the glenohumeral joint, bicipital tendinitis, cervical radiculopathy, and referred pain from the chest.

Trochanteric bursitis is the result of inflammation at the insertion of the gluteal muscles at the greater trochanter. It produces lateral thigh pain, which is often worse when the patient lies on the affected side. Women seem to be more prone to develop this condition, perhaps because of increased traction of the gluteal muscles as a result of the relatively broader female pelvis. Other potential risk factors include weight gain, local trauma, overuse activities such as jogging, and leg-length discrepancies (primarily on the side with the longer leg). These factors are thought to lead to increased tension of the gluteus maximus on the iliotibial band, producing bursal inflammation. The differential diagnosis of trochanteric bursitis includes lumbar radiculopathy (particularly of the L1 and L2 nerve roots), meralgia paresthetica (i.e., entrapment of the lateral cutaneous nerve of the thigh as it passes under the inguinal ligament), true hip joint disease, and intra-abdominal pathologic processes. Other bursitis syndromes are less common and listed in Table 9.2.

Septic bursitis is treated with a combination of serial aspirations of the infected bursa and antibiotics, initially directed against *S. aureus* and then adjusted depending on the results of bursal fluid cultures. Recurrent septic bursitis may need surgical excision of the bursa. The approach to nonseptic bursitis should include rest, local heat, and unless contraindicated by peptic ulcer disease, renal disease, or advanced age, nonsteroidal anti-inflammatory drugs (NSAIDs).

The most effective approach usually is local injection of a corticosteroid. Superficial bursae with obvious swelling should be aspirated before the corticosteroid is injected. For deep bursae, such as the subacromial or trochanteric bursae, aspiration yields little or no fluid, and direct injection of a corticosteroid without attempted aspiration is reasonable. Caution is advised in attempted aspiration or injection of the iliopsoas bursa, the ischiogluteal bursa, and the gastrocnemius-semimembranosus bursa (i.e., Baker cyst). These bursae lie close to important neural and vascular structures, and aspiration under ultrasound guidance is recommended.

表 9.1 非关节软组织疾病与关节疾病的鉴别

临床表现	非关节软组织疾病	关节疾病
活动受限	主动>被动	主动=被动
关节表面摩擦感（结构损伤）	0	+/0
压痛		
滑膜型（梭形肿胀）	0	+
局部	+	0
肿胀		
滑膜型（梭形肿胀）	0	+
局部	+/0	0

+，存在，0，不存在

表 9.2 滑囊炎综合征

部位	症状	体征
肩峰下滑囊炎	肩痛	肩峰下压痛
鹰嘴滑囊炎	肘痛	鹰嘴压痛肿胀
髂耻滑囊炎	腹股沟痛	腹股沟区域压痛
转子滑囊炎	外侧髋痛	大转子压痛
髌前滑囊炎	前膝痛	髌骨上方压痛肿胀
髌下滑囊炎	前膝痛	髌腱外侧或内侧压痛肿胀
鹅足滑囊炎	内侧膝痛	近端胫骨中部压痛（膝关节线下方）
坐骨结节滑囊炎	臀部痛	坐骨棘压痛（臀沟处）
跟骨后滑囊炎	足跟痛	跟腱插入处与跟骨之间的压痛肿胀
跟骨滑囊炎	足跟痛	足跟垫中心压痛

动的机械性受限，表现为主动和被动活动均受影响。非关节性疾病更显著地影响主动活动而非被动活动。

临床症状包括滑囊部位的疼痛、局部发热和肿胀，这些症状在活动时加重，休息时减轻。滑囊炎表现为主动和被动活动均出现疼痛，这与肌腱炎不同；肌腱炎中疼痛仅在主动活动时出现。然而，对于许多患者来说，滑囊炎和肌腱炎是同时存在的。

肌肉拉伤或扭伤通常是由于先前活动不当导致，通过以在肌肉收缩时出现疼痛以及活动受限来诊断。慢性肌筋膜疼痛的临床症状更为不特异，其特征是非解剖位置分布，并且与受影响区域的痛觉过敏有关。

纤维肌痛综合征的特征是广泛性疼痛和许多其他症状，包括失眠、认知功能障碍、抑郁、焦虑、反复头痛、头晕、疲劳、晨僵、四肢感觉异常、肠易激综合征和膀胱易激综合征。

诊断和治疗

化脓性滑囊炎

浅表滑囊炎，尤其是鹰嘴滑囊炎、髌前和偶有的髌下滑囊炎等，比深部滑囊炎更容易感染或出现晶体沉积，这可能是通过皮下组织有机体直接扩散所致。于感染的浅表滑囊分离出金黄色葡萄球菌最常见。当出现蜂窝织炎、红斑、发热和外周白细胞增多时，应怀疑脓毒性滑囊炎。通常需要对肿胀的滑囊进行穿刺来确诊和排除皮下滑囊感染。对于滑囊液应评估细胞计数、革兰氏染色和进行培养，并检查晶体。

非化脓性滑囊炎

非化脓性滑囊炎通常与相关肢体的过度使用有关，出现于肢体突然或不习惯的重复性活动之后。最常见的两种滑囊炎是肩峰下滑囊炎和转子滑囊炎（表 9.2）。

肩峰下滑囊炎是肩部疼痛（特别是在上臂外侧或三角肌疼痛）最常见的原因，在手臂外展时加剧。这是由肩袖肌腱在肩峰和肱骨头之间受压引起的炎症。由于肩袖形成肩峰下滑囊的底部，因此这个位置的滑囊炎通常由肩袖肌腱炎引起。偶尔情况下，肩峰下滑囊炎或肩袖肌腱炎是由肩锁关节的骨刺压迫肩袖肌腱引起的。鉴别诊断包括肩袖撕裂、肱盂关节内病变、二头肌肌腱炎、颈神经根病和胸部的牵涉痛。

转子滑囊炎是臀肌在大转子插入处发生炎症的结果。该病表现为大腿外侧疼痛，当患者躺在患侧时通常更明显。女性似乎更容易发生这种状况，可能是因为女性骨盆相对较宽，臀肌的牵引力增加。其他潜在的风险因素包括体重增加、局部外伤、过度活动（如慢跑）和腿长不等（主要是在腿较长的一侧）。这些因素会增加臀大肌对髂胫束的张力，从而产生滑囊炎症。转子滑囊炎的鉴别诊断包括腰椎神经根病（特别是 L1 和 L2 神经根病）、感觉异常性骨痛（即大腿外侧皮神经在穿过腹股沟韧带时受压）、真正的髋关节疾病和腹腔内病变。其他滑囊炎综合征较少见，在表 9.2 中列出。

化脓性滑囊炎的治疗方案结合多次穿刺抽吸受感染的滑囊和抗生素治疗，初始经验性针对金黄色葡萄球菌，随后根据滑囊液培养结果进行调整。复发性脓毒性滑囊炎可能需要手术切除滑囊。非化脓性滑囊炎的处理应包括休息、局部热敷，除非有消化性溃疡病、肾脏疾病或高龄禁忌，否则应使用非甾体抗炎药（NSAID）。

最有效的方法通常是局部注射皮质类固醇。在注射皮质类固醇之前，应对明显肿胀的浅表滑囊进行穿刺。对于深部滑囊，如肩峰下滑囊或大转子滑囊，穿刺几乎没有或没有液体，可直接注射皮质类固醇而不尝试穿刺。在尝试穿刺或注射髂腰肌滑囊、臀肌滑囊和腓肠肌-半膜肌滑囊（即，贝克囊肿）时要小心，因为这些滑囊靠近重要的神经和血管结构，建议在超声引导下进行穿刺。

TABLE 9.3 Tendinitis Syndromes

Location	Symptom	Finding
Extensor pollicis brevis and abductor pollicis longus (de Quervain tenosynovitis)	Wrist pain	Pain on ulnar deviation of the wrist, with the thumb grasped by the remaining four fingers (i.e., Finkelstein test)
Flexor tendons of fingers	Triggering or locking of fingers in flexion	Tender nodule on flexor tendon on palm over metacarpal joint
Medial epicondyle	Elbow pain	Tenderness of medial epicondyle
Lateral epicondyle	Elbow pain	Tenderness of lateral epicondyle
Bicipital tendon	Shoulder pain	Tenderness along bicipital groove
Patella	Knee pain	Tenderness at insertion of patellar tendon
Achilles	Heel pain	Tender Achilles tendon
Tibialis posterior	Medial ankle pain	Tenderness under medial malleolus with resisted inversion of ankle
Peroneal	Lateral midfoot or ankle pain	Tenderness under lateral malleolus with passive inversion

TABLE 9.4 2011 American College of Rheumatology Fibromyalgia Diagnostic Criteria Modification

Criteria
1. 0 to 19 pain locations on the widespread pain index (WPI)
2. 6 self-reported symptoms, including difficulty sleeping, fatigue, poor cognition, headache, depression and abdominal pain. 0–3 points for fatigue, cognition, and sleep; 1 point for abdominal pain, headache, and depression
3. Symptoms are present for at least 3 months
4. Exclusion of other explanation for the pain
Total score is calculated by adding WPI and self-reported symptom score; 12–13 is generally indicative of fibromyalgia. There has been a 2016 modification to this score to minimize misclassification of regional pain disorders.

Somatic symptoms may include muscle pain or weakness, irritable bowel syndrome, fatigue or tiredness, cognitive or memory problems, headache, numbness or tingling, dizziness, insomnia, depression, nervousness, seizures, abdominal pain or cramps (especially upper abdomen), constipation, diarrhea, nausea, vomiting, fever, dry mouth, itching, chest pain, wheezing, Raynaud's phenomenon, hives or welts, tinnitus, hearing difficulties, heartburn, oral ulcers, loss of or change in taste, dry eyes, blurred vision, shortness of breath, loss of appetite, rash, sun sensitivity, easy bruising, hair loss, frequent or painful urination, and bladder spasms.

Tendinitis

Most tendinitis syndromes are the result of inflammation in the tendon sheath. Overuse with microscopic tearing of the tendon is the most common risk factor for tendinitis. Tendon compression by an osteophyte may occur, such as in the rotator cuff tendon compressed by an osteophyte originating from the acromioclavicular joint.

A common form of tendinitis is lateral epicondylitis, also known as *tennis elbow* (Table 9.3). This is a common overuse syndrome among tennis players, but it can be seen in many other settings requiring repetitive extension of the forearm (e.g., painting overhead). The diagnosis is confirmed by exclusion of elbow joint pathology and the finding of local tenderness at the lateral epicondyle, which is typically exacerbated by forearm extension against resistance. Enthesopathies such as Achilles tendinitis and peroneal and posterior tibial tendinitis may occur in the setting of an underlying seronegative arthropathy such as Reiter disease or psoriatic arthritis. A history and clinical evaluation for these disorders should be pursued for the appropriate patient.

Therapy for tendinitis—NSAIDs, local heat, and corticosteroid injection—is similar to that for bursitis. Rest, physical therapy, occupational therapy, and occasionally ergonomic modification are useful adjuncts. The goal of corticosteroid injection in tendinitis is to infiltrate the tendon sheath rather than the tendon itself because direct injection into a tendon may result in rupture of the tendon. Corticosteroid injection of the Achilles tendon should be avoided because of the propensity of this tendon to rupture. Surgical management of tendinitis is indicated only after failure of conservative treatment. For example, chronic impingement of the supraspinatus tendon that is refractory to conservative treatment may require subacromial decompression.

Fibromyalgia Syndrome

Descriptions of fibromyalgia syndrome exist far back in the medical literature, but it remains a diagnosis of exclusion due to the lack of objective diagnostic or pathologic findings. Fibromyalgia syndrome as defined by the American College of Rheumatology (ACR) 1990 definition for use in clinical trials is a chronic, widespread pain condition with characteristic tender points on physical examination, often associated with a constellation of symptoms such as fatigue, sleep disturbance, headache, irritable bowel syndrome, and mood disorders. In 2010, the ACR developed preliminary diagnostic criteria based only on symptoms because of well-documented issues with the tender point examination (Table 9.4). These criteria do not require a tender point examination, but they provide a scale for measuring the severity of symptoms that are characteristic of fibromyalgia and show good correlation with the 1990 ACR criteria.

The clinical presentation of fibromyalgia syndrome is an insidious onset of chronic, diffuse, poorly localized musculoskeletal pain, typically accompanied by fatigue and sleep disturbance. The physical examination reveals a normal musculoskeletal system, with no deformity or synovitis. However, widespread tenderness occurs, especially at tendon insertion sites, indicating a general reduction in the pain threshold.

Approximately one third of the patients identify antecedent trauma as a precipitant for their symptoms, one third of patients describe a viral prodrome, and one third have no clear precipitant. A variety of less typical presentations has been described, including a predominantly neuropathic presentation with paresthesias (i.e., numbness and tingling) in a nondermatomal distribution, an arthralgic rather than myalgic presentation, and an axial skeletal manifestation resembling degenerative disk disease. Many patients may have undergone invasive diagnostic tests and, in some cases, inappropriate procedures such as carpal tunnel release or cervical or lumbar laminectomies.

Conditions that should be considered in the differential diagnosis of fibromyalgia syndrome include polymyalgia rheumatica (in older patients), hypothyroidism, polymyositis, and early systemic lupus erythematosus or rheumatoid arthritis. However, symptoms are exhibited for many months or years without evidence of other signs or symptoms of an underlying connective tissue disease, making other possible diagnoses unlikely.

表 9.3 　肌腱炎综合征

部位	症状	体征
拇短伸肌腱和拇长外展肌腱（de Quervain 腱鞘炎）	腕痛	拇指被其余四指抓握后手向尺侧偏斜时出现桡骨茎突处疼痛（即 Finkelstein 测试）
手指屈肌腱	手指屈曲时触发或锁住手指	掌骨关节掌侧屈肌腱上有压痛结节
内上髁	肘痛	内上髁压痛
外上髁	肘痛	外上髁压痛
肱二头肌腱	肩痛	沿肱二头肌沟的压痛
髌骨	膝痛	髌腱附着处压痛
跟腱	足跟痛	跟腱压痛
胫后肌	内踝痛	内踝下方压痛，伴踝内翻受阻
腓骨肌	足中外侧或踝痛	外踝下方压痛，伴踝被动内翻

表 9.4 　2011 年美国风湿病学会纤维肌痛诊断标准修订

标准
1. 在广泛性疼痛指数（WPI）上有 0～19 个疼痛部位。
2. 6 种自我报告的症状，包括睡眠困难、疲劳、认知障碍、头痛、抑郁和腹痛。疲劳、认知障碍和睡眠困难每项得 0～3 分；腹痛、头痛和抑郁各得 1 分。
3. 症状至少存在 3 个月。
4. 排除其他疼痛原因。
   总得分通过 WPI 和自我报告的症状得分相加计算；12～13 分通常表示纤维肌痛。2016 年对该评分进行了修订，以减少区域性疼痛性疾病的误诊。

躯体症状可能包括肌肉疼痛或无力、肠易激综合征、疲劳或倦怠、认知或记忆问题、头痛、麻木或刺痛、头晕、失眠、抑郁、紧张、癫痫、腹痛或痉挛（特别是上腹部）、便秘、腹泻、恶心、呕吐、发热、口干、瘙痒、胸痛、喘息、雷诺现象、荨麻疹或风疹、耳鸣、听力困难、胃灼热、口腔溃疡、味觉丧失或改变、眼干、视物模糊、呼吸急促、食欲减退、皮疹、对阳光敏感、容易瘀伤、脱发、尿频或排尿疼痛，以及膀胱痉挛。

肌腱炎

大多数肌腱炎综合征由腱鞘内炎症引起。过度使用导致肌腱微撕裂是肌腱炎最常见的危险因素。肌腱可能因骨刺的压迫而受压，例如肩袖肌腱可能被源于肩锁关节的骨刺压迫。

常见的肌腱炎是外上髁炎，也称网球肘（表 9.3）。这是网球运动员中常见的过度使用综合征，在需要反复伸展前臂的其他运动中也可以发生（如头顶绘画）。其通过排除肘关节病变，并在外侧髁发现局部压痛，且在前臂伸展及发生抗阻运动时疼痛加剧来进行确诊。在潜在的血清阴性关节病如 Reiter 病或银屑病关节炎的情况下，可能发生跟腱炎、腓骨和胫后肌腱炎等附着点疾病。应针对相关患者进行这些疾病的病史和临床评估。

肌腱炎的治疗，如 NSAID、局部热敷和皮质类固醇注射，与治疗滑囊炎相似。休息、物理疗法、职业治疗，以及偶尔的人体工程学改造都是有用的辅助手段。肌腱炎皮质类固醇注射的目标是经腱鞘渗透而非经肌腱本身，因为直接注射到肌腱可能会导致肌腱断裂。应避免对跟腱进行皮质类固醇注射，因为这种肌腱容易断裂。只有在保守治疗失败后才考虑外科治疗。例如，冈上肌腱慢性撞击若对保守治疗无效，可能需要进行肩峰下减压手术。

纤维肌痛综合征

纤维肌痛综合征的描述在医学文献中可以追溯到较早时期，但由于缺乏客观的诊断或病理学发现，它依然被视为一种排除性诊断。根据美国风湿病学会（ACR）1990 年用于临床试验的定义，纤维肌痛综合征是一种慢性、广泛的疼痛，体格检查时有特征性的压痛点，通常与疲劳、睡眠障碍、头痛、肠易激综合征和情绪障碍等一系列症状相关。2010 年，由于对压痛点检查存在的问题，ACR 制定了仅基于症状的初步诊断标准（表 9.4）。这些标准不要求进行压痛点检查，但它们提供了一个衡量纤维肌痛特征性症状严重程度的量表，并与 1990 年 ACR 标准有很好的相关性。

纤维肌痛综合征以慢性、弥漫性、定位不明确的肌肉骨骼疼痛为临床表现，隐匿性发作，通常伴有疲劳和睡眠障碍。体格检查显示肌肉骨骼系统正常，没有畸形或滑膜炎。然而，患者会出现广泛的压痛，特别是在肌腱附着点，表明疼痛阈值普遍降低。

大约 1/3 的患者认为先前的创伤是他们症状的诱因，1/3 的患者表述有病毒感染的前驱症状，还有 1/3 的患者没有明显的诱因。已经报道了本病各种不典型的表现，包括以感觉异常（即麻木和刺痛）为主的神经表现（呈非皮肤节段分布），关节痛而非肌痛的表现，以及类似于退行性椎间盘病的中轴骨骼表现。许多患者可能已经进行了有创性诊断检查，甚至进行了不恰当的操作，如腕管减压术或颈椎或腰椎椎板切除术。

纤维肌痛综合征的鉴别诊断应考虑风湿性多肌痛（老年患者）、甲状腺功能减退、多发性肌炎及早期系统性红斑狼疮或类风湿关节炎。然而，症状出现数月甚至数年后没有其他潜在结缔组织病的迹象或症状，使得其他诊断的可能性不大。

Results of laboratory and radiographic studies are usually normal for patients with fibromyalgia syndrome. Exclusion of other conditions, such as osteoarthritis, rheumatoid arthritis, and systemic lupus erythematosus, by radiography, erythrocyte sedimentation rate, assays for rheumatoid factor or antinuclear antibody, and other tests is no longer considered necessary for the diagnosis of fibromyalgia syndrome. Fibromyalgia should be diagnosed on the basis of positive criteria.

The treatment of fibromyalgia includes reassurance that the condition is not a progressive, crippling, or life-threatening entity. A combination of treatment options, including medication and physical measures, is helpful for most patients. Medications found to be helpful in short-term, double-blind, placebo-controlled trials include amitriptyline and cyclobenzaprine. Low doses of these medications (e.g., 10 to 30 mg of amitriptyline, 10 to 30 mg of cyclobenzaprine) are moderately effective and generally well tolerated. Studies have shown that newer antidepressants of the serotonin-norepinephrine reuptake inhibitor group (e.g., duloxetine, venlafaxine, bupropion) and $\alpha_2\delta$ ligands (e.g., gabapentin, pregabalin) are also effective, particularly in combination with low doses of tricyclic agents. There is currently significant interest among patients regarding the use of cannabinoids for the management of chronic pain but very little data to support their use. However, there is evidence that chronic opioids are not indicated in these patients due to the high risk of dependence, tolerance, and possible worsening of hyperalgesia in these patients.

Patients should be encouraged to take an active role in the management of their condition. If possible, they should begin a progressive, low-level aerobic exercise program to improve muscular fitness and provide a sense of well-being. Cognitive behavioral therapy has been shown to improved function significantly. Adherence, compliance, and access to these modalities are limitations in patients. A combination approach is effective for most patients in alleviating symptoms, although a small minority of patients requires more intensive treatment strategies, such as psychiatric treatment or referral to a pain center.

SUGGESTED READINGS

Goldenberg DL, Burkhardt C, Crofford L: Management of fibromyalgia syndrome, J Am Med Assoc 292:2388–2395, 2004.

Littlejohn GO: Balanced treatments for fibromyalgia, Arthritis Rheum 50:2725–2729, 2004.

纤维肌痛综合征患者的实验室和影像学检查结果通常是正常的。不再认为必须通过放射学检查、红细胞沉降率、类风湿因子或抗核抗体检测以及其他检查来排除其他疾病，如骨关节炎、类风湿关节炎和系统性红斑狼疮。纤维肌痛应该根据其标准来诊断。

纤维肌痛治疗中需要让患者理解该状况不是一个进展性、致残性或危及生命的状况。包括药物治疗和物理措施在内的一系列治疗选择对大多数患者都有帮助。在短期、双盲、安慰剂对照试验中发现有效的药物包括阿米替林和环苯扎林。低剂量应用这些药物（如 10～30 mg 阿米替林，10～30 mg 环苯扎林）具有中等疗效，通常耐受性良好。研究表明，新型抗抑郁药血清素-去甲肾上腺素再摄取抑制剂类药物（如度洛西汀、文拉法辛、安非他酮）和 $\alpha_2\delta$ 配体类药物（如加巴喷丁、普瑞巴林）同样有效，特别是与低剂量的三环类制剂联合使用时。目前，患者乐于接受使用大麻治疗慢性疼痛，但支持应用的数据尚少。然而，有证据表明，由于药物依赖、耐受性以及可能会加剧患者痛觉过敏的高风险，长期应用阿片类药物在这些患者中并不适用。

应鼓励患者积极参与自身疾病管理。推荐这些患者开始循序渐进的低强度有氧运动，以提高肌肉健康并改善自身状态。认知行为疗法已被证明能显著改善功能。患者依从性以及治疗的可及性是主要限制因素。对于大多数患者来说，综合治疗方法在缓解症状方面有效，尽管少部分患者需要强化治疗，如精神科治疗或转诊至疼痛中心。

推荐阅读

Goldenberg DL, Burkhardt C, Crofford L: Management of fibromyalgia syndrome, J Am Med Assoc 292:2388–2395, 2004.

Littlejohn GO: Balanced treatments for fibromyalgia, Arthritis Rheum 50:2725–2729, 2004.

10

Rheumatic Manifestations of Systemic Disorders and Sjögren's Syndrome

Andreea Coca, Ghaith Noaiseh

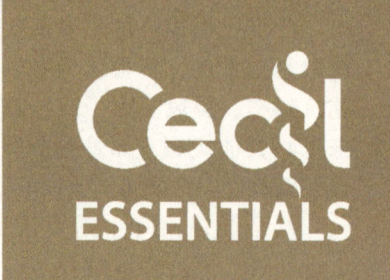

INTRODUCTION

Rheumatologic manifestations may herald a variety of systemic conditions, including malignancy, endocrinopathy, and hematologic disorders (Tables 10.1 and 10.2). Musculoskeletal symptoms can precede or follow the diagnosis of these diseases. Patients may complain of joint or muscle pain, joint swelling, rashes, and many other symptoms.

RHEUMATOLOGIC PARANEOPLASTIC MANIFESTATIONS

Cancer has a myriad of presentations, and paraneoplastic rheumatologic manifestations are not uncommon. They can vary from musculoskeletal conditions to vascular involvement (leukocytoclastic vasculitis), myositis, systemic lupus erythematosus (SLE)–like symptoms, and scleroderma. The pathophysiologic mechanisms of musculoskeletal symptoms in a patient with cancer are often unknown and remain speculative. The association is presumed if there is a close temporal relationship between the diagnosis of a malignancy and the onset of musculoskeletal symptoms or the rheumatic syndrome resolves after successful treatment of the malignancy. In many cases, however, the association may be coincidental.

Cancer may directly invade articular or periarticular structures and mimic rheumatic syndromes, as in chondrosarcoma, giant cell tumor, and osteogenic sarcoma. Musculoskeletal symptoms can occur as paraneoplastic phenomena without direct involvement by the tumor, as in dermatomyositis (DM) in patients with ovarian cancer.

The incidence of malignancy with rheumatic manifestations is unclear, but musculoskeletal symptoms occur more frequently with hematologic malignancies than with solid tumors. No single laboratory test can confirm the diagnosis of a rheumatic illness in a patient with cancer. All patients with rheumatologic syndromes should be evaluated with a thorough history, physical examination, and age-appropriate malignancy screening.

Hypertrophic Osteoarthropathy

Hypertrophic osteoarthropathy (HOA) is characterized by digital clubbing, periostitis of the long bones, and arthritis. Arthritis is most prominent in large joints, and periostitis develops mostly at the distal ends of the femur, tibia, and radius. The primary form of HOA (primary pachydermoperiostosis) is usually a self-limited disease of childhood. The secondary form may be generalized or localized and is mainly associated with lung cancer and suppurative lung disease.

HOA is also associated with cardiovascular disease (e.g., cyanotic congenital heart disease, infective endocarditis), hepatobiliary disorders (e.g., liver cirrhosis, primary biliary cirrhosis), and gastrointestinal disease (e.g., inflammatory bowel disease, celiac disease). Periostitis without digital clubbing can be seen in thyroid acropachy, hypervitaminosis A, fluorosis, venous stasis, hyperphosphatemia, and sarcoidosis. Isolated chronic digital clubbing, which is mainly associated with pleuropulmonary disease, does not seem to cause HOA.

The pathogenesis of HOA remains elusive, although several possible mechanisms have been proposed, including platelet derived growth factor and vascular derived growth factor.

HOA is usually accompanied by bone and joint pain associated with periarticular periostitis. The pain is usually exacerbated by dependency and relieved with limb elevation. Typical signs of periostitis include periosteal new bone along the distal ends of long bones, which can be seen on plain radiographs. When periostitis is not obvious on plain radiography, a bone scan is useful to demonstrate early evidence of disease. Radiologic evaluation of the thorax is important because of the association between HOA and lung neoplasms.

In many cases, symptomatic management with nonsteroidal anti-inflammatory drugs or other analgesics while treating the underlying disorder provides significant relief of symptoms. In refractory cases, bisphosphonates such as pamidronate and zoledronic acid have been reported to be effective.

Rheumatoid Arthritis–like Polyarthritis

Inflammatory rheumatoid arthritis–like syndrome has been associated with solid neoplasms and hematologic malignancies. Clinical characteristics associated with this paraneoplastic syndrome include acute onset, asymmetrical disease frequently involving the lower extremities, synovitis in large joints that spares the wrists and hands without bony erosion, and negative results for rheumatoid factor and cyclic citrullinated peptide antibody. However, these features are not specific and may be confused with elder-onset rheumatoid arthritis, seronegative rheumatoid arthritis, spondyloarthropathy, and remitting seronegative symmetrical synovitis with pitting edema (RS3PE).

Remitting Seronegative Symmetrical Synovitis With Pitting Edema

RS3PE manifests with sudden onset of polyarthritis, pitting edema, and prominent constitutional symptoms. More than one half of the RS3PE cases are associated with malignancy, including hematologic and solid tumors. The evaluation of the patient presenting with RS3PE should prompt an age-appropriate malignancy work-up.

Eosinophilic Fasciitis

Eosinophilic fasciitis can be easily mistaken for scleroderma, presenting with puffy skin, sometimes indurated, progressing towards significant subcutaneous thickening, with characteristic peripheral eosinophilia. It can be seen in the setting of a variety of hematologic malignant disorders.

系统性疾病的风湿性表现和干燥综合征

金月波 译　何菁 李茹 审校　栗占国 通审

引言

风湿性表现可能预示着多种系统性疾病，包括恶性肿瘤、内分泌疾病和血液病（表10.1和10.2）。肌肉骨骼症状的出现可以先于或晚于这些疾病的诊断。患者可能会主诉关节或肌肉疼痛、关节肿胀、皮疹以及很多其他症状。

风湿性副肿瘤表现

癌症有多种表现形式，副肿瘤的风湿性表现并不少见。这些表现从肌肉骨骼疾病到血管受累（如白细胞破碎性血管炎）、肌炎、系统性红斑狼疮（SLE）样症状和硬皮病等不一而足。癌症患者肌肉骨骼症状的病理生理机制通常不明，仍然只能推测。如果恶性肿瘤的诊断与肌肉骨骼症状的出现有密切的时间关系，或者在成功治疗恶性肿瘤后风湿性综合征得到缓解，则推测两者之间有关系。然而，在许多情况下，这种关联可能存在偶然性。

癌症可能直接侵袭关节或关节周围结构，表现出风湿性综合征的症状，如软骨肉瘤、巨细胞瘤和成骨肉瘤。肌肉骨骼症状也可以作为副肿瘤现象出现，而没有肿瘤的直接参与，如卵巢癌患者的皮肌炎（DM）。

具有风湿性表现的恶性肿瘤的发病率尚不清楚，但肌肉骨骼症状在血液恶性肿瘤中比实体瘤中更常见。没有单一的实验室检测能够确认癌症患者的风湿性疾病诊断。所有风湿性综合征患者都应进行全面的病史采集、体格检查和适龄的恶性肿瘤筛查。

肥厚性骨关节病

肥厚性骨关节病（HOA）的特征是杵状指、长骨的骨膜炎和关节炎。关节炎在大关节中最为显著，骨膜炎主要发生在股骨、胫骨和桡骨的远端。原发性HOA（原发性厚皮性骨膜病）通常是儿童自限性疾病。继发性HOA可能是全身性或局灶性的，主要与肺癌和化脓性肺病有关。

HOA还与心血管疾病（如发绀型先天性心脏病、感染性心内膜炎）、肝胆疾病（如肝硬化、原发性胆汁性肝硬化）和胃肠道疾病（如炎症性肠病、乳糜泻）相关。甲状腺肢端病变、维生素A过量、氟中毒、静脉淤滞、高磷血症和结节病中可见到没有杵状指的骨膜炎。孤立的慢性杵状指主要与胸膜肺疾病有关，似乎不会引起HOA。

HOA的发病机制尚不清楚，尽管已经提出了几种可能的机制，包括血小板衍生生长因子和血管衍生生长因子。

HOA通常伴有与关节周围骨膜炎相关的骨和关节疼痛。疼痛通常因肢体活动而加剧，抬高肢体可以缓解。典型的骨膜炎表现包括长骨远端的骨膜新生骨，可于放射线平片中显示。当放射线平片上骨膜炎不明显时，骨扫描有助于提供疾病的早期证据。由于HOA与肺部肿瘤有关，胸部的放射学评估很重要。

在许多情况下，在治疗潜在疾病的同时，通过非甾体抗炎药或其他止痛药对症治疗，可以显著缓解症状。在难治性病例中，双膦酸盐如帕米膦酸盐和唑来膦酸盐被报道有效。

类风湿关节炎样多关节炎

炎性类风湿关节炎样综合征与实体肿瘤和血液恶性肿瘤有关。这种副肿瘤综合征的临床特点包括急性发作和非对称性，常累及下肢的大关节滑膜炎，而不累及腕关节和手关节，且没有骨侵蚀，类风湿因子和抗环瓜氨酸肽抗体阴性。然而，这些特征并不特异，可能与老年发病的类风湿关节炎、血清阴性类风湿关节炎、脊柱关节炎和缓解性血清阴性对称性滑膜炎伴凹陷性水肿（RS3PE）混淆。

缓解性血清阴性对称性滑膜炎伴凹陷性水肿

RS3PE表现为突然发作的多关节炎、凹陷性水肿和显著的全身症状。超过一半的RS3PE病例与恶性肿瘤有关，包括血液恶性肿瘤和实体肿瘤。RS3PE患者应积极排查年龄相关的恶性肿瘤。

嗜酸细胞性筋膜炎

嗜酸细胞性筋膜炎很容易被误诊为硬皮病，表现为皮肤肿胀，有时硬化，进展出明显的皮下增厚，具有特征性的外周血嗜酸性粒细胞增多。它可以在多种血液恶性疾病的背景下出现。

TABLE 10.1 Systemic Conditions Associated With Rheumatic Manifestations

Malignancies
- Myelodysplasia
- Lymphoma
- Leukemia

Paraneoplastic Rheumatologic Disorders
- RS3PE
- Eosinophilic fasciitis
- Hypertrophic osteoarthropathy

Hematologic Disorders
- Hemophilia
- Sickle cell disease
- Thalassemia

Endocrinopathies
- Diabetes
- Hypothyroidism
- Hyperthyroidism
- Hyperparathyroidism
- Acromegaly

Gastrointestinal Disorders
- Whipple disease
- Hemochromatosis
- Primary biliary cirrhosis

Miscellaneous
- Multiple myeloma
- Amyloidosis
- HIV-related rheumatologic disorders
- Sarcoidosis

TABLE 10.2 Musculoskeletal Manifestations of Endocrine Disease

Endocrine Disease	Musculoskeletal Manifestations
Diabetes mellitus	Carpal tunnel syndrome
	Charcot arthropathy
	Adhesive capsulitis
	Cheiroarthropathy
	Diabetic amyotrophy
	Diabetic muscle infarction
Hypothyroidism	Proximal myopathy
	Joint effusions
	Carpal tunnel syndrome
	Chondrocalcinosis
Hyperthyroidism	Myopathy
	Osteoporosis
	Thyroid acropachy
Hyperparathyroidism	Myopathy
	Erosive arthritis
	Chondrocalcinosis
Hypoparathyroidism	Muscle cramps
	Soft tissue calcifications
	Spondyloarthropathy
Acromegaly	Carpal tunnel syndrome
	Myopathy
	Raynaud's phenomenon
	Premature osteoarthritis
Cushing syndrome	Myopathy
	Osteoporosis
	Avascular necrosis

Rheumatologic Complications of Checkpoint Inhibitor Immunotherapy

Immune checkpoint inhibitors (ICIs) are the most commonly used type of cancer immunotherapy. They work by blocking inhibitory molecules on the T cells, resulting in heightened T-cell mediated immune response against malignancy. Unfortunately, they have a variety of side effects, the musculoskeletal ones being among the predominant ones.

Inflammatory arthritis can present in a pattern similar to rheumatoid arthritis or a seronegative spondyloarthropathy. Joint damage can be severe and erosions are common. For the most part, the work-up is normal, although inflammatory markers can be elevated. Mild inflammatory arthritis responds to NSAIDs. In cases of severe arthritis, oral corticosteroids are warranted as well as anti-tumor necrosis factor (TNF) agents.

Sjögren's syndrome (SS)–like presentation manifests primarily with significant ocular and mucosal dryness. Most patients do not exhibit autoantibodies. The distinction from SS is based on minor salivary gland biopsy, which demonstrates a diffuse T cell lymphocytic infiltrate and acinar injury, a pattern distinct from SS.

Polymyalgia rheumatica and giant cell arthritis have been described following treatment with ICIs. PMR symptoms are typical, and temporal artery biopsy pathology is under distinguishable between users or nonusers of ICIs.

DM and polymyositis (PM) have also been described, with proximal muscle weakness, elevated muscle enzymes and pathognomonic abnormalities of the electromyography (EMG) and MRI images. Monotherapy with oral steroids has generally been very effective.

Immune checkpoint inhibitors can also modulate the underlying systemic autoimmune diseases. In patients with rheumatoid arthritis or psoriasis, up to 30% of them can flare during treatment. However, discontinuation of systemic immunosuppression is not recommended, and patients should continue the treatment.

Systemic Autoimmune Diseases and Malignancy
Lupus-like Syndrome

Antinuclear antibodies (ANAs) can be seen in patients with solid neoplasms (e.g., gastric, cervical, and breast carcinomas, testicular seminoma), lymphomas, or myelodysplastic disorders, but the significance of these autoantibodies is poorly understood. It is not clinically indicated to search for an underlying malignancy in a patient with typical SLE. However, lupus-like autoantibodies and unexplained Coombs-positive hemolytic anemia or thrombocytopenia without clinical signs of rheumatic disease warrant further investigation for an occult neoplasm.

Raynaud's Phenomenon and Scleroderma-like Syndrome

The sudden onset of Raynaud's phenomenon and scleroderma-like syndrome can herald an underlying tumor such as hematologic malignancies and carcinomas of the liver, ovary, testis, bladder, breast, or stomach. Scleroderma-like skin changes may also occur in patients with osteosclerotic myeloma with *p*olyneuropathy, *o*rganomegaly, *e*ndocrinopathy, *m*onoclonal gammopathy, and *s*kin abnormalities (i.e., POEMS syndrome) and in those with carcinoid tumors.

Characteristics that suggest secondary Raynaud's phenomenon include age at onset older than 50 years, symptom asymmetry, symptoms that persist year-round, and rapid digital ulceration and necrosis. Secondary Raynaud's is also suggested by scleroderma-like syndromes

表 10.1 与风湿性表现相关的系统性疾病

恶性肿瘤
骨髓增生异常综合征
淋巴瘤
白血病

副肿瘤性风湿病
RS3PE（缓解性血清阴性对称性滑膜炎伴凹陷性水肿）
嗜酸细胞性筋膜炎
肥厚性骨关节病

血液系统疾病
血友病
镰状细胞病
地中海贫血

内分泌疾病
糖尿病
甲状腺功能减退症
甲状腺功能亢进症
甲状旁腺功能亢进症
肢端肥大症

胃肠道疾病
惠普尔病
血色病
原发性胆汁性肝硬化

其他
多发性骨髓瘤
淀粉样变性
HIV相关风湿病性异常
结节病

表 10.2 内分泌疾病的肌肉骨骼表现

内分泌疾病	肌肉骨骼表现
糖尿病	腕管综合征 Charcot 关节病 粘连性关节囊炎 手关节病 糖尿病性肌萎缩 糖尿病性肌肉梗死
甲状腺功能减退症	近端肌病 关节积液 腕管综合征 软骨钙化
甲状腺功能亢进症	肌病 骨质疏松 甲状腺肢端肥大症
甲状旁腺功能亢进症	肌病 侵蚀性关节炎 软骨钙化
甲状旁腺功能减退症	肌肉痉挛 软组织钙化 脊柱关节病
肢端肥大症	腕管综合征 肌病 雷诺现象 早发性骨关节炎
库欣综合征	肌病 骨质疏松 缺血性骨坏死

检查点抑制剂免疫治疗的风湿并发症

免疫检查点抑制剂（ICI）是最常用的癌症免疫疗法。它们通过阻断T细胞上的抑制分子，增强T细胞介导的对恶性肿瘤的免疫应答。但是它们有很多副作用，其中肌肉骨骼副作用突出。

炎性关节炎的表现类似于类风湿关节炎或血清阴性脊柱关节炎。关节损伤可能很严重，常见骨侵蚀。大多数情况下，检查结果正常，尽管炎性标志物可能升高。轻度炎性关节炎对NSAID有反应。在严重关节炎的情况下，需要口服糖皮质激素以及抗肿瘤坏死因子（TNF）药物。

干燥综合征（SS）样表现主要表现为显著的眼部和黏膜干燥。大多数患者没有自身抗体。与SS的区别在于小唾液腺活检，显示弥漫性T淋巴细胞浸润和腺泡损伤，这种模式与SS不同。

已有报道风湿性多肌痛（PMR）和巨细胞动脉炎在接受ICI治疗后出现。PMR症状典型，颞动脉活检病理在使用与未使用ICI的患者之间并无区别。

皮肌炎（DM）和多发性肌炎（PM）也有描述，表现为近端肌肉无力、肌酶升高以及肌电图（EMG）和MRI影像的特征性病理异常。

口服类固醇激素单药治疗通常非常有效。

免疫检查点抑制剂还可以调控潜在的系统性自身免疫性疾病。在类风湿关节炎或银屑病患者中，多达30%的患者在治疗期间可能出现疾病加重。然而，不建议停用系统性免疫抑制治疗，患者应继续接受治疗。

系统性自身免疫性疾病与恶性肿瘤

狼疮样综合征

抗核抗体（ANA）可见于实体肿瘤（如胃癌、宫颈癌和乳腺癌、睾丸精原细胞瘤）、淋巴瘤或骨髓增生异常综合征的患者，但这些自身抗体的意义尚不清楚。在典型SLE患者中没有临床指征去寻找潜在的恶性肿瘤。然而，没有风湿性临床表现但有狼疮样自身抗体和不明原因的Coombs阳性溶血性贫血或血小板减少症的患者需要进一步排查隐匿性肿瘤。

雷诺现象和硬皮病样综合征

雷诺现象和硬皮病样综合征的突然发病可能预示着潜在的肿瘤，如血液恶性肿瘤和肝、卵巢、睾丸、膀胱、乳腺或胃的癌症。患有POEMS综合征（即骨硬化性骨髓瘤伴多发性神经病、器官肿大、内分泌疾病、单克隆免疫球蛋白病和皮肤异常）的患者以及患有类癌肿瘤的患者可能会出现硬皮病样皮肤改变。

提示继发性雷诺现象的特征包括发病年龄大于50岁、症状不对称、症状全年持续以及指端溃疡和坏死的迅速发生。在年龄大于50岁、皮肤硬化快速进展或

in patients older than 50 years, rapid progression of skin sclerosis, or a poor response to therapy. The lack of Raynaud's phenomenon can be another distinguishing characteristic of paraneoplastic scleroderma-like syndrome because Raynaud's phenomenon occurs in approximately 95% of cases of systemic sclerosis.

Vasculitides
Vasculitis is rarely associated with malignancy and is most commonly seen in patients with lymphoproliferative disorders and myelodysplastic syndrome. Cutaneous leukocytoclastic vasculitis is the most common manifestation of paraneoplastic vasculitis. Although clinical presentations of paraneoplastic vasculitides are indistinguishable from those of the idiopathic condition, a chronic, relapsing disease with cytopenias and poor response to conventional treatment suggests a hidden malignancy.

Inflammatory Myopathies
The association between inflammatory myopathies and malignancies has been well established. DM and PM have an increased risk for malignancy, primarily solid tumors. Most malignancies are ovarian, lung, and stomach, primarily seen in the Western population. Differentiating between malignancy or not-malignancy-associated DM or PM can be very challenging, because CPK levels and muscle biopsy findings are similar. Immediately after diagnosis, all patients should undergo age-appropriate malignancy screening. This screening should be repeated every 3 to 5 years, regardless of disease activity. The suspicion for malignancy should be significantly increased in treatment-resistant myositis. The association of anti-P1 55/P1 40 antibodies has been described as highly predictive of cancer-associated DM.

Malignancies Associated With TNF Inhibitors
Adalimumab and etanercept have been on the market since the late 1990s and widely used in a variety of systemic and organ-specific autoimmune diseases. The most common malignancy reported was Hodgkin's and non-Hodgkin's lymphomas. There is an increased risk for nonmelanoma skin cancer but no evidence of other malignancies.

HEMATOLOGIC DISORDERS WITH RHEUMATIC MANIFESTATIONS

Hemophilia
Acute, painful hemophilic arthropathy of the knees, elbows, and ankles is the most common manifestation of hemophilia. Repeated episodes of hemarthrosis result in synovial proliferation and chronic inflammation, causing chronic hemophilic arthropathy. This is characterized by joint deformity, fibrous ankylosis, and osteophyte overgrowth. Radiography typically shows degenerative arthritis. Besides prompt administration of factor concentrate replacement, acute hemarthrosis must be treated conservatively with cold applications and joint immobilization followed by a structured physical therapy program. Aspiration (after factor replacement) is needed only if concomitant septic arthritis is suspected or the joint is very tense.

Sickle Cell Disease
Musculoskeletal complications of sickle cell disease include painful crises, arthropathy, dactylitis, osteonecrosis, and osteomyelitis. Sickle cell crisis is the most common musculoskeletal feature, and it can produce painful arthritis of the large joints and noninflammatory joint effusions adjacent to areas of bony crisis. Osteonecrosis of the femoral head, shoulder, and tibial plateau may result from repeated local bone ischemia or infarct.

Dactylitis manifesting as bilateral, painful, swollen hands or feet (i.e., hand-foot syndrome) may be the first manifestation of the disease in infants and young children. It can be associated with fever and leukocytosis, believed to be secondary to local bone marrow ischemia. Treatment is supportive. Increased risk of septic arthritis and osteomyelitis, most often due to *Salmonella* species, has been associated with hemoglobinopathies.

Endocrine Disorders
Endocrine diseases usually manifest with diffuse, poorly defined musculoskeletal symptoms and joint pain that is more often periarticular. Clinical suspicion of endocrinopathy is by far the most important diagnostic step. Routine clinical laboratory tests such as erythrocyte sedimentation rate (ESR), C-reactive protein (CRP), ANA, rheumatoid factor, and uric acid level are usually not helpful. Radiographs often raise the suspicion of an endocrinopathy and are pathognomonic in advanced disease.

Diabetes
One of the most common musculoskeletal complications of diabetes is diabetic cheiroarthropathy (i.e., diabetic hand syndrome). It is characterized by insidious development of waxy thickening of the skin of the fingers and hands and by flexion contractures of the metacarpophalangeal joints and interphalangeal joints. Patients cannot press the palms together completely without a gap with the wrists fully flexed (i.e., prayer sign). Although this syndrome is associated with long duration of diabetes and poor glycemic control, it may develop before the onset of overt diabetes and mimic sclerodactyly.

Dupuytren contracture and stenosing flexor tenosynovitis (i.e., trigger finger) may be identified. People with diabetes are more prone to develop carpal tunnel syndrome. Diabetic periarthritis of the shoulders (i.e., adhesive capsulitis or frozen shoulder) is more common in patients with diabetes, especially in women with a long history of diabetes. Capsulitis is characterized by staged progression of pain and restriction of shoulder motion.

Patients with long-standing, poorly controlled diabetes may develop a painless, swollen, deformed joint known as a Charcot joint or neuropathic arthropathy. Tarsal, metatarsophalangeal, and tarsometatarsal joints are most commonly involved, and it can be confused with osteomyelitis on radiographs.

Diffuse idiopathic skeletal hyperostosis (DISH) is seen in up to 20% of diabetic patients, who are typically obese and older than 50 years. It is associated with neck and back stiffness rather than pain. Lateral radiographic views of the spine show four or more contiguously fused vertebrae, the result of flowing ossification of the anterior longitudinal ligament without involvement of apophyseal (facet) joints.

Diabetic amyotrophy (i.e., diabetic lumbosacral radiculoplexus neuropathy) is remarkable for acute or subacute onset of severe hip, buttock, or thigh pain followed by progressive weakness of the affected extremity. It occurs typically in older male patients who have relatively well-controlled diabetes.

Diabetic muscle infarction occurs in long-standing insulin-dependent diabetes. It presents with sudden onset of pain and swelling in the calf, mimicking deep venous thrombosis. CK levels might be elevated. A biopsy is often necessary to rule out other possible etiologies.

Thyroid Disease
Hypothyroidism is primarily associated with myxedematous arthropathy, primarily affecting the large joints with swelling and stiffness. Synovial fluid analysis reveals a noninflammatory fluid and radiographs are generally normal. Other common rheumatologic manifestations are carpal tunnel, nonspecific arthralgia, and a myositis-like picture with proximal muscle weakness and elevated CK.

对治疗反应不佳的患者中，硬皮病样综合征也可提示继发性雷诺现象。缺乏雷诺现象是排除副肿瘤性硬皮病样综合征的另一个特征，因为大约 95% 的系统性硬化症病例中都会出现雷诺现象。

血管炎

血管炎与恶性肿瘤的关联很少见，最常见于患有淋巴增殖性疾病和骨髓增生异常综合征的患者中。皮肤白细胞破碎性血管炎是副肿瘤性血管炎的最常见表现。尽管副肿瘤性血管炎的临床表现与特发性病症难以区分，但慢性、复发性疾病伴有血细胞减少且对传统治疗反应差提示背后存在恶性肿瘤。

炎性肌病

炎性肌病与恶性肿瘤之间的关联已得到充分证实。DM 和 PM 的恶性肿瘤风险增加，主要是实体肿瘤。大多数恶性肿瘤是卵巢癌、肺癌和胃癌，主要见于西方人群。区分恶性肿瘤和非恶性肿瘤相关的 DM 或 PM 非常具有挑战性，因为 CPK 水平和肌肉活检结果均相似。确诊后，无论疾病活动度如何，所有患者均应接受与其年龄相应的恶性肿瘤筛查。这种筛查应每 3～5 年重复一次。在疗效不佳的肌炎中，应显著提高对恶性肿瘤的怀疑度。抗 Pl 55/Pl 40 抗体已被发现对癌症相关 DM 具有高度预测价值。

TNF 抑制剂相关恶性肿瘤

自 20 世纪 90 年代末上市以来，阿达木单抗和依那西普广泛用于多种系统性和器官特异性自身免疫性疾病。最常见的恶性肿瘤报告是霍奇金和非霍奇金淋巴瘤。非黑色素瘤皮肤癌的风险增加，但没有证据表明其他恶性肿瘤风险增加。

血液系统疾病的风湿性表现

血友病

膝关节、肘关节和踝关节急性疼痛的血友病性关节病是血友病最常见的表现。反复的关节出血导致滑膜增生和慢性炎症，造成慢性血友病性关节病，其特征是关节畸形、纤维性强直和骨赘增生。X 线通常显示退行性关节炎。除了及时给予凝血因子浓缩物替代治疗外，急性关节出血必须通过冷敷和关节制动进行保守治疗，然后进行有计划的物理疗法。只有在怀疑伴有化脓性关节炎或关节腔张力很大时，才需要关节腔穿刺（在凝血因子替代治疗后）。

镰状细胞病

镰状细胞病的肌肉骨骼并发症包括疼痛危象、关节病、指/趾炎、骨坏死和骨髓炎。镰状细胞危象是最常见的肌肉骨骼表现，可导致大关节的疼痛性关节炎和骨危象区域附近的非炎症性关节积液。反复的局部骨缺血或梗死可能导致股骨头、肩部和胫骨平台的骨坏死。

指/趾炎表现为婴幼儿的手或足对称性的疼痛、肿胀（即手足综合征），可能是疾病的首发症状。它可能伴有发热和白细胞增多，被认为是局部骨髓缺血的继发表现。治疗为支持性的。感染性关节炎和骨髓炎的风险增加与血红蛋白病有关，最常见的病原体是沙门菌属。

内分泌疾病的风湿性表现

内分泌疾病通常表现为弥漫性、难以解释的肌肉骨骼症状和更多发生在关节周围的关节痛。对内分泌疾病的临床疑诊是目前最重要的诊断步骤。常规临床实验室检测如红细胞沉降率（ESR）、C 反应蛋白（CRP）、抗核抗体（ANA）、类风湿因子和尿酸水平通常没有帮助。X 线检查常能发现可疑的内分泌疾病，并在疾病进展期具有病理特征性。

糖尿病

糖尿病最常见的肌肉骨骼并发症之一是糖尿病性手关节病（即糖尿病手综合征）。其特征是隐匿进展的手指和手部皮肤的蜡样增厚，以及掌指关节和指间关节的屈曲挛缩。患者在完全弯曲手腕时，无法完全合拢手掌（即祈祷征）。尽管这种综合征与糖尿病病程长和血糖控制不佳有关，但它可能在明显糖尿病发病前即出现并模拟硬皮病。

糖尿病患者可出现 Dupuytren 挛缩和狭窄性屈肌腱鞘炎（即扳机指）；更容易发生腕管综合征。糖尿病性肩周炎（即粘连性关节囊炎或冻结肩）在糖尿病患者中更为常见，尤其是有长期糖尿病病史的女性。关节囊炎的特点是疼痛和肩关节活动受限的分阶段进展。

病程长、控制不佳的糖尿病患者可能会出现无痛性肿胀、变形的关节，称为 Charcot 关节或神经病性关节病。跗骨、跖趾关节和跗跖关节最常受累，并且在放射影像上可能与骨髓炎混淆。

弥漫性特发性骨肥厚（DISH）见于多达 20% 的糖尿病患者，典型患者肥胖且年龄超过 50 岁。其特点是颈部和背部僵硬，而非疼痛。脊柱的侧面放射影像显示 4 个或更多连续融合的椎骨，这是前纵韧带流动性骨化的结果，而不涉及棘突关节（关节突关节）。

糖尿病性肌萎缩（即糖尿病性腰骶根丛神经病）以急性或亚急性发作的严重髋部、臀区或大腿疼痛为特征，随后出现受累肢体的进行性无力。它通常发生在糖尿病控制相对较好的老年男性患者中。

糖尿病性肌肉梗死发生在长期依赖胰岛素的糖尿病患者中。表现为小腿突然疼痛和肿胀，类似于深静脉血栓形成，CK 水平可能升高，通常需要进行活检以排除其他可能的病因。

甲状腺疾病

甲状腺功能减退主要与黏液水肿性关节病有关，主要影响大关节，表现为肿胀和僵硬。滑液分析提示非炎症性液体，而 X 线通常正常。其他常见的风湿性表现包括腕管综合征、非特异性关节痛，以及近端肌无力和 CK 升高的肌炎样症状。

Hyperthyroidism is associated with pain and proximal muscle weakness in up to 70% of hyperthyroid patients. Osteoporosis is likely the most common musculoskeletal manifestation of thyroid disease.

Thyroid acropachy is a rare manifestation of Graves' disease presenting with swelling of the hands, digital cramping, and periostitis. It is more likely to occur in patients already having other complications of Graves' disease, primarily ophthalmopathy.

Parathyroid Disease

The most common rheumatologic manifestations of primary hyperparathyroidism include pain, proximal muscle weakness, chondrocalcinosis, tendon ruptures, and osteoporosis. Long-standing uncontrolled hyperparathyroidism leads to osteitis fibrosis cystica, primarily seen in end-stage renal disease. Radiographs are characteristic, with subperiosteal resorption and resorption of the tuft of the distal phalanx. Occasionally, erosions can be seen, making it easy to confuse it with rheumatoid arthritis. Secondary hyperparathyroidism is the leading cause of renal osteodystrophy in chronic kidney disease.

Acromegaly

Acromegaly is often associated with joint pain, mostly secondary to degenerative disease affecting the weight-bearing joints, including the spine. Radiographs are characteristic and include periosteal apposition of tubular bones, deformation of the epiphysis, and chondrocalcinosis. In addition, acromegaly can also be associated with carpal tunnel and proximal muscle weakness. Overgrowth of cartilage initially produces joint space widening, but it may eventually lead to severe osteoarthritis with pain, limited range of motion, and deformity.

GASTROINTESTINAL DISEASES WITH RHEUMATIC MANIFESTATIONS

Whipple Disease

Whipple disease is a rare, multisystem disease that most often affects the gastrointestinal tract, caused by an infection with *Tropheryma whippelii*. Musculoskeletal symptoms can precede the diagnosis by years. Intermittent migratory oligoarthritis of large joints is typical, but some patients may have a florid polyarthritis. Synovial fluid is usually inflammatory with predominant mononuclear cells. Radiographs are often normal.

Hemochromatosis

Hemochromatosis is one of the most common genetic diseases among people of northern European ancestry, and it is frequently associated with osteoarthritis-like arthropathy, chondrocalcinosis, and osteoporosis. The second and third metacarpophalangeal joints of both hands are typically involved, and hook-like osteophytes on the radial side of the metacarpal are characteristic in radiographs, the "iron-fist" sign. Chondrocalcinosis of the wrist and knee is very common in patients with hemochromatosis. Acute attacks of pseudogout can be a predominant clinical manifestation. There is no effective treatment, and regular phlebotomies are not effective.

MISCELLANEOUS DISORDERS

Multiple Myeloma

Rheumatologic manifestations of multiple myeloma include bone pain resulting from lytic bone lesions, pathologic fractures, and osteoporosis. Thoracolumbar pain in the setting of hypercalcemia, renal insufficiency, and anemia suggest the possibility of multiple myeloma. Multiple myeloma can manifest atypically and mimic specific autoimmune disorders such as SS and SLE.

Amyloidosis

Amyloidosis is a disorder of protein folding in which insoluble fibrillar proteins are deposited in the extracellular space in one or more organs, disrupting tissue structure and function. The clinical manifestations and prevalence depend on the type of amyloidosis. The amyloid protein can be identified as apple green birefringence on Congo red staining of an abdominal fat pad aspiration or rectal mucosal biopsy specimen.

Systemic light-chain (AL) amyloidosis is one of the most common forms of systemic amyloidosis. Amyloid proteins derived from monoclonal light chains can invade the synovium, producing rheumatoid arthritis–like symptoms. Joint stiffness is more pronounced in amyloid arthropathy, and deposition of amyloid protein at the glenohumeral joint produces enlargement of the anterior shoulder, called the *shoulder pad sign*. Amyloid deposition in the blood vessels can manifest as claudication and symptoms similar to those of temporal arteritis. Deposition in the muscles may also lead to weakness or pain, presenting with a myositis-like picture or muscle pseudohypertrophy.

Systemic AA amyloidosis (formerly known as secondary amyloidosis) can complicate any chronic inflammatory disorder. The most common rheumatologic diseases complicated by a systemic AA amyloidosis are rheumatoid arthritis, juvenile idiopathic arthritis and ankylosing spondylitis.

Human Immunodeficiency Virus Infection

There are a plethora of muscular skeletal manifestations associated with human immunodeficiency (HIV), either disease specific or secondary to highly active antiretroviral therapy (ART). They range from arthralgias and arthritis to inflammatory myositis, sarcoidosis, rheumatoid arthritis, SLE, SS, zidovudine-associated myopathy, osteopenia, osteomalacia, and osteomyelitis.

HIV-associated arthritis is seronegative polyarticular noninflammatory arthritis, primarily affecting the weight-bearing joints. It is a self-limiting condition, responding to conservative management. Rarely, it requires NSAIDs or low-dose corticosteroids for symptoms relief.

The incidence of reactive arthritis has been drastically reduced since introduction of ART. The presentation is classical, with enthesopathy, plantar fasciitis, dactylitis, and inflammatory synovial fluid. However, it can be associated with severe erosive arthritis, which is generally not seen in non-HIV-related reactive arthritis.

Muscle involvement in HIV is common. It can present with inflammatory or noninflammatory myopathy. Prior to ART, the patient was more likely to develop PM, nemaline rod (rod like structures in muscle cells) myopathy and HIV wasting syndrome. Posttreatment, mitochondrial myopathy and rhabdomyolysis are more commonly seen. The most common bone diseases seen in HIV patients are osteoporosis and avascular necrosis, especially in patients that have a very low CD4 count.

Sarcoidosis

Clinical features of sarcoidosis can mimic those of many acute and chronic rheumatic diseases. Acute sarcoidosis (also called Löfgren syndrome) manifests with fever, erythema nodosum, hilar lymphadenopathy, and acute polyarthritis, almost invariably involving the ankles and knees. The arthritis is usually self-limited and tends to be nondeforming and nonerosive.

Chronic sarcoid arthropathy is less common and usually associated with active multisystemic disease. Osseous involvement can be focal or

在多达 70% 的甲状腺功能亢进症（甲亢）患者中，甲状腺功能亢进症与疼痛和近端肌无力有关。骨质疏松症可能是甲状腺疾病最常见的肌肉骨骼表现。

甲状腺肢端肥大症是 Graves 病的罕见表现，表现为手部肿胀、手指痉挛和骨膜炎。它更有可能发生在已经有 Graves 病其他并发症（主要是眼病）的患者中。

甲状旁腺疾病

原发性甲状旁腺功能亢进症最常见的风湿性表现包括疼痛、近端肌肉无力、软骨钙质沉着、肌腱断裂和骨质疏松。长期控制不佳的甲状旁腺功能亢进症会导致纤维囊性骨炎，主要见于终末期肾病患者。放射影像具有特征性，表现为骨膜下吸收和远端指骨吸收。偶尔可以看到侵蚀性病变，容易与类风湿关节炎混淆。继发性甲状旁腺功能亢进症是慢性肾病中肾性骨营养不良的主要原因。

肢端肥大症

肢端肥大症常与关节疼痛相关，主要继发于影响负重关节（包括脊柱）的退行性疾病。放射影像具有特征性，包括管状骨的骨膜增生、骨骺变形和软骨钙质沉着。此外，肢端肥大症还可能与腕管综合征和近端肌肉无力相关。软骨的过度生长最初导致关节间隙增宽，但最终可能导致严重的骨关节炎，伴有疼痛、活动受限和畸形。

胃肠道疾病的风湿性表现

惠普尔病

惠普尔病是一种罕见的多系统疾病，最常影响胃肠道，由惠普尔养障体感染引起。肌肉骨骼症状可能在确诊前数年出现。典型表现为大关节的间歇性游走性寡关节炎，但一些患者可能有急性多关节炎。滑液通常为炎性，主要为单个核细胞。X 线通常正常。

血色病

血色病是北欧祖先人群中最常见的遗传病之一，通常与类似骨关节炎的关节病、软骨钙化和骨质疏松有关。典型表现为双手第二和第三掌指关节受累，X 线特征为掌骨桡侧钩样骨赘，称为"铁拳"征。腕和膝的软骨钙质沉着在血色病患者中非常常见。假性痛风的急性发作可能是主要的临床表现。没有有效的治疗方法，定期放血无效。

其他疾病

多发性骨髓瘤

多发性骨髓瘤的风湿性表现包括溶骨性疼痛、病理性骨折和骨质疏松。伴有高钙血症、肾功能不全和贫血的胸腰椎痛提示可能存在多发性骨髓瘤。多发性骨髓瘤可表现为非典型形式，并模拟特定的自身免疫性疾病，如干燥综合征和系统性红斑狼疮。

淀粉样变性

淀粉样变性是一种蛋白质折叠障碍，表现为不可溶性纤维状蛋白沉积在一个或多个器官的细胞外间隙中，破坏组织结构和功能。临床表现和患病率取决于淀粉样蛋白的类型。淀粉样蛋白在腹部脂肪垫抽吸或直肠黏膜活检标本的刚果红染色中显示为苹果绿双折射。

系统性轻链（AL）型淀粉样变性是最常见的系统性淀粉样变性形式之一。由单克隆轻链衍生的淀粉样蛋白可侵入滑膜，产生类似类风湿关节炎的症状。淀粉样变性关节病中关节僵硬更为明显，淀粉样蛋白在肩关节的沉积可导致前肩肿大，称为肩垫征。淀粉样蛋白在血管中的沉积可表现为跛行和类似颞动脉炎的症状。淀粉样蛋白在肌肉中的沉积也可能导致无力或疼痛，表现为类似肌炎的症状或肌肉假性肥大。

系统性 AA 型淀粉样变性（以前称为继发性淀粉样变性）可以并发任何慢性炎症性疾病。最常见的与系统性 AA 型淀粉样变性并发的风湿病包括类风湿关节炎、幼年特发性关节炎和强直性脊柱炎。

人类免疫缺陷病毒感染

与人类免疫缺陷病毒（HIV）感染（艾滋病）相关的肌肉骨骼表现种类繁多，既有疾病特异性的，也有继发于高度活跃的抗逆转录病毒治疗（ART）的。表现从关节痛和关节炎到肌炎、结节病、类风湿关节炎、系统性红斑狼疮、干燥综合征、齐多夫定相关的肌病、骨量减少、骨软化和骨髓炎等。

HIV 感染相关关节炎是一种血清阴性的非炎症性多关节炎，主要影响负重关节。它是一种自限性疾病，通过保守治疗可缓解，很少需要使用 NSAID 或低剂量皮质类固醇来缓解症状。

反应性关节炎的发生率自 ART 问世以来显著降低。其典型临床表现包括附着点病、跖筋膜炎、指炎和炎性滑液。然而，它可能与严重的侵蚀性关节炎有关，这在非 HIV 相关的反应性关节炎中通常见不到。

HIV 感染患者肌肉受累常见，表现为炎性或非炎性肌病。在 ART 之前，患者更可能发展为多发性肌炎（PM）、杆状体（肌肉细胞中的杆状结构）肌病和 HIV 消耗综合征。治疗后，更常见的是线粒体肌病和横纹肌溶解症。HIV 感染患者中最常见的骨病是骨质疏松和缺血性骨坏死，尤其是在 CD4 计数非常低的患者中。

结节病

结节病的临床表现可以模拟许多急性和慢性风湿病。急性结节病（也称为 Löfgren 综合征）表现为发热、结节性红斑、肺门淋巴结病和急性多关节炎，几乎总是累及踝关节和膝关节。关节炎通常是自限性的，倾向于非畸形和非侵蚀性。

慢性结节病性关节病较少见，其通常与活动性的多系统疾病相关。骨骼受累可以是局灶性或弥漫性的，约

generalized and occurs in about 5% of patients with sarcoidosis. Bone cysts are usually asymptomatic, but they can manifest in the phalanges with sausage-like fingers or pseudoclubbing. Focal osteolytic changes can lead to pathologic fractures. Sarcoid muscle involvement is often asymptomatic, but it may manifest with proximal pain, progressive weakness, or atrophy

SJÖGREN'S SYNDROME

Definition and Epidemiology

SS is a chronic systemic autoimmune disease characterized by lymphocytic infiltration of salivary and lacrimal glands that leads to mucosal dryness and salivary gland enlargement, and by autoantibody production. Extra-glandular manifestations occur in 25% to 30% of patients and may occur as the presenting feature or during the evolution of the disease.

Prevalence is approximately 0.1% to 0.6% of the general population. SS is mostly a disease of middle-aged women, but it can affect people of all ages. The female-to-male ratio is at least 9:1. SS can occur as a primary disorder or can be associated with other autoimmune diseases such as rheumatoid arthritis and SLE.

Pathogenesis

The pathogenesis of SS is not fully understood. Autoimmune epithelitis is the most widely accepted model of autoimmunity in SS, in which the glandular epithelial cells (EC) act as a main orchestrator of the inflammatory response and not just an innocent bystander that is damaged by surrounding inflammation. In a genetically predisposed subject (e.g., HLA-DR3-DQ1-positive), outside triggers, such as sialotropic viruses or hormonal factors, activate EC, which then act as nonprofessional antigen presenting cells by expressing MHC I and II molecules and toll-like receptors, secreting cytokines and chemokines necessary to attract other inflammatory cells and activating both innate and adaptive immunity. Altogether, these steps promote a vicious cycle perpetuating immune system activation. Activated macrophages and dendritic cells produce type I interferon, leading to local tissue damage. Inflammatory milieu attracts and activates T and B lymphocytes to form lymphocytic foci. In fact, the presence of lymphocytic infiltration around the epithelial structures of salivary glands and other affected tissues is the histopathologic hallmark of SS.

Additionally, EC are among inflammatory cells that produce B-cell activating factor (BAFF or BLyS), a pivotal molecule that promotes B-cell maturation, proliferation, and survival. B-cell hyperactivity in SS is a key feature of the disease highlighted by presence of specific autoantibodies such as anti-Ro/SSA and anti-La/SSB antibodies, nonspecific hypergammaglobulinemia, presence of monoclonal gammopathy, and development of non-Hodgkin's lymphoma. Moreover, antibody production is essential for the formation of immune complexes (IC), which can lead to complement activation and tissue damage, or vasculitis, when deposited in the capillaries of certain organs such as the skin, kidneys, and peripheral nerves.

To summarize, immunopathogenesis of SS is thought to result from either lymphocytic infiltration of target tissue epithelia leading to progressive functional impairment or IC-mediated complement activation and tissue damage.

Clinical Presentation

Patients typically present with insidious onset of sicca syndrome (persistent dry eyes and dry mouth). Decreased tear flow leads to epithelial damage of cornea and conjunctiva, a condition known as keratoconjunctivitis sicca. Grittiness, foreign body sensation, photophobia, and formation of thick secretions in the inner canthus can occur. Untreated cases can lead to corneal ulcerations, scarring, bacterial infections, and visual impairment.

Occasionally, patients may deny dry mouth but report difficulty swallowing dry food. Exam may reveal absence of a normal salivary pool under the tongue, dry and sticky mucosa, gingival recession, and dental caries. Atrophic oral candidiasis is a less recognized complication and usually presents with burning mouth syndrome and atrophied papillae on the tongue surface with or without angular cheilitis in the absence of classic whitish exudate. Upper respiratory tract involvement may lead to nasal dryness, recurrent nonallergic rhinitis and sinusitis, and dry cough. Vaginal dryness associated with dyspareunia and dry skin may also occur. Salivary gland enlargement is seen in about 30% to 40% of patients, classically presenting as painless unilateral or bilateral parotid gland enlargement, which spontaneously resolves 2 to 3 weeks later. Other common presentations include arthralgia, myalgia, fatigue, and malaise.

SS can overlap with several nonrheumatic autoimmune diseases, such as Hashimoto thyroiditis and celiac disease. In addition to SS-specific symptoms, patients may have a plethora of extraglandular manifestations, summarized in Table 10.3.

Placental transmission of maternal anti-SSA/Ro and anti-SSB/La may lead to neonatal disease. Female patients with SS or SLE planning a family who have anti-Ro/La antibodies should be counselled about this risk to the neonate, which occurs in approximately 2% to 5% of cases.

Sjögren's Syndrome and Non-Hodgkin Lymphomas

Compared to the general population, SS patients have a 15- to 20-fold increased risk of developing lymphomas, usually mucosa-associated lymphoid tissue (MALT) B-cell lymphoma. Interestingly, lymphoma typically develops in organs where the disease is active, such as salivary glands. Persistent unilateral parotid gland enlargement in SS is alarming and requires additional work-up. Other risk factors associated with lymphoma development include palpable purpura, splenomegaly, lymphadenopathy, positive rheumatoid factor, positive serum cryoglobulins, C4 hypocomplementemia, lymphopenia, and monoclonal gammopathy. Patients who exhibit one or several risk factors need to be closely monitored.

Laboratory Findings

Antinuclear antibodies and rheumatoid factor are seen in up to 80% and 50% of cases, respectively. When present, patients may be erroneously diagnosed with SLE or RA. Anti-SSA/Ro, and anti-SSB/La antibodies are present in 60% to 80% and 30% to 40% of SS patients, respectively. Hypergammaglobulinemia, anemia of chronic disease, and elevated ESR (related to hypergammaglobulinemia) are commonly encountered. CRP is usually normal. Lymphopenia, neutropenia, and thrombocytopenia may also occur. Serum cryoglobulins and monoclonal gammopathy are present in 10% and 15%, respectively. Complement levels C3 and C4 may be decreased as markers of disease activity but low C4 may occasionally be congenital.

Diagnosis

In the clinically appropriate context, such as presence of sicca symptoms or an extraglandular manifestation, the diagnosis is made based on objective demonstration of glandular dysfunction *and* presence of autoimmunity as assessed by elevated serum anti SSA/Ro or a positive minor salivary gland biopsy. Importantly, absence of sicca symptoms does *not* rule out SS.

Various tests are used to assess for glandular dysfunction. To confirm keratoconjunctivitis sicca, the Schirmer test measures tear flow over a 5-minute period using standardized paper strips; 5 mm or less

在5%的结节病患者中出现。骨囊肿通常无症状，但可以在指骨上表现为香肠样手指或假性杵状指。局灶性溶骨性改变可导致病理性骨折。结节病肌肉受累通常是无症状的，但可能表现为近端疼痛、进行性无力或萎缩。

干燥综合征

定义和流行病学

干燥综合征（SS）是一种慢性系统性自身免疫性疾病，特征是唾液腺和泪腺的淋巴细胞浸润，导致黏膜干燥和唾液腺肿大，以及自身抗体的产生。大约25%～30%的患者会出现腺外表现，这些表现可以作为疾病的首发症状或在疾病进展过程中出现。

SS在普通人群中的患病率约为0.1%～0.6%。该病主要影响中年女性，但可发生在任何年龄段。女性与男性的比例至少为9：1。SS可以作为一种原发性疾病，也可以并发于其他自身免疫性疾病（如类风湿关节炎和系统性红斑狼疮）。

发病机制

SS的发病机制尚不完全清楚。自身免疫性上皮炎是SS最广为接受的自身免疫模型，其中腺上皮细胞（EC）并非周围炎症的无辜受害者，而是炎症反应的主导者。在遗传易感个体（如HLA-DR3-DQ1阳性）中，外界触发因素（如唾液腺病毒或性激素因素）激活EC，这些EC作为非专职性抗原提呈细胞，通过表达MHC Ⅰ和Ⅱ分子以及Toll样受体，分泌吸引其他炎症细胞并激活先天和适应性免疫所需的细胞因子和趋化因子。这些步骤共同促进了免疫系统持续激活的恶性循环。激活的巨噬细胞和树突状细胞产生Ⅰ型干扰素，导致局部组织损伤。炎症环境吸引并激活T和B淋巴细胞，形成淋巴细胞浸润灶。实际上，唾液腺和其他受累组织的上皮结构周围的淋巴细胞浸润是SS的组织病理学特征。

此外，EC也是一种炎症细胞，能够产生B细胞激活因子（BAFF或BLyS），这是一种促进B细胞成熟、增殖和存活的关键分子。B细胞过度活化是SS的关键特征，尤其表现为特异性自身抗体（如抗SSA/Ro和抗SSB/La抗体）的存在、非特异性高丙种球蛋白血症、单克隆丙种球蛋白病的出现，以及非霍奇金淋巴瘤的发生。此外，抗体产生对于免疫复合物（IC）的形成至关重要，当IC在特定器官（如皮肤、肾脏和周围神经）的毛细血管中沉积时，会导致补体激活和组织损伤或血管炎。

总之，SS的免疫发病机制被认为是由淋巴细胞对靶组织上皮的浸润导致的进行性功能损害或IC介导的补体激活和组织损伤所致。

临床表现

患者通常表现为隐匿起病的干燥综合征（持续的眼干和口干）。泪液分泌减少导致角膜和结膜上皮损伤，称为角结膜干燥症。患者可能会出现眼部磨砂感、异物感、畏光、内眦分泌物增多等症状。如不及时治疗，可能导致角膜溃疡、瘢痕、细菌感染和视力受损。

有时，患者可能否认口干，但主诉吞咽干燥食物困难。检查可能发现舌下正常唾液池消失、口腔黏膜干燥和发黏、牙龈萎缩和龋齿。萎缩性口腔念珠菌病是一个很少被发现的并发症，通常表现为口腔烧灼感和舌面乳头萎缩，伴或不伴口角炎，没有经典的白色渗出物。上呼吸道受累可能导致鼻腔干燥、反复非过敏性鼻炎和鼻窦炎以及干咳。还可能出现与性交痛相关的阴道干燥和皮肤干燥。约30%～40%的患者出现唾液腺肿大，典型表现为无痛性单侧或双侧腮腺肿大，通常在2～3周后自行消退。其他常见表现包括关节痛、肌痛、疲劳和不适感。

SS可与几种非风湿性自身免疫性疾病重叠，如桥本甲状腺炎和乳糜泻。除了SS特异性症状外，患者还可能有多种腺外表现，见表10.3。

母体抗SSA/Ro和抗SSB/La抗体的胎盘传递可能导致新生儿疾病。有生育计划的女性SS或SLE患者如果有抗Ro/La抗体，应进行新生儿风险咨询，这种风险约为2%～5%。

干燥综合征与非霍奇金淋巴瘤

与一般人群相比，SS患者发生淋巴瘤的风险增加了15～20倍，通常是黏膜相关淋巴组织（MALT）B细胞淋巴瘤。有趣的是，淋巴瘤通常在疾病活跃的器官中发生，如唾液腺。需要警惕SS患者的持续性单侧腮腺肿大，有必要进一步检查。与淋巴瘤发生相关的其他危险因素包括可触及的紫癜、脾大、淋巴结病、类风湿因子阳性、血清冷球蛋白阳性、C4补体降低、淋巴细胞减少和单克隆丙种球蛋白病。出现一个或多个危险因素的患者需要密切监测。

实验室检查

抗核抗体和类风湿因子分别在多达80%和50%的病例中出现。如果存在，患者可能被误诊为SLE或RA。抗SSA/Ro和抗SSB/La抗体分别在60%～80%和30%～40%的SS患者中出现。高丙种球蛋白血症、慢性病贫血和由于高丙种球蛋白血症引起的ESR升高很常见。CRP通常正常。还可能出现淋巴细胞减少、中性粒细胞减少和血小板减少。血清冷球蛋白和单克隆丙种球蛋白分别存在于10%和15%的病例中。补体C3和C4水平可能降低，作为疾病活动的标志，但低C4有时可能是先天性的。

诊断

在干燥症状或腺外表现的临床前提下，存在腺体功能障碍的客观证据和自身免疫（通过血清抗SSA/Ro抗体升高或小唾液腺活检阳性）可诊断SS。重要的是，干燥症状的缺失并不能排除SS。

有多种检测用于评估腺体功能障碍。为了确认角结膜干燥症，Schirmer试验使用标准化的纸条测量5 min内的泪液流量；润湿5 mm或更少代表客观干燥。这是

TABLE 10.3 Systemic Manifestations of Sjögren's Syndrome

System	Clinical Manifestations
Constitutional	Fever
	Fatigue
Cutaneous	Purpura: hypergammaglobulinemic or cryoglobulinemia-associated leukocytoclastic vasculitis
	Annular erythema (photosensitive, indistinguishable from subacute cutaneous lupus erythematosus)
	Urticaria
	Xeroderma
Musculoskeletal	Arthralgia and myalgia
	Nonerosive arthritis (mimicking rheumatoid arthritis)
	Inflammatory myopathy
Pulmonary	Obstructive pattern on pulmonary function testing
	Interstitial lung disease (nonspecific, usual and lymphocytic interstitial pneumonia)
	Cryptogenic organizing pneumonia
	Bronchiectasis
Renal	Interstitial nephritis
	Renal tubular acidosis (typically type I, less commonly type II)
	Cryoglobulin-mediated membranoproliferative glomerulonephritis
Central nervous system	Multiple sclerosis-like syndrome
	Transverse myelitis
	Cognitive dysfunction
Peripheral nervous system	Axonal sensory polyneuropathy
	Sensorimotor polyneuropathy
	Small fiber neuropathy
	Autonomic neuropathy
	Ganglionopathy
	Chronic inflammatory demyelinating polyneuropathy
	Cranial neuropathies (usually trigeminal neuralgia)
	Mononeuritis multiplex (vasculitis-associated)
Hepatobiliary	Autoimmune cholangitis
Vascular	Raynaud's phenomenon (without digital tip ulcerations)
	Vasculitis (affecting small vessels, usually in skin, kidney, and nerves)
Reticuloendothelial	Lymphadenopathy
	Splenomegaly
Lymphoproliferative	Non-Hodgkin's lymphoma, usually marginal-zone histologic type, particularly mucosa-associated lymphoid tissue (MALT)-related lymphoma

focal lymphocytic sialadenitis, which is foci of 50 or more lymphocytes clustered around normal appearing salivary tissue (periepithelial infiltrates) (Fig. 10.1).

Classification Criteria

2016 ACR/EULAR classification criteria are listed in Table 10.4. Although designed for research purposes and not considered diagnostic criteria, they can be helpful as a diagnostic framework in patients suspected to have SS. These classification criteria are applicable to any patient with at least one item of the following:

1. A symptom of ocular or oral dryness (persistent dry eyes >3 months, recurrent sensation of sand or gravel in the eyes, using tear substitutes >3 times daily, persistent dry mouth >3 months, or need to drink liquids to aid in swallowing dry food)
2. Suspicion of SS based on presence of a suggestive body organ involvement or abnormal laboratory testing as listed in the ESSDAI (European League Against Rheumatism SS Disease Activity Index) tool. Examples include prominent parotid swelling, recent diagnosis of axonal sensory polyneuropathy, significant neutropenia, hypergammaglobulinemia, and hypocomplementemia.

Objective dryness testing should be performed after holding anticholinergic medications for adequate period of time.

Exclusion criteria include history of head and neck radiation therapy, polymerase chain reaction (PCR)–confirmed active hepatitis C infection, AIDS, sarcoidosis, amyloidosis, graft-versus-host disease, and IgG4-related disease.

Differential Diagnosis

The differential diagnosis of SS includes etiologies that can cause sicca symptoms and or lacrimal/salivary gland enlargement. Numerous medications with anticholinergic properties, including over-the-counter products, may lead to dry eyes and mouth. Anxiety, depression or aging may also lead to sicca symptoms. Diffuse infiltrative lymphadenopathy syndrome associated with HIV and infiltrative diseases such as sarcoidosis can cause dry mouth and parotid swelling. IgG4-related disease is associated with sicca complaints and persistent lacrimal and salivary gland swelling. Sialadenosis (or sialosis) is a persistent, usually painless, bilateral swelling of parotid glands, associated with alcoholism, obesity, diabetes mellitus, chronic liver disease, and eating disorders. Histologic findings include fatty infiltrates and minimal inflammatory cells. Fibromyalgia syndrome may lead to sicca symptoms, along with fatigue and musculoskeletal pain.

Management

The goal of therapy in SS is to prevent complications and alleviate symptoms. Topical and systemic pharmacologic therapies can improve sicca symptoms, but therapeutic agents able to induce remission or alter the course of the disease are not yet available. Immunosuppressive medications are usually used in patients with severe systemic involvement. Treatment of sicca syndrome is summarized in Table 10.5.

Oral disease-modifying antirheumatic drugs (such as azathioprine and methotrexate) do not appear to be effective, although hydroxychloroquine is frequently used to treat arthralgia, rashes, and fatigue. Cyclophosphamide may be used with severe body organ involvement such as vasculitic neuropathies or glomerulonephritis. Currently, use of biologic therapies in SS is experimental; however, rituximab has been used in severe thrombocytopenia, interstitial lung disease, vasculitic neuropathies, and non-Hodgkin's lymphoma.

of wetting confirms objective dryness. It is a simple test that can be performed routinely in the clinic. A normal Schirmer test does not rule out dry eyes. Slit-lamp examination of the ocular surface, using vital dye drops such as Lissamine green and fluorescein, assesses severity of ocular damage by staining devitalized spots. Unstimulated salivary flow can be measured by asking the patient to spit into a container for 5 to 15 minutes; a saliva flow rate of 0.1 mL/min or less confirms objective dryness. Diagnostic labial salivary gland biopsy is usually performed by harvesting four to six minor glands from the inner mucosa of the lower lip. The classical histological feature is

表 10.3	干燥综合征的系统表现
系统	临床表现
全身性	发热 疲劳
皮肤	紫癜：高丙种球蛋白血症或冷球蛋白血症相关性白细胞破碎性血管炎 环形红斑（光敏性，无法与亚急性皮肤型红斑狼疮区分） 荨麻疹 干皮症
肌肉骨骼	关节痛和肌痛 非侵蚀性关节炎（模拟类风湿关节炎） 炎性肌病
肺部	肺功能检查显示阻塞性通气障碍 间质性肺病（非特异性、普通型和淋巴细胞性间质性肺炎） 隐源性机化性肺炎 支气管扩张症
肾脏	间质性肾炎 肾小管酸中毒（典型为 I 型，较少见 II 型） 冷球蛋白介导的膜增殖性肾小球肾炎
中枢神经系统	多发性硬化样综合征 横贯性脊髓炎 认知功能障碍
周围神经系统	轴索性感觉性多发性神经病 感觉运动性多发性神经病 小纤维神经病 自主神经病 神经节病 慢性炎症性脱髓鞘性多发性神经病 脑神经病（通常为三叉神经痛） 多发性单神经炎（血管炎相关）
肝胆	自身免疫性胆管炎
血管	雷诺现象（无指尖溃疡） 血管炎（通常影响皮肤、肾脏和神经的小血管）
网状内皮系统	淋巴结病 脾大
淋巴增殖性	非霍奇金淋巴瘤，通常为边缘区组织学类型，特别是与黏膜相关淋巴组织（MALT）相关的淋巴瘤

一个简单的测试，可以在门诊常规进行。Schirmer 试验正常并不能排除干眼症。可用裂隙灯检查眼表，采用丽丝胺绿和荧光素染料来染色无活性斑点，以评估眼损伤的严重程度。非刺激性唾液流量可以通过让患者将唾液吐到一个容器中 5～15 min 来测量；唾液流率 ≤ 0.1 ml/min 代表客观干燥。诊断性唇腺活检通常通过从下唇内黏膜采集 4～6 个小腺体来进行。经典的组织学特征是灶性淋巴细胞性腮腺炎，即有 ≥ 50 个淋巴细胞聚集在外观正常的唾液组织周围形成淋巴细胞灶（上皮周围浸润）（图 10.1）。

分类标准

2016 年 ACR/EULAR 分类标准如表 10.4 所示。虽然是为研究目的而设计，并非诊断标准，但它们可以作为诊断 SS 的框架。这些分类标准适用于具有以下至少一项的患者：

1. 眼部或口腔干燥症状（持续眼干 > 3 个月，眼中反复砂砾感，每天使用人工泪液 > 3 次，持续口干 > 3 个月，或需要饮用液体来帮助吞咽干燥食物）。

2. 基于 ESSDAI（European League Against Rheumatism SS Disease Activity Index）工具中列出的器官受累或实验室检查异常而疑诊 SS，包括明显的腮腺肿大、近期诊断的轴索感觉性多神经病、中性粒细胞显著减少、高丙种球蛋白血症和低补体血症。

客观的干燥检查应在停止使用抗胆碱能药物足够长时间后进行。

排除标准包括头颈部放射性治疗史、PCR 确认的活动性丙型肝炎感染、艾滋病、结节病、淀粉样变性、移植物抗宿主病和 IgG4 相关疾病。

鉴别诊断

SS 的鉴别诊断包括可能导致干燥症状和（或）泪腺/唾液腺肿大的病因。许多具有抗胆碱能特性的药物，包括非处方药，可能导致眼干和口干。焦虑、抑郁或年老也可能导致干燥症状。与 HIV 相关的弥漫性浸润性淋巴结病综合征和结节病等浸润性疾病可能导致口干和腮腺肿大。IgG4 相关疾病与干燥主诉和持续的泪腺和唾液腺肿大有关。唾液腺病（或唾液腺炎）是一种持续的、通常无痛性的双侧腮腺肿大，常与酒精中毒、肥胖、糖尿病、慢性肝病和饮食失调有关。组织学检查显示脂肪浸润和极少的炎症细胞。纤维肌痛综合征可能导致干燥症状，伴有疲劳和肌肉骨骼疼痛。

治疗

SS 的治疗目标是预防并发症和缓解症状。局部和全身药物治疗可以改善干燥症状，但尚无能够诱导缓解或改变疾病进程的治疗药物。免疫抑制药物通常用于有严重系统受累的患者。干燥综合征的治疗总结见表 10.5。

口服改善病情的抗风湿药（如硫唑嘌呤和甲氨蝶呤）似乎无效，尽管羟氯喹常用于治疗关节痛、皮疹和疲劳。对于严重的器官受累如血管炎性神经病或肾小球肾炎，可以使用环磷酰胺。目前，SS 中生物制剂的使用是试验性的；然而，利妥昔单抗已用于治疗严重的血小板减少、间质性肺病、血管炎性神经病和非霍奇金淋巴瘤。

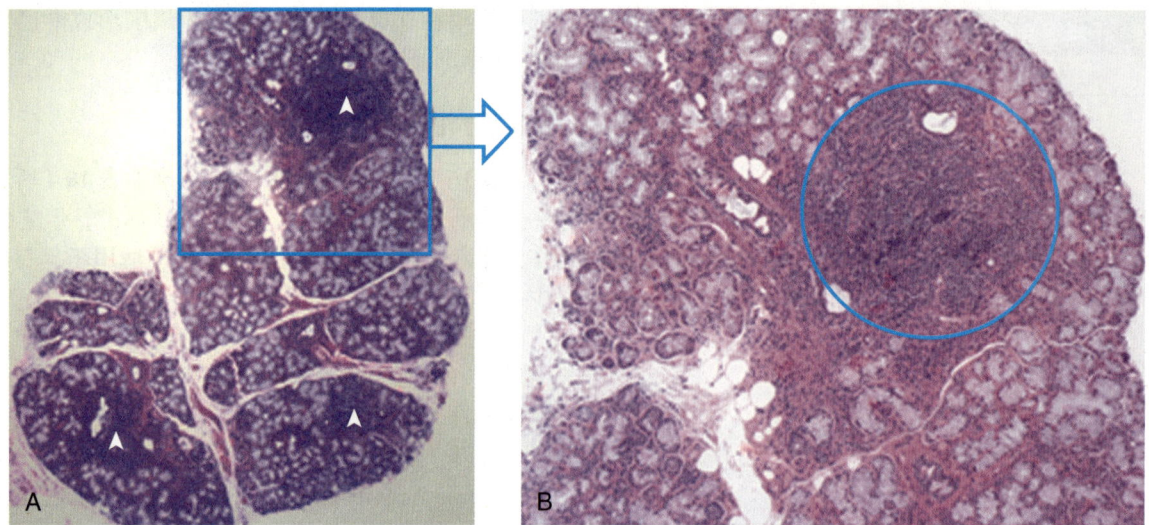

Fig. 10.1 (A) Low magnification. Cross-section of a labial minor salivary gland in SS patient revealing focal lymphocytic sialadenitis. Three lymphocytic foci, each *(triangles)* with >50 lymphocytes adjacent to normal-appearing glandular tissue. (B) High magnification. Several hundred lymphocytes forming a lymphocytic focus.

TABLE 10.4 2016 ACR/EULAR Classification Criteria of Primary Sjögren's Syndrome

Item	Score
Labial salivary gland with focal lymphocytic sialadenitis and focus score of ≥1 foci/4 mm²	3
Positive anti-SSA/Ro	3
Ocular staining score ≥5 in any eye	1
Schirmer test ≤5 mm/5 min in any eye	1
Unstimulated salivary flow rate ≤0.1 mL/min	1

A score ≥4 points classifies a patient as having SS.

TABLE 10.5 Management of Sicca Syndrome in Patients With Sjögren's Syndrome

Treatment of dry eyes	Avoid dry environment
	Moisture chamber goggles/glasses
	Artificial tears (preservative free if used more than four times daily)
	Lubricating gels (at bedtime)
	Tear drainage duct plugging (reversible) or cautery (irreversible)
	Topical anti-inflammatory therapy (cyclosporine, lifitegrast, corticosteroids)
Treatment of dry mouth	Avoid or discontinue medications with anticholinergic properties, when possible
	Optimize oral hygiene (regular brushing, flossing)
	Sugar-free lozenges (to stimulate saliva)
	Artificial saliva
	Fluoride-based topical products
	Oral secretagogues (pilocarpine, cevimeline)

SUGGESTED READINGS

Brito-Zerón P, Baldini C, Bootsma H, et al: Sjögren syndrome, Nat Rev Dis Primers 2:16047, 2016.

Chakravarty SD, Markenson JA: Rheumatic manifestations of endocrine disease, Curr Opin Rheumatol 25(1):37–43, 2013.

Cordner S, De Ceulaer K: Musculoskeletal manifestations of hemoglobinopathies, Curr Opin Rheumatol 15:44–47, 2003.

Goules AV, Tzioufas AG: Lymphomagenesis in Sjögren's syndrome: predictive biomarkers towards precision medicine, Autoimmun Rev 18(2):137–143, 2019.

Ravindran V, Anoop P: Rheumatologic manifestations of benign and malignant haematological disorders, Clin Rheumatol 30:1143–1149, 2011.

Vivino FB, Bunya VY, Massaro-Giordano G, et al: Sjögren's syndrome: an update on disease pathogenesis, clinical manifestations and treatment, Clin Immunol 203:81–121, 2019.

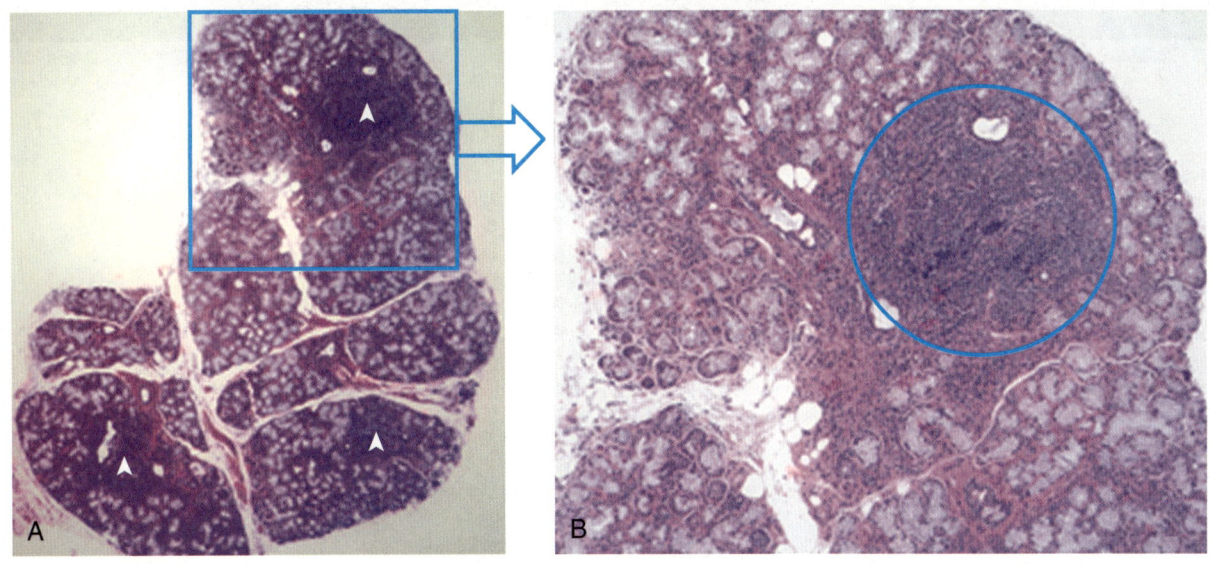

图 10.1 （A）低倍放大。干燥综合征（SS）患者唇腺的截面，显示灶性淋巴细胞性唾液腺炎。3 个淋巴细胞灶，每个灶（三角形标记）有超过 50 个淋巴细胞，邻近外观正常的腺体组织。（B）高倍放大。数百个淋巴细胞形成 1 个淋巴细胞灶

表 10.4　2016 ACR/EULAR 原发性干燥综合征的分类标准	
项目	得分
唇腺灶性淋巴细胞性唾液腺炎，且灶性指数 ≥ 1 灶 / 4 平方毫米	3
抗 SSA/Ro 抗体阳性	3
任何一只眼睛的眼表染色评分 ≥ 5	1
任何一只眼睛的 Schirmer 试验 ≤ 5 mm/5 min	1
非刺激性唾液流率 ≤ 0.1 ml/min	1

总分 ≥ 4 分可将患者分类为干燥综合征。

表 10.5　干燥综合征患者的干燥症状管理	
眼干的治疗	避免干燥环境
	使用湿目镜 / 护目镜
	人工泪液（若每日使用超过 4 次，建议使用无防腐剂的）
	润滑凝胶（睡前使用）
	泪道栓塞（可逆）或烧灼（不可逆）
	局部抗炎治疗（环孢素、立他司特、皮质类固醇）
口干的治疗	避免或停用具有抗胆碱能性质的药物（若可能）
	改善口腔卫生（规律刷牙、使用牙线）
	无糖含片（刺激唾液分泌）
	人工唾液
	含氟的局部产品
	口服分泌刺激剂（匹罗卡品、西维美林）

推荐阅读

Brito-Zerón P, Baldini C, Bootsma H, et al: Sjögren syndrome, Nat Rev Dis Primers 2:16047, 2016.

Chakravarty SD, Markenson JA: Rheumatic manifestations of endocrine disease, Curr Opin Rheumatol 25(1):37–43, 2013.

Cordner S, De Ceulaer K: Musculoskeletal manifestations of hemoglobinopathies, Curr Opin Rheumatol 15:44–47, 2003.

Goules AV, Tzioufas AG: Lymphomagenesis in Sjögren's syndrome: predictive biomarkers towards precision medicine, Autoimmun Rev 18(2):137–143, 2019.

Ravindran V, Anoop P: Rheumatologic manifestations of benign and malignant haematological disorders, Clin Rheumatol 30:1143–1149, 2011.

Vivino FB, Bunya VY, Massaro-Giordano G, et al: Sjogren's syndrome: an update on disease pathogenesis, clinical manifestations and treatment, Clin Immunol 203:81–121, 2019.

索引 Index

A

Abatacept, for rheumatoid arthritis, 20t
Acetaminophen
　　for osteoarthritis, 102
Achilles tendinitis, 110
Acromegaly
　　rheumatic manifestations of, 120
Acute gouty attack, 84-88, 88f
Acute phase proteins, rheumatic disease and, 8-10
Acute phase reactants, in rheumatoid arthritis, 18
Adalimumab
　　for rheumatoid arthritis, 20t
　　for spondyloarthritis, 32
Allopurinol
　　for gout, 92
　　for prevention of tumor lysis syndrome, 92
Amitriptyline, for fibromyalgia syndrome, 112
Amyloidosis
　　rheumatic manifestations of, 120
Anakinra, for rheumatoid arthritis, 20t
Anemia
　　in systemic lupus erythematosus, 38
Aneurysm (s)
　　coronary artery, in Kawasaki disease, 78
Angiotensin-receptor blockers (ARBs)
　　for Raynaud's phenomenon, 66
Ankylosing spondylitis
　　clinical features of, 28-30
Anterior uveitis, spondyloarthritis and, 28, 30f
Anti-cyclic citrullinated peptide (anti-CCP) antibodies, in rheumatoid arthritis, 16-18
Antidepressants, for fibromyalgia syndrome, 112
Antineutrophil cytoplasmic antibodies (ANCAs), 72-76
　　associated vasculitides with, 72
Antinuclear antibodies (ANAs)
　　low specificity of, 8
　　in systemic lupus erythematosus, 42
Antiphospholipid antibodies (APAs), in systemic lupus erythematosus, 38
Anxiety
　　in systemic lupus erythematosus, 54
Aortitis
　　in giant cellarteritis, 80
　　spondyloarthritis and, 28
Apatite-associated arthropathy, 94
Arrhythmias
　　in systemic sclerosis, 62
Arthralgias, in systemic lupus erythematosus, 40
Arthritis
　　crystal-induced, 4
　　differentiating features of, 6t
　　evaluation of, 4
　　　　biopsy in, 10
　　　　laboratory testing for, 8-10, 8t
　　　　musculoskeletal history and examination of, 4, 6t, 8f
　　　　radiographic studies in, 10
　　　　summary of, 10
　　in sarcoidosis, 120
　　in sickle cell disease, 118
　　viral, 18
Arthritis mutilans, 32

Page numbers followed by "f" indicate figures, "t" indicate tables, and "b" indicate boxes.

A

阿巴西普，治疗类风湿关节炎，21t
对乙酰氨基酚
　　骨关节炎，103
跟腱炎，111
肢端肥大症
　　风湿性表现，121
急性痛风发作，85-89，89f
急性期蛋白，风湿性疾病，9-11
急性期反应物，见于类风湿关节炎，19
阿达木单抗
　　类风湿关节炎，21t
　　脊柱关节炎，33
别嘌呤醇
　　痛风，93
　　肿瘤溶解综合征，93
阿米替林，治疗纤维肌痛综合征，113
淀粉样变性
　　风湿性表现，121
阿那白滞素，治疗类风湿关节炎，21t
贫血
　　系统性红斑狼疮，39
动脉瘤
　　冠状动脉瘤，见于川崎病，79
血管紧张素受体阻滞剂（ARB）
　　雷诺现象，67
强直性脊柱炎
　　临床特征，29-31
前葡萄膜炎，脊柱关节炎，29，31f
抗环瓜氨酸肽抗体（anti-CCP），见于类风湿关节炎，17-19
抗抑郁药，治疗纤维肌痛综合征，113
抗中性粒细胞胞质抗体（ANCA），73-77
　　ANCA相关性血管炎，73
抗核抗体（ANA）
　　特异性低，9
　　系统性红斑狼疮，43
抗磷脂抗体，见于系统性红斑狼疮，39
焦虑
　　系统性红斑狼疮，55
主动脉炎
　　巨细胞性动脉炎，81
　　脊柱关节炎，29
磷灰石相关性关节病，95
心律失常
　　系统性硬化症，63
关节痛，见于系统性红斑狼疮，41
关节炎
　　晶体诱发的关节炎，5
　　鉴别特征，7t
　　评估，5
　　　　活检，11
　　　　实验室检查，9-11，9t
　　　　肌肉骨骼病史和检查，5，7t，9f
　　　　影像学检查，11
　　　　总结，11
　　结节病，121
　　镰状细胞病，119
　　病毒性关节炎，19
毁损型关节炎，33

页码数字中，"f"代表"图"，"t"代表"表格"，"b"代表"框"。

Articular disease, differentiating nonarticular soft tissue disorders from, 108t
Aspirin
  for Kawasaki disease, 80
Autoantibodies
  anti-cyclic citrullinated peptide antibodies, in rheumatoid arthritis, 16-18
  in systemic lupus erythematosus, 42, 48t

B

Baker cyst, 16
Bamboo spine, 30
Bleomycin
  scleroderma-like effects of, 66t
Bone
  health of, systemic lupus erythematosus and, 52
Bone mineral density
  osteoarthritis and, 96
Boutonnière deformity, in rheumatoid arthritis, 16
Bursitis, 106, 108t

C

Calcium-channel blockers, for Raynaud's phenomenon, 66
Calcium oxalate deposition disease, 94
Calcium pyrophosphate dehydrate, in osteoarthritis, 100
Calcium pyrophosphate dihydrate deposition disease, 90f, 92-94
Capsaicin, topical, for osteoarthritis, 102
Cardiovascular disease (CVD)
  systemic lupus erythematosus and, 52
Carpal tunnel syndrome
  in diabetes, 118
  in rheumatoid arthritis, 16
Catastrophic antiphospholipid syndrome, 52
Certolizumab, for rheumatoid arthritis, 20t
Cervical spine, subluxation of, in rheumatoid arthritis, 16
Charcot joint, 118
Cheiroarthropathy, diabetic, 118
Chlamydia trachomatis
  infection, reactive arthritis secondary to, 26
Chondrocalcinosis, 10, 92
  in hemochromatosis, 120
Chondroitin sulfate, for osteoarthritis, 102
Chronic gout, clinical features of, 88
Churg-Strauss syndrome, 72
Circinate balanitis, 30, 30f
Cirrhosis
  primary biliary, 114
Clubbing
  in hypertrophicosteoarthropathy, 114
Colchicine
  in calcium pyrophosphate dihydrate, 92-94
  for gout, 90
Conjunctivitis, in spondyloarthritis, 30
Coronary artery, aneurysms of, in Kawasaki disease, 78
Corticosteroids
  for bursitis, 108
  fluorinated, 42-46
  for gout, 90
  immunosuppression and, for systemic sclerosis and, 68
  intra-articular
    for gout, 90
    for osteoarthritis, 102
    for tendinitis, 110
C-reactive protein
  in rheumatic disease, 8-10
  in rheumatoid arthritis, 18
Crohn's disease
  spondyloarthritis and, 30

关节疾病，与非关节软组织疾病鉴别，109t
阿司匹林
  川崎病，81
自身抗体
  抗环瓜氨酸肽抗体，见于类风湿关节炎，17-19
  系统性红斑狼疮，43，49t

B

腘窝囊肿，17
竹节状脊柱，31
博来霉素
  硬皮病样疾病，67t
骨骼
  骨骼健康，系统性红斑狼疮，53
骨密度
  骨关节炎，97
纽扣花畸形，见于类风湿关节炎，17
滑囊炎，107，109t

C

钙通道阻滞剂，治疗雷诺现象，67
草酸钙沉积病，95
焦磷酸钙脱水，见于骨关节炎，101
二羟焦磷酸钙沉积病，91f，93-95
辣椒素，局部应用，治疗骨关节炎，103
心血管疾病（CVD）
  系统性红斑狼疮，53
腕管综合征
  糖尿病，119
  类风湿关节炎，17
灾难性抗磷脂综合征，53
赛妥珠单抗，治疗类风湿关节炎，21t
颈椎，半脱位，见于类风湿关节炎，17
Charcot 关节，119
糖尿病性手关节病，119
沙眼衣原体
  感染，诱发反应性关节炎，27
软骨钙质沉着，11，93
  血色病，121
硫酸软骨素，治疗骨关节炎，103
慢性痛风，临床特征，89
Churg-Strauss 综合征，73
环状龟头炎，31，31f
肝硬化
  原发性胆汁性肝硬化，115
杵状指
  肥厚性骨关节病，115
秋水仙碱
  二羟焦磷酸钙沉积病，93-95
  痛风，91
结膜炎，见于脊柱关节炎，31
冠状动脉瘤，见于川崎病，79
皮质类固醇
  滑囊炎，109
  氟化皮质类固醇，43-47
  痛风（糖皮质激素），91
  联合免疫抑制剂，治疗系统性硬化症，69
  关节腔内注射用于
    痛风（糖皮质激素），91
    骨关节炎，103
    肌腱炎，111
C 反应蛋白
  风湿性疾病，9-11
  类风湿关节炎，19
克罗恩病
  脊柱关节炎，31

Crystal arthropathies, 84-94
Cyclobenzaprine, for fibromyalgia syndrome, 112
Cyclooxygenase-2 (COX-2)
    for osteoarthritis, 102
Cyclophosphamide
    for premature ovarian failure, 80
    for systemic lupus erythematosus, 48
    for systemic sclerosis, 68
    for vasculitides, ANCA-associated, 78
Cytokines
    in rheumatoid arthritis, 14

D

Dactylitis, 28
    in sickle cell disease, 118
Depression
    in fibromyalgia syndrome, 108
    in systemic lupus erythematosus, 54
Diabetes
    rheumatic manifestations of, 118
Diastolic dysfunction
    in systemic sclerosis, 62
Diffuse idiopathic skeletal hyperostosis (DISH), 118
Digital ulcerations, systemic sclerosis and, 66
Disease-modifying antirheumatic drug (DMARD) therapy, for rheumatoid arthritis, 20, 20t
Drug-induced lupus, 42

E

Education, in gout, 92
Endocrine disease
    musculoskeletal manifestations of, 116t
Enteropathic arthritis, 30
Enthesitis, spondyloarthritis and, 26
Enthesopathies, 110
Eosinophilia-myalgia syndrome, 66t
Eosinophilic fasciitis, 64, 114
Erythrocyte sedimentation rate
    in rheumatic disease, 8-10
    in rheumatoid arthritis, 18
Estrogen
    osteoarthritis and, 96
Etanercept, 32
    for rheumatoid arthritis, 20t
Exercise
    in fibromyalgia syndrome, 112
    in rheumatoid arthritis, 18

F

Fatigue
    in systemic lupus erythematosus, 36-38, 54
Febuxostat, for gout, 90
Felty syndrome, 16
Fibromyalgia, 106
Fibromyalgia syndrome, 108-112, 110t

G

Gadolinium, 66t
Giant cell arteritis (GCA), 78
Glucocorticoids
    for spondyloarthritis, 32
Glucosamine, for osteoarthritis, 102
Golimumab, for rheumatoid arthritis, 20t
Gout, 6t, 84-92
    clinical features of, 86-88
    diagnosis of, 88-90, 90f
    differential diagnosis of, 90

晶体性关节病，85-95
环苯扎林，治疗纤维肌痛综合征，113
环氧合酶-2（COX-2）
    骨关节炎，103
环磷酰胺
    卵巢早衰，81
    系统性红斑狼疮，49
    系统性硬化症，69
    ANCA相关性血管炎，79
细胞因子
    类风湿关节炎，15

D

指/趾炎，29
    镰状细胞病，119
抑郁
    纤维肌痛综合征，109
    系统性红斑狼疮，55
糖尿病
    风湿性表现，119
舒张功能障碍
    系统性硬化症，63
弥漫性特发性骨肥厚（DISH），119
指溃疡，系统性硬化症，67
改善病情抗风湿药（DMARD），治疗类风湿关节炎，21，21t

药物性狼疮，43

E

教育，对痛风患者，93
内分泌疾病
    肌肉骨骼表现，117t
肠病性关节炎，31
附着点炎，见于脊柱关节炎，27
附着点疾病，111
嗜酸细胞增多性肌痛综合征，67t
嗜酸细胞性筋膜炎，65，115
红细胞沉降率
    风湿性疾病，9-11
    类风湿关节炎，19
雌激素
    骨关节炎，97
依那西普，33
    类风湿关节炎，21t
运动/锻炼
    纤维肌痛综合征，113
    类风湿关节炎，19

F

疲劳
    系统性红斑狼疮，37-39，55
非布司他，治疗痛风，91
Felty综合征，17
纤维肌痛，107
纤维肌痛综合征，109-113，111t

G

钆，67t
巨细胞动脉炎（GCA），79
糖皮质激素
    脊柱关节炎，33
葡萄糖胺，治疗骨关节炎，103
戈利木单抗，治疗类风湿关节炎，21t
痛风，7t，85-93
    临床特征，87-89
    诊断，89-91，91f
    鉴别诊断，91

epidemiology of, 84
pathogenesis of, 84-86
radiologic features of, 88-90
in transplantation patients, 90
treatment for
    acute, 90
    intercritical and chronic, 90-92
Graft-*versus*-host disease (GVHD)
    vs. systemic sclerosis, 66t

H

Hemarthrosis, in hemophilia, 118
Hemochromatosis
    rheumatic manifestations of, 120
Hemophilia
    rheumatic manifestations of, 118
Henoch-Schönlein purpura (HSP), 72, 76, 76f
    leukocytoclastic vasculitis in, 74
Hepatitis B
    polyarteritis nodosa in, 72, 76-78
Hepatitis C, polyarteritis nodosa in, 72, 76-78
Hormone therapy
    systemic lupus erythematosus and, 50
Human immunodeficiency virus (HIV), polyarteritis nodosa in, 76-78
Human immunodeficiency virus (HIV) infection, 120
Human leukocyte antigen (HLA)
    B27, spondyloarthritis and, 26
Hyaluronate, intra-articular, for osteoarthritis, 102
Hydroxychloroquine, for rheumatoid arthritis, 20t
Hyperostosis, diffuse idiopathic skeletal, 118
Hyperparathyroidism
    musculoskeletal manifestations of, 120
Hyperthyroidism, 120
Hypertrophicosteoarthropathy (HOA), 114
Hyperuricemia
    asymptomatic, 84
    causes of, 86t
    pathophysiology of, 84
    treatment of, inpatients without gout, 92

I

Immune checkpoint inhibitors (ICIs), 116
Infections
    rheumatoid arthritis and, 22
Inflammatory arthritis, 4, 26. *See also* Arthritis
    synovial fluid analysis in, 8
Inflammatory joint diseases, osteoarthritis and, 96
Inflammatory myopathies, 118
Inflammatory spine pain, spondyloarthritis and, 28
Infliximab, 32
    for rheumatoid arthritis, 20t
International Society of Nephrology/Renal Pathology Society (ISN/RPS), 38
Interstitial lung diseases (ILD)
    rheumatoid arthritis with, 16
    in systemic sclerosis, 62, 68
Intravenous immunoglobulin (IVIG), 80

J

Jaccoud arthropathy, 38
Joint replacement surgery, for rheumatoid arthritis, 22

K

Kawasaki disease, 78
Keratoconjunctivitis sicca, in systemic lupus erythematosus, 40
Keratodermablennorrhagicum, 30, 30f

流行病学，85
发病机制，85-87
影像学特征，89-91
移植患者，91
治疗
    急性痛风，91
    间歇期和慢性痛风，91-93
移植物抗宿主病（GVHD）
    系统性硬化症，67t

H

关节出血，见于血友病，119
血色病
    风湿性表现，121
血友病
    风湿性表现，119
过敏性紫癜（HSP），73，77，77f
    白细胞破碎性血管炎，75
乙型肝炎
    结节性多动脉炎，73，77-79
丙型肝炎，结节性多动脉炎，73，77-79
激素治疗
    系统性红斑狼疮，51
人类免疫缺陷病毒（HIV），结节性多动脉炎，77-79
人类免疫缺陷病毒（HIV）感染，121
人类白细胞抗原（HLA）
    HLA-B27，脊柱关节炎，27
透明质酸，关节内注射，治疗骨关节炎，103
羟氯喹，治疗类风湿关节炎，21t
弥漫性特发性骨肥厚，119
甲状旁腺功能亢进症
    肌肉骨骼表现，121
甲状腺功能亢进症，121
肥厚性骨关节病（HOA），115
高尿酸血症
    无症状性高尿酸血症，85
    病因，87t
    病理生理学，85
    治疗，无痛风患者，93

I

免疫检查点抑制剂（ICI），117
感染
    类风湿关节炎，23
炎症性关节炎，5，27；参见关节炎
    滑液分析，9
炎症性关节疾病，骨关节炎，97
炎性肌病，119
炎性脊柱疼痛，脊柱关节炎，29
英夫利昔单抗，33
    类风湿关节炎，21t
国际肾脏病学会/肾脏病理学学会（ISN/RPS），39
间质性肺病（ILD）
    类风湿关节炎，17
    系统性硬化症，63，69
静脉注射免疫球蛋白（IVIG），81

J

Jaccoud 关节病，39
关节置换术，治疗类风湿关节炎，23

K

川崎病，79
干燥性角结膜炎，见于系统性红斑狼疮，41
脓溢性皮肤角化病，31，31f

L

Leflunomide, for rheumatoid arthritis, 20t
Leukocytoclastic vasculitis, 74, 118
Leukopenia
    in systemic lupus erythematosus, 38
Libman-Sacks endocarditis, 38
Lifestyle modifications
    in gout, 92
Linear scleroderma, 64
Lower extremity osteoarthritis, 96
Lung cancer
    hypertrophic osteoarthropathy in, 114
Lung transplantation
    for interstitial lung disease, in systemic sclerosis, 68
Lupus anticoagulant, 52
    digital ulcerations associated with, 66-68
Lupus nephritis, 38
Lupus-like syndrome, 116

M

Magnetic resonance imaging (MRI)
    of rheumatic disease, 10
Malignancy
    systemic lupus erythematosus and, 54
Methotrexate
    for rheumatoid arthritis, 20t
    teratogenicity of, 80
Microscopic polyangiitis (MPA), 72
Microtophi, 84-86
Mixed connective tissue disease (MCTD), 46-48
    systemic sclerosis and, 64
Monoclonal gammopathy, systemic sclerosis and, 64
Morphea, 64, 66t
Multiple myeloma
    rheumatic manifestations of, 120
Musculoskeletal system
    anatomic structures of, 8f
Myocarditis
    in systemic lupus erythematosus, 38
Myopathy(ies)
    bland, systemic sclerosis and, 64, 68
Myositis
    acute inflammatory, 6

N

Nail thickening, in reactive arthritis, 30
Neonatal lupus, 42-46
Nephrogenic systemic fibrosis, 64
Nephrolithiasis
    in gout, 92
Neuropathic arthropathy, 118
Nitroglycerin
    topical, for Raynaud's phenomenon, 66
Nodules, rheumatoid, 16
Non-Hodgkin's lymphomas
    in systemic lupus erythematosus, 54
Nonseptic bursitis, 108
Nonsteroidal anti-inflammatory drugs (NSAIDs)
    for bursitis, 108
    for calcium pyrophosphate dihydrate, 92-94
    for gout, 90
    for osteoarthritis, 102
    for reactive arthritis, 32-34
    for rheumatoid arthritis, 22
    for spondyloarthritis, 32
    for tendinitis, 110
Non-urate-lowering prophylactic therapy, 92

L

来氟米特，治疗类风湿关节炎，21t
白细胞破碎性血管炎，75，119
白细胞减少
    系统性红斑狼疮，39
利布曼-塞克斯心内膜炎，39
生活方式调整
    痛风，93
线状硬皮病，65
下肢骨关节炎，97
肺癌
    肥厚性骨关节病，115
肺移植
    间质性肺病，见于系统性硬化症，69
狼疮抗凝物，53
    指溃疡，67-69
狼疮性肾炎，39
狼疮样综合征，117

M

磁共振成像（MRI）
    风湿性疾病，11
恶性肿瘤
    系统性红斑狼疮，55
甲氨蝶呤
    类风湿关节炎，21t
    致畸性，81
显微镜下多血管炎（MPA），73
微痛风石，85-87
混合性结缔组织病（MCTD），47-49
    系统性硬化症，65
单克隆丙种球蛋白病，系统性硬化症，65
硬斑病，65，67t
多发性骨髓瘤
    风湿性表现，121
肌肉骨骼系统
    解剖结构，9f
心肌炎
    系统性红斑狼疮，39
肌病
    轻度，系统性硬化症，65，69
肌炎
    急性炎症性肌炎，7

N

指甲增厚，见于反应性关节炎，31
新生儿狼疮，43-47
肾源性系统性纤维化，65
肾结石
    痛风，93
神经病性关节病，119
硝酸甘油
    局部使用治疗雷诺现象，67
类风湿结节，17
非霍奇金淋巴瘤
    系统性红斑狼疮，55
非化脓性滑囊炎，109
非甾体抗炎药（NSAID）
    滑囊炎，109
    二羟焦磷酸钙沉积病，93-95
    痛风，91
    骨关节炎，103
    反应性关节炎，33-35
    类风湿关节炎，23
    脊柱关节炎，33
    肌腱炎，111
非降尿酸预防性治疗，93

O

Obesity
  osteoarthritis and, 96
Occupational therapy, for rheumatoid arthritis, 18
Opioids
  for osteoarthritis, 102
Oral ulcerations, in systemic lupus erythematosus, 38
Orthopedic surgery, for spondyloarthritis, 32
Osteoarthritis, 4, 6t, 96-104
  clinical presentation of, 100
  definition and epidemiology of, 96
  diagnosis and differential diagnosis of, 100-102
  lower extremity, 96
  pathologic factors of, 96-100, 98f-100f
  prognosis of, 104
  secondary, 96
  treatment for, 102-104
Osteolysis, 32
Osteomyelitis
  in sickle cell disease, 118
Osteopenia
  glucocorticoid therapy causing, 80
Osteophyte, in osteoarthritis, 96
Osteoporosis
  glucocorticoid therapy causing, 80
  rheumatoid arthritis and, 22
Overlap syndrome, systemic lupus erythematosus and, 46-48

P

Pain
  in osteoarthritis, 100
Pannus, 14-16
Parathyroid disease, 120
Pericarditis
  rheumatoid arthritis with, 16
  in systemic lupus erythematosus, 38
Peripheral joint disease, spondyloarthritis and, 28
Physical therapy
  for rheumatoid arthritis, 18
  for spondyloarthritis, 32
  for systemic sclerosis, 68
Plasmapheresis
  for vasculitides, ANCA-associated, 78
Pneumocystis jirovecii pneumonia
  glucocorticoid therapy and, 80
Podagra, 88
Polyarteritis nodosa (PAN), 76-78
Polymyalgia rheumatica (PMR), 72, 116
Pregnancy
  systemic lupus erythematosus and, 50
Probenecid, for gout, 92
Prostacyclin analog, 68
Psoriatic arthritis, 26, 30
Pulmonary fibrosis
  in spondyloarthritis, 28
Pulmonary hypertension
  in systemic sclerosis, 62, 68
Purine metabolism, 84, 86f

R

Range of motion, assessment of, 106-108
Raynaud's disease, systemic sclerosis and, 64
Raynaud's phenomenon, 38, 116-118
  in systemic sclerosis, 60-62, 66-68
Reactive arthritis, 6t, 26, 30-34, 30f
Remitting seronegative symmetrical synovitis, with pitting edema, 114
Renal crisis, in scleroderma, 60
Renal osteodystrophy, 120

O

肥胖症
　骨关节炎，97
作业疗法，治疗类风湿关节炎，19
阿片类药物
　骨关节炎，103
口腔溃疡，见于系统性红斑狼疮，39
矫形外科手术，治疗脊柱关节炎，33
骨关节炎，5，7t，97-105
　临床表现，101
　定义和流行病学，97
　诊断和鉴别诊断，101-103
　下肢骨关节炎，97
　病理因素，97-101，99f-101f
　预后，105
　继发性骨关节炎，97
　治疗，103-105
骨溶解，33
骨髓炎
　镰状细胞病，119
骨量减少
　糖皮质激素治疗引起的骨量减少，81
骨赘，见于骨关节炎，97
骨质疏松
　糖皮质激素治疗引起的骨质疏松，81
　类风湿关节炎，23
重叠综合征，系统性红斑狼疮，47-49

P

疼痛
　骨关节炎，101
血管翳，15-17
甲状旁腺疾病，121
心包炎
　类风湿关节炎，17
　系统性红斑狼疮，39
外周关节疾病，脊柱关节炎，29
物理疗法
　类风湿关节炎，19
　脊柱关节炎，33
　系统性硬化症，69
血浆置换
　ANCA相关性血管炎，79
肺孢子菌肺炎
　糖皮质激素治疗，81
足痛风，89
结节性多动脉炎（PAN），77-79
风湿性多肌痛（PMR），73，117
妊娠
　系统性红斑狼疮，51
丙磺舒，治疗痛风，93
前列环素类似物，69
银屑病关节炎，27，31
肺纤维化
　脊柱关节炎，29
肺动脉高压
　系统性硬化症，63，69
嘌呤代谢，85，87f

R

关节活动范围评估，107-109
雷诺病，系统性硬化症，65
雷诺现象，39，117-119
　系统性硬化症，61-63，67-69
反应性关节炎，7t，27，31-35，31f
缓解性血清阴性对称性滑膜炎伴凹陷性水肿，115
肾危象，见于硬皮病，61
肾性骨营养不良，121

Rheumatic disease, approach to, 2-10
    biopsy in, 10
    laboratory testing for, 8-10, 8t
    musculoskeletal history and examination in, 4, 6t, 8f
    radiographic studies in, 10
    summary of, 10
Rheumatic manifestations, of systemic disorders, 114-126, 116t
Rheumatoid arthritis, 6t, 12-24, 30
    classification criteria for, 18t
    clinical presentation of, 16, 16t
    definition of, 12
    diagnosis and differential diagnosis of, 16-18
    epidemiology of, 12
    etiology of, 12
    genetics of, 12
    pathogenesis of, 12-16, 14f
    pathology of, 12-16
    prognosis of, 22
    treatment of, 18-22
Rheumatoid arthritis-like polyarthritis, 114-116
Rheumatoid arthritis-like syndrome, 116-118
Rheumatoid factor, 8
    rheumatoid arthritis and, 18
Rheumatoid nodules, 16
Rituximab
    for rheumatoid arthritis, 20t

S

Sacroiliac joints, inflammation of, spondyloarthritis and, 26
Sacroiliitis, 30, 32f
Sarcoidosis
    rheumatic manifestations of, 120-122
Scleroderma, 58
Scleroderma renal crisis (SRC), 62, 68
Scleroderma sine scleroderma, 60
Scleroderma-like syndrome, 116-118
Scleromyxedema, systemic sclerosis and, 64
Secondary antiphospholipid syndrome, systemic lupus erythematosus and, 52, 52t
Secondary osteoarthritis, 96
Septic arthritis, 4, 6t
    gout and, 88
    in sickle cell disease, 118
Septic bursitis, 108
Shared epitope, 12
Shoulder pad sign, 120
Sickle cell disease
    rheumatic manifestations of, 118
Sjögren's syndrome, 122-124
    classification criteria for, 124, 126t
    clinical presentation of, 122, 124t
    definition and epidemiology of, 122
    diagnosis of, 122-124, 126f
    differential diagnosis of, 124
    laboratory findings of, 122
    management for, 124, 126t
    non-Hodgkin lymphomas and, 122
    pathogenesis of, 122
    rheumatoid arthritis and, 18
    in systemic lupus erythematosus, 40
Skin, in Sjögren's syndrome, 122
Small bowel dysmotility, systemic sclerosis and, 68
Soft tissue disorders, nonarticular, 106-112
    bursitis, 106, 108t
    clinical presentation of, 106-108
    diagnosis and treatment of, 108-112
    epidemiology of, 106
    etiologic factors of, 106
    fibromyalgia syndrome, 110-112, 110t

风湿性疾病，3-11
    活检，11
    实验室检查，9-11，9t
    肌肉骨骼病史和检查，5，7t，9f
    影像学检查，11
    总结，11
风湿性表现，系统性疾病，115-127，117t
类风湿关节炎（RA），7t，13-25，31
    分类标准，19t
    临床表现，17，17t
    定义，13
    诊断和鉴别诊断，17-19
    流行病学，13
    病因，13
    遗传学，13
    发病机制，13-17，15f
    病理学，13-17
    预后，23
    治疗，19-23
类风湿关节炎样多关节炎，115-117
类风湿关节炎样综合征，117-119
类风湿因子，9
    类风湿关节炎，19
类风湿结节，17
利妥昔单抗
    类风湿关节炎，21t

S

骶髂关节炎症，脊柱关节炎，27
骶髂关节炎，31，33f
结节病
    风湿性表现，121-123
硬皮病，59
硬皮病肾危象（SRC），63，69
无硬皮的硬皮病，61
硬皮病样综合征，117-119
硬化性黏液性水肿，系统性硬化症，65
继发性抗磷脂综合征，系统性红斑狼疮，53，53t

继发性骨关节炎，97
化脓性关节炎，5，7t
    痛风，89
    镰状细胞病，119
化脓性滑囊炎，109
共享表位，13
肩垫征，121
镰状细胞病
    风湿性表现，119
干燥综合征，123-125
    分类标准，125，127t
    临床表现，123，125t
    定义和流行病学，123
    诊断，123-125，127f
    鉴别诊断，125
    实验室检查，123
    治疗，125，127t
    非霍奇金淋巴瘤，123
    发病机制，123
    类风湿关节炎，19
    系统性红斑狼疮，41
皮肤，干燥综合征，123
小肠动力障碍，系统性硬化症，69
非关节软组织疾病，107-113
    滑囊炎，107，109t
    临床表现，107-109
    诊断和治疗，109-113
    流行病学，107
    病因，107
    纤维肌痛综合征，111-113，111t

pathogenesis of, 106
tendinitis, 110, 110t
Spinal cord compression
   in rheumatoid arthritis, 16
   in spondyloarthritis, 28
Spine, inflammation of,spondyloarthritis and, 26
Spondylitis, 30
Spondyloarthritis, 26-34
   clinical presentation of, 28-30
   comparison of, 28t
   definition of, 26
   diagnosis and differential diagnosis of, 30-32
   pathology of, 26-28
   peripheral arthritis of, 28
   radiographic, 30
   summary of, 34
   treatment for, 32-34
   undifferentiated, 28
Spondyloarthropathy, 6t
Sulfasalazine
   for rheumatoid arthritis, 20t
Swan-neck deformity, in rheumatoid arthritis, 16
Symmetrical polyarthropathy,spondyloarthritis and, 28
Synovial fluid analysis, 8, 8t
   in calcium pyrophosphate dihydrate, 92
   in gout, 88
   in osteoarthritis, 100
   in rheumatoid arthritis, 18
Synovitis
   palpable, rheumatoid arthritis and, 4
   in rheumatoid arthritis, 16
Systemic lupus erythematosus (SLE), 6t, 36-56
   bone health and, 52
   cardiovascular disease and, 52
   classification of, 40-42, 42t-48t
   clinical presentation of, 36-40, 40t
   definition of, 36
   diagnosis and differential diagnosis of, 40-48
   epidemiology of, 36
   malignancy and, 54
   overlap syndrome and, 46-48
   pathology of, 36
   prognosis of, 50
   secondary antiphospholipid syndrome and, 52, 52t
   treatment for, 48, 50t
Systemic Lupus International Collaborating Clinics (SLICC), 40-42
   classification criteria for, 44t
Systemic sclerosis (SSc), 58-70
   clinical presentation of, 58-64, 62t, 64f
   diagnosis and differential diagnosis of, 64
   epidemiology of, 58
   mimics of, 64, 66t
   pathology of, 58, 60f
   peripheral vascular involvement in, 60-62
   renal crisis in, 62
   treatment for, 64-68

T

Takayasu's arteritis, 78
Temporal arteritis, 78
Tendinitis, 110, 110t
Tennis elbow, 110
Tenosynovitis, in rheumatoid arthritis, 16
Thrombocytopenia
   in systemic lupus erythematosus, 38
Thyroid disease, 118-120
Tocilizumab, for rheumatoid arthritis, 20t
Tofacitinib, for rheumatoid arthritis, 20
Tophus, 88

发病机制，107
肌腱炎，111，111t
脊髓压迫
   类风湿关节炎，17
   脊柱关节炎，29
脊柱炎，脊柱关节炎，27
脊柱炎，31
脊柱关节炎，27-35
   临床表现，29-31
   比较，29t
   定义，27
   诊断和鉴别诊断，31-33
   病理学，27-29
   外周关节炎，29
   影像学，31
   总结，35
   治疗，33-35
   未分化脊柱关节炎，29
脊柱关节病，7t
柳氮磺吡啶
   类风湿关节炎，21t
天鹅颈畸形，见于类风湿关节炎，17
对称性多关节病，脊柱关节炎，29
滑液分析，9，9t
   二羟焦磷酸钙，93
   痛风，89
   骨关节炎，101
   类风湿关节炎，19
滑膜炎
   可触及的滑膜炎，类风湿关节炎，5
   类风湿关节炎，17
系统性红斑狼疮（SLE），7t，37-57
   骨骼健康，53
   心血管疾病，53
   分类，41-43，43t-49t
   临床表现，37-41，41t
   定义，37
   诊断和鉴别诊断，41-49
   流行病学，37
   恶性肿瘤，55
   重叠综合征，47-49
   病理学，37
   预后，51
   继发性抗磷脂综合征，53，53t
   治疗，49，51t
系统性红斑狼疮国际临床协作组（SLICC），41-43
   分类标准，45t
系统性硬化症（SSc），59-71
   临床表现，59-65，63t，65f
   诊断和鉴别诊断，65
   流行病学，59
   硬皮病样疾病，65，67t
   病理学，59，61f
   外周血管受累，61-63
   肾危象，63
   治疗，65-69

T

大动脉炎，79
颞动脉炎，79
肌腱炎，111，111t
网球肘，111
腱鞘炎，见于类风湿关节炎，17
血小板减少
   系统性红斑狼疮，39
甲状腺疾病，119-121
托珠单抗，治疗类风湿关节炎，21t
托法替布，治疗类风湿关节炎，21
痛风石，89

Total joint replacement, for osteoarthritis, 102-104
Trochanteric bursitis, 108
L-Tryptophan, eosinophilia-myalgia syndrome from, 66t
Tumor necrosis factor (TNF) inhibitors
 malignancies associated with, 118
 for Takayasuarteritis, 80
Tumor necrosis factor-α (TNF-α)
 blockers, for spondyloarthritis, 32
 inhibitors, for rheumatoid arthritis, 20

U

Ulcerative colitis (UC)
 spondyloarthritis and, 30
Undifferentiated connective tissue disease, 46-48
Urate-lowering therapy (ULT), 90-92
Urethritis
 reactive arthritis associated with, 30
Uric acid, 84
Uricolytic therapy, 92
Uricostatic therapy, 90-92
Uricosuric therapy, 92
Ustekinumab, 32

V

Vaccinations
 rheumatoid arthritis and, 22
Vaccines
 systemic lupus erythematosus and, 54
Vasculitides, 118
Vasculitis
 leukocytoclastic, 74
 of rheumatoid arthritis, 16
 systemic, 72-82
  clinical presentation and diagnosis of, 74-78, 76t
  definition of, 72
  epidemiology of, 72
  large vessel, 72
  medium vessel, 72
  pathology of, 72-74, 74f
  small vessel, 72
  types of, 72, 74f
Vinyl chloride, scleroderma-like effects of, 66t

W

Warfarin, 52
Wegener's granulomatosis, 72, 74f
Whipple disease, 120

全关节置换，治疗骨关节炎，103-105
转子滑囊炎，109
L-色氨酸，嗜酸细胞增多性肌痛综合征，67t
肿瘤坏死因子（TNF）抑制剂
 相关恶性肿瘤，119
 大动脉炎，81
肿瘤坏死因子-α（TNF-α）
 TNF-α阻滞剂，治疗脊柱关节炎，33
 TNF-α抑制剂，治疗类风湿关节炎，21

U

溃疡性结肠炎（UC）
 脊柱关节炎，31
未分化结缔组织病，47-49
降尿酸治疗（ULT），91-93
尿道炎
 反应性关节炎，31
尿酸，85
尿酸溶解治疗，93
抑制尿酸合成治疗，91-93
促进尿酸排泄治疗，93
乌司奴单抗，33

V

疫苗接种
 类风湿关节炎，23
疫苗
 系统性红斑狼疮，55
血管炎，119
血管炎
 白细胞破碎性血管炎，75
 类风湿关节炎，17
 系统性血管炎，73-83
  临床表现和诊断，75-79，77t
  定义，73
  流行病学，73
  大血管血管炎，73
  中等血管血管炎，73
  病理学，73-75，75f
  小血管血管炎，73
  分类，73，75f
氯乙烯，硬皮病样疾病，67t

W

华法林，53
韦格纳肉芽肿，73，75f
惠普尔病，121